Urology at Michigan:
The Origin Story

Copyright © 2020 by the Regents of the University of Michigan
Some rights reserved

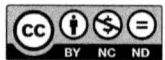

This work is licensed under the Creative Commons Attribution-NonCommercial-NoDerivatives 4.0 International License. To view a copy of this license, visit http://creativecommons.org/licenses/by-nc-nd/4.0/ or send a letter to Creative Commons, PO Box 1866, Mountain View, California, 94042, USA.

Published in the United States of America by
Michigan Publishing
Manufactured in the United States of America

DOI: http://dx.doi.org/10.3998/mpub9470414

ISBN 978-1-60785-523-1 (paper)
ISBN 978-1-60785-524-8 (e-book)
ISBN 978-1-60785-634-4 (OA)

An imprint of Michigan Publishing, Maize Books serves the publishing needs of the University of Michigan community by making high-quality scholarship widely available in print and online. It represents a new model for authors seeking to share their work within and beyond the academy, offering streamlined selection, production, and distribution processes. Maize Books is intended as a complement to more formal modes of publication in a wide range of disciplinary areas.

http://www.maizebooks.org

Urology at Michigan: The Origin Story

Emergence of a Medical Subspecialty and Its Deployment at the University of Michigan

David A. Bloom, Julian Wan, John W. Konnak, Dev S. Pardanani, and Meidee Goh

Contents

PREFACE — vii

PART I
An Ancient Medical Specialty Reiterated and the University of Michigan — 1

    Introduction to a Medical Specialty — 3

    Medical Education, Practice, and the University of Michigan in Early America — 17

    The Department of Medicine and Surgery, Moses Gunn, and Civil War — 27

    A Medical School Hospital and Scientific Curriculum — 40

    Victor Vaughan's Time — 48

PART II
A New Medical Subspecialty in North America and Ann Arbor — 57

    Origin Claims for Genitourinary Surgery in North America — 59

    The Bumpy Path to Charles de Nancrede and the Fulltime Salary Model — 77

    Challenges and Changes in a New Century — 87

Cyrenus Darling and Ira Dean Loree   94

The Post-Flexnerian Decade and Hugh Cabot   100

PART III
The Roaring Twenties, Ann Arbor, and Hugh Cabot   119

Hugh Cabot: Family and Early Career   121

Hugh Cabot Comes to Ann Arbor, 1919   135

Hugh Cabot, President Burton, and 1920   143

Dean Cabot, 1921   151

Hugh Cabot, 1922–1926   160

Hugh Cabot, 1927–1930   179

The Medical School after Cabot   201

Cabot after Michigan   207

The Curious Connection of Howard Kelly to the
University of Michigan   221

Epilogue   226

Index   228

Preface

The story of the practice and discipline of urology at the University of Michigan was last told 20 years ago just after the Urology Section in the Medical School Department of Surgery emerged as a full-fledged department alongside its sibling disciplines of Neurosurgery and Orthopaedic Surgery on July 1, 2001. Much happened in the next 20 years to justify a new rendition of the story and additionally much more has been learned about the earlier times. Urology is a microcosm of modern specialized health care, but its story is also of particular interest for its ancient root as the single designated medical subspecialty set apart by the Hippocratic Oath 2,400 years ago from all other parts of medical care and education.

The progression of skills and ideas, as well as stories of the people who advanced primitive healing arts to nineteenth-century genitourinary practice and then to twentieth-century urology, will be recounted as a primer on this field. We want to reinforce this part of medical historical literacy for new generations of learners while refreshing it for veterans. Just as urology training programs have had to provide basic surgical education for resident trainees, since most medical schools no longer reliably impart basic surgical skills, medical cultural literacy also must be taught, by default after medical school, in graduate medical educational levels of residency training and through continuing medical education for practitioners.

No story is ever complete in its recollections of the past. An author has only partial relevant knowledge of any story, and the myriad other details of the cultural and physical soups that surrounded those facts are mostly lost to historical recollection. Lucky historians recover, reconstruct, or resuscitate useful information, but all stories are mainly narratives of imagination and facts, whether *true facts* or otherwise. Don Coffey, the great urological scientist at Johns Hopkins Medical School, used to instruct his research trainees: "You have to learn to tell the difference between facts and true facts." Historical studies no less than scientific investigations aim to discern truth, although the sciences may strive to reduce facts and observations to laws and principles, whereas historical understanding is broadened by context. Stories, even as particular as this one of a single academic urology unit, are enriched by the context of their people, events, and circumstances. For example, it's inconceivable to consider urology at Michigan without understanding the roles of early founders and university leaders in shaping the institution, the political tensions of the times, relationships with state and community, and the generous philanthropy that built and sustains the school, its faculty, and its programs.

No less important are certain individuals such as Moses Gunn, present at the start of the University of Michigan Medical School in 1848, and any appreciation of Gunn requires the context of the Civil War. Tension between the clinical enterprise, so essential to medical education, and the other two elements of medical academia, teaching and research, first manifested at Michigan with Gunn, driving his practice to Detroit and ultimately to Chicago. The mission balance dilemma continues to perplex medical schools today. Victor Vaughan was another towering figure at the University of Michigan from his awkward arrival in 1874 to the end of his life in 1927. His big career opportunity came with the Rose-Douglas controversy, when he was the right person in the right place, and throughout the years that followed the homeopathy issue bubbled to the top, collapsed, and resurfaced again. These stories are interwoven deeply in the Michigan urology narrative just as all medical specialties and academic organizational structures have their own relevant intersecting stories.

The small detail of a *genito-urinary surgery* title on a University of Michigan Hospital letterhead from 1919 (on next page) signaled the transition from a small clinical practice of genitourinary surgery to modern academic urology. Hugh Cabot was the reason for that transition, as the Konnak and Pardanani book slyly reveals, with the section "Why is Hugh Cabot included?" While it was a well-known fact that the Cabot era began in the 1920 academic year, the letter just mentioned and other documents to follow show the true fact of his actual arrival in Ann Arbor and work in the medical school to have begun in the autumn term of 1919.

The contentious Cabot decade that followed defined urology at Michigan for the next century and brought the first two urology trainees to Ann Arbor: Charles Huggins would win a Nobel Prize in medicine for his work with prostate cancer, and Reed Nesbit would achieve nearly equivalent international prominence for clinical innovation and postgraduate education. Nesbit led Michigan's first *Section of Urology* within the Department of Surgery and his fifth successor, Jim Montie, inaugurated an independent Department of Urology, in concert with Dean Allen

Lichter and surgery chair Lazar Greenfield, in 2001. Over the next two decades, the Department of Urology became one of the leaders and best of academic urologic departments according to surveys, rankings, patient preferences, learners, and faculty recruits. With those relevant details, and many others, this story aims to be rich in contextual factors.

This volume entwines the stories of one medical subspecialty and a public university medical school within a single narrative. Other works probe the distinct stories of urology in America, the University of Michigan, and American medicine with far greater depth. Margaret and Nicholas Steneck's bicentennial edition of Howard Peckham's sesquicentennial work, *The Making of the University of Michigan*, is particularly

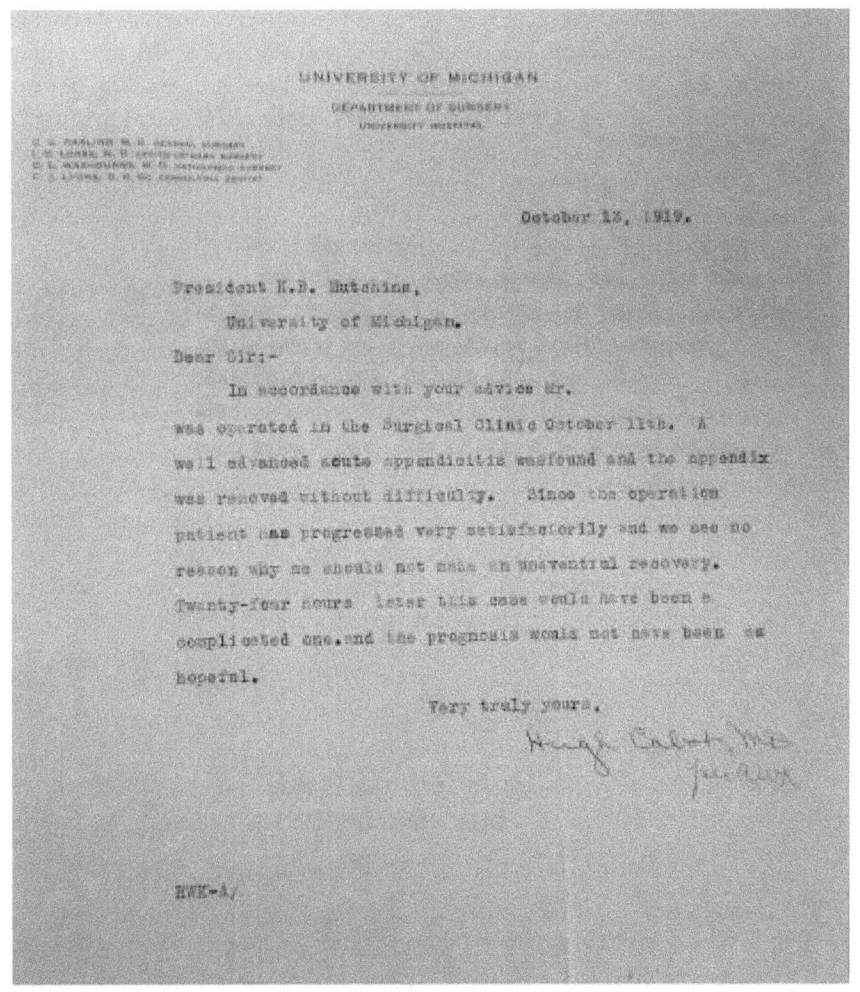

Surgery department letterhead, Bentley Library collection of President Hutchins' papers.

indispensable to understanding this institution and is a model that its urology story herein seeks to emulate. The Stenecks proposed, metaphorically, that this university began with a single strand that represented the university's foundational aim of teaching, to disseminate knowledge and embrace education at all levels. This strand thickened over time and was joined by a second strand, representing the knowledge itself, that must be interpreted, renewed, and rebutted, through exploration, criticism, research, and invention, while winding around the first strand of teaching. The Stenecks then added another part to the braid:

> Now there is a third strand wound with the other two. The University touches more than just its young students and faculty. It gives services to the State that help maintain it; it aids citizens who never enroll. These services began when its hospitals received perplexing cases from all over the State. It continued with the upgrading of high schools, the testing of municipal water supplies, with experiments in reforestation, testing programs for state highways. It supplied reading lists for club programs, lecture series for enlightenment, and musical concerts for entertainment. It expanded to research contracts for Michigan industries, development of new products for manufacture in Michigan, seminars for business executives, realtors and assessors, state college presidents, and refresher demonstrations for physicians and dentists. It provided radio and TV educational programs for all . . . Teaching—research—and service. These are the warp and woof of the University today.[1]

Public goods is a useful alternative for "service thread" and the public goods of the University of Michigan extend today far beyond the university and state to the world at large. Since the Middle Ages, universities have been the single entity in human society to attend consistently and dutifully, albeit imperfectly, to the future of our children and planet. The university, or *The Academy* as some would say, has extended over the past few centuries from small *Ivory Towers* that educated narrow subsets of learners to complex *multiversities* with broader aims such as those the Stenecks described.[i]

The magnificent University of Michigan library system, refreshed and reinvigorated under the recent leadership of Paul Courant, made this

---

i The Ivy Tower versus the Ivory Tower. These common metaphors are confusing. The Ivory Tower was applied to academia to imply rigidity, and the Ivy Tower refers to the comforting image of ivy-covered buildings and perhaps the Ivy League. In fact, the two metaphors are used interchangeably if not with precision. For example, a 1969 television show, *Judd for the Defense*, had an episode called "The View from the Ivy Tower."

book possible. The Special Collections team at the Graduate Library, the superb cadre at the Taubman Health Sciences Library, and experts at the Bentley Library, well-stewarded by Fran Blouin and now Terry McDonald, have been indispensable. The Bentley has been a primary work site, nearly on a daily basis for many stretches. Brian Williams has been my (David A. Bloom) go-to expert in historical research for nearly 30 years at the Bentley and to him the debt of this senior author is enormous. This work also stands on the shoulders of Horace Davenport, late dean of Michigan's medical narrative.[2] Joel Howell and Howard Markel have done much to illuminate the Michigan medical narrative. Joel and Dea Boster produced a beautifully documented book celebrating the 200th anniversary of the founding of the University of Michigan, *Medicine at Michigan*.[3] No less important is the contribution of the late John W. Konnak, professor of urology at Michigan along with Dev S. Pardanani, academic urologist now retired in Mumbai. One of the first inspirations of Jim Montie, after our transition to departmental status, was to commission Konnak and Pardanani to produce *A History of Urology at the University of Michigan*. That work serves as a "first draft" for the next approximation of the Michigan urology story and this volume begins that new iteration.[4] As we study the past, questions emerge, assumptions are challenged, new investigations are stimulated, and knowledge expands. In that sense, we have learned much in preparing this version of the Michigan Urology story.

The powerful idea of the division of labor plays out in health care, perhaps more than any other general field of endeavor, with such complexity that the lay public and entering medical students have only vague notions of what constitutes the field of urology. Novice physicians may not understand whether a patient needs a *nephrologist* or *urologist*. Emergency Department requests for *neurologists* are sometimes misdirected to *urologists* on call. Some confusion is understandable, given that the 24-member boards of the American Board of Medical Specialties encompass more than 175 areas of focused practice, often overlapping. Twenty-first-century physicians have many career possibilities and these continue to grow as new knowledge and technology create new subspecialties.

By the third year of medical school, a small number of students per class targets urology for residency training, appropriately so given the small fraction of urologists necessary to the medical workforce and the limited number of available training positions. The attraction of students to urology is often contingent on their positive experience with role models through shadowing or direct involvement with urologic health care of a family member, friend, or personal medical condition. Applicants to urology residency commonly recall endearing personalities and perceptions of joy at work as attractive features of the specialty. Some students are motivated by the mix of cutting-edge technology and patient care. The opportunity for long-term relationships with patients is another compelling feature. These attractive forces and others created today's global urologic workforce and built a century of urologic excellence at the University of Michigan, where the story of urology at its centennial is significant in its own right and reflects the development of modern urology everywhere else.

This recapitulation of the evolution of a single medical subspecialty and its development in a public university and medical school replays common themes of human behavior, noble or sometimes ignoble. The urge and need to educate future generations is the heart of the matter of the university and the medical profession. Methodologic observation and reasoning to create new knowledge and apply it rationally to human well-being and planetary sustainability (the latter becoming so clear in the twenty-first century) necessarily follows the educational mission closely. Kindness, collegiality, equality, freedom, teamwork, and discovery are attributes and adjectives that dignify the work of universities, but these are too often offset by envy, greed, unkindness, lurching leadership, personal aggrandizement, dishonesty, dogmatism, sectarianism, and nationalism. All these human characteristics are interwoven throughout history and inevitably will continue, but as we inform ourselves of the past we can better attain the good and navigate the negative.

A memorable thought came from surgical educator Edward Churchill (1916–1972) via his surgical intern, M. Judah Folkman (1933–2008), who recalled Churchill's opening lecture to his intern class on the first day of training at the Massachusetts General Hospital (MGH). The interns were chaffing at the bit to get into the operating rooms or at least in clinics or on wards to begin their lives' work, but Churchill seemed oblivious to their impatience as he spoke for more than an hour in a hot classroom that July in 1957, recalling the generations of the surgeons who had preceded him at the MGH. Churchill, Folkman explained, finally said something like this:

> I know you young men are anxious to roll up your sleeves and get to work. But if you don't understand the history of your field, those who came before you, and the place where you work, you will soon feel exploited.[5]

Exploited might be currently translated to *burned out*, but Churchill's idea is clear: a sense of history enhances meaning in one's work and belief in one's mission. Another relevant thought comes from professor Sarah Buss in the University of Michigan Philosophy Department who once explained that her students can't gain a deeper understanding of issues they consider in class without becoming less certain where they stand on those issues, paraphrasing Kieran Setiya:

> I aim to help them *gain* clarity, knowing that the result will often be a *loss* of certainty. The patience to ask and keep asking questions, without the reassurance of agreement or the availability of methods apt to elicit clarity, is the philosopher's gift. It is an expression of intellectual hope, and the repudiation of philosophy (or repudiation of reason) is a counsel of despair.[6]

My lesson from these points of view is that a rich sense of history and belief in one's culture will inoculate against this thing we call "burn out." Equally important is the ability to question "facts" and yet accept degrees of ambiguity and uncertainty as we work and learn. Once again, here is evidence that culture trumps strategy, metrics, structure, rules, or whatever else may be thrown your way. Buss's point fits in well with the modern organization, particularly so with her point of "the patience to ask and keep asking questions," an idea at the very center of *lean process engineering*, so effectively brought into the workplace by Toyota, taught here in North America through the Lean Enterprise Institute and championed for two decades at our health system at the University of Michigan by Jack Billi and Jeanne Kin.

Medical practice changed greatly in the 170 years since the University of Michigan opened its medical school, then called the Department of Medicine and Surgery. During its first half-century of medicine at the University of Michigan, genitourinary procedures were a sidebar of the work of general surgeons. Whatever might have been the first genitourinary operative procedures at Michigan's first University Hospital awaits discovery by some future historian, as does documentation of the earliest efforts back then to teach the knowledge and skills of the rudimentary specialty. Genitourinary surgery didn't become a distinct area of focused practice except in sporadic locations until the early twentieth century, but the clinical wizardry along with the rich educational and investigational components of modern urology is something substantially greater.

This story of a medical specialty, *genitourinary surgery*, and its current iteration *urology* at the University of Michigan begins with 10 intersecting narratives in two parts that form the roots of urology at the University of Michigan. This is followed by an inspection of Hugh Cabot and his era, plus a curious story related to Michigan and finally an epilogue to this portion of the story of Michigan Urology. Some names and anecdotes find their ways into more than one of these 10 intersecting narratives, and that is much of the fun of history, because it is not a simple chronology of people and events but rather a rich web of the narrative of humanity.

After this volume of our Michigan Urology origin story, the Konnak and Pardanani book will be revised and then the subsequent 20 years will be encapsulated in a narrative to tell our version of the first century of urology at the University of Michigan from its start with Hugh Cabot to the time of Ganesh Palapattu, current chair of the department.

Jim Montie rightly asked,

> Who is your audience for this work? Those with a desire and affection for historical perspectives, with particular association with UM urology OR urologists and trainees at UM OR a broad cross-section of urologists curious about urology at UM? I am thinking aloud and wondering if the depth of historical detail and length of the work will intimidate many of a potential audience? Are you hoping for a Michigan urologic counterpart to Churchill's *History of the English Speaking Peoples* that is a classic but not for the masses?
> (J. Montie, personal communication, March, 2019)

Jim's question sharpened my ambition to claim all the audiences he postulated. This work is intended for the centennial audience, friends of the Department of Urology, new trainees and faculty over the next 10–20 years, and a small audience of those curious about urological and medical history. Ultimately, this is an attempt of the writers to personally reconcile our work, our institution, and place in the world, much as the quotes above from the Stenecks, Edward Churchill via Folkman, and Buss indicated. Winston Churchill's *History of the English Speaking Peoples* came in at around 510,000 words. Much of it was dictated by Churchill during his baths starting in 1937 and finally published in 1956–1958. Political opponent Clement Attlee said the title should have been *Things in History that Interested Me*, and probably few readers of the bestseller persevered through each sentence in the entire four volumes.[ii]

The Michigan Urology Story has no grand scale or expectations, and someday may be enriched by further detail as well as further pruning. This first section, the Michigan Urology Origin Story can be easily set aside after the preface by those impatient for the details of the first century of Michigan Urology (1919–2020) to appear after that century concludes.

---

ii The Churchill Project at Hillsdale College also lists his complete speeches at 5,200,000 words, the six-volume *Second World War* at 1,600,000 words, his collected essays at 860,000 words, *The World Crisis* at 824,000 words, *Marlborough: His Life and Times* at 779,000 words, *Lord Randolph Churchill* at 278,000 words, and *The River War* at 200,000 words.

True facts are elusive and, as should be clear by now in this preface, this work could not have been accomplished alone. Sandra Heskett and our researchers, Katie Baxter and Sarah Streit, made this work come together. Martha Bloom offered endless proofreading and support for the keyboard time and research behind this story. Fran Blouin, Terry McDonald, Marschall Runge, and the University of Michigan Press provided the framework for this study. Anne Duderstadt and Mary Banks helped provide wonderful factual detail. My colleagues in the Urology Department and my successor as chair, Ganesh Palapattu, extended the time and resources for this work to come together. The Schlesinger Library at Radcliffe and Sarah Hutcheon helped enormously finding documents on the Cabot Story. Scott Podolsky and his amazing team at the Countway Library at Harvard inspired recollection of Humphrey Bogart in *Casablanca* (1942) when he said to Claude Rains, "I think this is the beginning of a beautiful friendship." Many other colleagues and friends also contributed, and we hope to account for them in our references and acknowledgments. We expect most readers will deal with this text selectively and recurrently, as it attempts to be, for now, a deep contextual story of urology at the University of Michigan.

David A. Bloom, for the entire UM Urology team
2020

Notes

1 H. H. Peckham, *The Making of the University of Michigan 1817–1992*. Edited and updated by M. L. Steneck and N. H. Steneck (Ann Arbor: University of Michigan Press, 1967, 1994), 1–2.
2 H. W. Davenport, *Not Just Any Medical School* (Ann Arbor: University of Michigan Press, 1999); H. W. Davenport, *Fifty Years of Medicine at the University of Michigan 1891–1941* (Ann Arbor: University of Michigan Press, 1986).
3 D. H. Boster and J. D. Howell, *Medicine at Michigan* (Ann Arbor: University of Michigan Press, 2017).
4 J. W. Konnak and D. S. Pardanani, *A History of Urology at the University of Michigan 1920–2001* (Ann Arbor: University of Michigan Department of Urology, 2002).
5 Personal communication to David A. Bloom from Judah Folkman, Boston, c. 2003 or 2004—Victor Vaughan Society trip.
6 P.c. Sarah Buss, November 13, 2018. Kieran Setiya, "Monk Justice" in *London Review of Books* 40.16 (Aug 30, 2018).

PART I

An Ancient Medical Specialty Reiterated and the University of Michigan

Introduction to a Medical Specialty

Humans, like most primates and other mammals, have keen interest in urine and recognize changes in its characteristics not only personally but also as observant bystanders or as sympathetic healers trying to offer diagnosis, prognosis, and remedy. Visual inspection of urine, uroscopy, was one of the earliest medical practices. Logical approaches to understanding disease and finding remedies were evident in ancient Asian traditions, notably Ayurvedic and traditional Chinese medicine. The *Sushruta Samhita* text in early India as well as the *Huang Ti Nei Ching Su Wen* of ancient China considered matters of urine inspection as well as dysfunctions and treatments, specifically urinary retention and catheterization. The Code of Hammurabi and the Edwin Smith Papyrus of Egypt made no mention of catheterization, although likely it was part of the skill sets of some practitioners.[1]

The most complete known medical system of the past, the Hippocratic School in the fourth to fifth century BCE, encompassed nearly all parts of health care of the time, including physical examination, history taking, pulse characterization, uroscopy, dietary practice, education, and professional standards. A single specific therapeutic exclusion, "cutting for stone," was left to the acknowledged experts in that art, lithotomists, but little evidence of their ancient work remains. Bladder stones were so common a problem and their therapeutic solutions so fraught that this separate cadre of specialists filled a necessary need. In those ancient days, long before anesthesia, analgesia, antisepsis, and antibiotics, lithotomy was a grim matter, understandable only as an alternative to living with the daily misery of bladder stones. Lithotomy worked well enough when it was successful, but it was a horrific experience, with terrible morbidity and very high mortality. Incredibly, lithotomy was performed solely by perineal routes. The work of lithotomists changed little over the ensuing two millennia until new technology and a verifiable expanding scientific basis of medical knowledge in the nineteenth century set the stage for suprapubic lithotomy. Technology and subspecialty medicine of the twentieth century provided the previously unimaginable reality of safe and tolerable modern noninvasive lithotomy.[i]

The Hippocratic school functioned around a health spa on the island of Cos, just off the coast of modern-day Turkey, and delivered nearly the entire range of medical practice and education for its time, except for that single "urologic" exclusion. Uroscopy, in contrast to lithotomy, was well within the Hippocratic domain, and urine examination was fundamental to *diagnosis* and, more importantly, *prognosis*. Useful treatments for most diseases being few and far between, knowledge of a patient's fate, with respect to recovery or death, was valuable information. The Hippocratic School reflected much of the intellectual excitement of the Ioanian Enchantment and the professional values listed in the *Hippocratic Oath* endure today.[ii,2]

Four centuries after Hippocrates, Galen contributed importantly to medicine in general and urology in particular, endorsing uroscopy and lithotomy and conducting investigations (often through vivisection) that contributed to understanding urinary tract function.[3]

The *Golden Age of Islamic Medicine* brought important concepts to health care, now mainly reflected in extant writings of the times and archeological remnants. The ancient Hippocratic example of places for the sick extended over the ensuing centuries to eighth-century specialized leprosaria, Baghdad's first general hospital in 805, specialized tents on battlefields to care for wounded, and mobile hospitals carried by camels. A hospital in 872, in an area that is now Old Cairo, included care for mental illness. Al-Razi's hospital in Baghdad opened in the late ninth century with 25 physicians of different sorts including surgeons, oculists, and bonesetters, whose numbers and specialties grew at the hospital until it was destroyed along with the rest of the city by the Mongolian invasion of 1258.[4] No specific lithotomists have been identified for that time, but it is safe to assume that bladder stones were prevalent and somehow cared for by some practitioners. The Nuri Hospital in Damascus, founded in mid-twelfth century, persisted into the fifteenth century. On

---

i The phrase cutting for stone persists across millennia, notably in the title of Abraham Verghese's novel of 2009, one of the great and most authentic medical narratives. A. Verghese. *Cutting For Stone* (New York: Knopf, 2009).

ii Ioanian enchantment was the title of the first chapter in the remarkable book; E. O. Wilson, *Consilience* (New York: Knopf, 1998).

the Iberian Peninsula, Córdoba alone was said to have had 50 major hospitals offering military and specialized care. Some of these facilities, called *bimaristans*, were carefully planned and highly organized to include medical schools, dispensaries, physicians, nurses, libraries, specialties, administrators, and high standards. Philanthropy played roles in building and supporting many of these, along with other funding models. Tschanz described and illustrated the Bimaristan Argun in Aleppo, Syria, founded in the mid-fourteenth century and functioning as a hospital into the early twentieth century, although little remains now in early twenty-first century, given the gross destruction of that Syrian civil war. The urological work throughout these eras and geographies has been largely lost in history.

Urinary tract catheterization has had a long and parallel course with uroscopy and lithotomy, the latter being a far more complex intervention, while urethral catheterization for urinary retention is far more generalizable. Early Greek and Roman practitioners described urinary retention and relief by catheterization. Avicenna (980–1037), the famed Muslim philosopher, Koranic scholar, physician, and author of *The Canon of Medicine*, discussed intermittent bladder catheterization and advised doing it gently with lubrication by soft cheese. He used flexible and rigid catheters and warned against catheterization in the presence of inflammation. Avicenna believed in cleanliness, even to the point of handwashing when applying leeches, and presumably used the same hygienic principle in the rest of his work.[5] Abulcasis of Córdoba (936–1013) employed bladder irrigation through urethral catheters and recommended a silver catheter for urinary retention due to bladder calculus. Silver catheter technology advanced on the other side of the Atlantic centuries later with a flexible version invented by Benjamin Franklin.[6]

Uroscopy, like lithotomy, changed little for most of the 2,500 years after Hippocrates with only incremental refinements in details of urine color, odor, sediment, and taste. Fanciful color gradients, specified in uroscopy charts and standard bottles on shelves, were linked to imagined prognoses and remedies. The printing press in 1450 disseminated uroscopy charts and methodologies to wide audiences and *Hortus Sanitatis*, Jacob Meydenbach's incunabulum printed in Mainz in 1491, for example, shows doctors and students in a uroscopy clinic studying urine samples in glass matulas and pointing to standard samples on the shelves. Twin boys, presumably patients, are fighting in the foreground while two women and one young man are shown, also in the foreground, carrying wicker baskets with urine specimens to the clinic, presumably on a fee-for-service basis. [Figure on next page.]

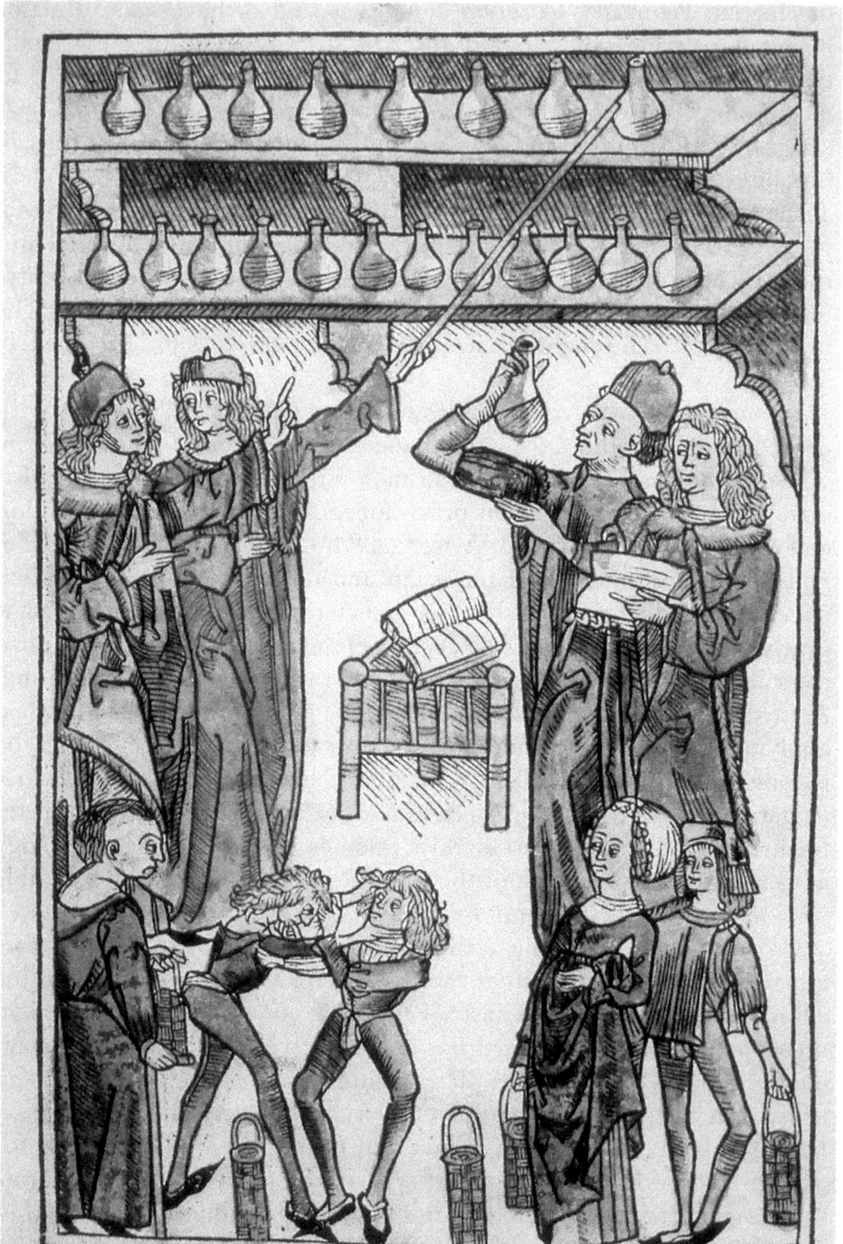

Uroscopy chart. *Hortus Sanitatis*. 1491, Mainz. Courtesy Dick Wolfe, Countway Library.

Genitourinary anatomic illustration with fairly accurate speculations of relevant physiology came to a high level of detail and accuracy during the curiously short academic career of Vesalius (1514–1564), anatomist and educator in Italy. He teamed up with Johan van Calcar and other illustrators to produce extraordinary illustrated anatomical texts that made anatomical learning feasible for students as well as liberating practitioners from cadaveric study. Vesalius corrected the inaccurate Galenic conclusions of renal position, described the lateral differences of gonadal vasculature, comprehended the valvular nature of the ureterovesical junction, understood prostatic anatomy better than any predecessors, and had sophisticated recognition of penile genital physiology. The productive work of Vesalius lasted only six years from the time of his medical degree at the University of Padua in 1537 to the publication in 1543 of his magnum opus *De Humani Corporis Fabrica* with its 273 spectacular illustrations, after which he accepted the position of imperial physician in the court of Emperor Charles V and ended his scholarly work.

The well-known Shakespearian reference in *Henry IV*, written in 1597–1598, finds Sir John Falstaff asking his page what a uroscopist said about the urine sample delivered in a flask called matula. This may be the first written allusion to the common error in which a physician foolishly confuses a laboratory test for the actual patient:

> SIR JOHN Sirrah, you giant, what says the doctor to my water?
> PAGE He said, sir, the water itself was a good healthy water; but for the party that owed it, he might have more diseases that he knew for.[7]

Soon after Shakespeare lampooned uroscopy, the Royal College of Surgeons passed a statute in 1601 to prohibit uroscopic examination by members of its college, *in absentia* of patients.[8] Speculative uroscopy, sometimes called *uromancy*, inspired Petrus Forestus, a well-regarded Dutch physician, to write a book with stories of charlatanism and uroscopic pranks on physicians, such as substitution of urine samples from barnyard animals for legitimate samples of patients. The exhausting title, in the James Hart translation of 1623, explains the book without sarcastic restraint:

> The Arraignment of Urines: Wherein are Set downe the manifold errors and abuses of ignorant Urine-monging Empirickes, cozening Quacksalvers, women-physicians, and the like stuffe: Confining the urines within their owne lists and limits; and adding such Caveats and Cautions to the inspection and judgement of Diseases by the same as have not hitherto by any beene observed.

Thomas Brian, a graduate of Cambridge University and medical practitioner, similarly criticized the uroscopy industry in *The Pisse-Prophet* of 1637, a rare book with only nine copies of the extant 1655 edition.

William Harvey (1578–1657) refuted Galen's ancient idea of separate dual circulatory systems in *Exercitatio Anatomica de Motu Cordis et Sanguinis in Animalibus*, cleverly rushing to publication in Frankfurt during the city's annual book fair in 1628. This work was a forerunner to the broader understanding of human physiology that more fully emerged two and a half centuries later. Three years after Harvey died, microscopic studies of Marcello Malpighi (1628–1694) identified the missing piece of Harvey's postulated single circulatory system, the capillaries.[iii]

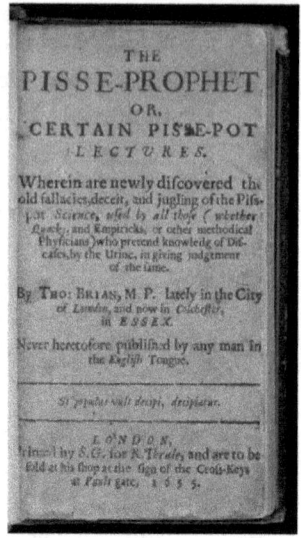

Brian cover, *Wikimedia*.

Just as uroscopy persisted throughout most of the second millennium, ancient lithotomy practices continued, untouched by isolated medical discoveries like Harvey's. The best known lithotomist was Jacques Beaulieu (1651–1720), a self-styled "monk," known as Frère Jacques, who traveled from town to town in Europe with "certificates of cures" and may have performed 5,000 perineal lithotomies.[9] Other itinerant lithotomists, long forgotten, similarly plied their trade with techniques from Hippocratic times, but left no written evidence. Lithotomy must have had enough anecdotal success, as well as effective marketing by flamboyant salesmen for the practice to continue, although it was mainly

---

iii Centuries later at the University of Michigan Medical School, professor of physiology Horace Davenport would challenge his students in their first physiology class: "What happened in 1623?" He promised that whoever got the correct answer would get an "A" and be exempted from examinations or attendance in the course. The obvious intent of the question was to identify the greatest human accomplishment of 1623. Many answers were forthcoming, according to a recollection of Joseph Weiss (MD, 1961), until another student, Nancy Zuzow, offered an answer that caught Davenport's interest: "Harvey's discovery of the circulation of the blood." Davenport acknowledged that she offered the only intelligent response of the day, but countered, "that publication occurred in 1628." The professor then supplied the answer he had sought: "1623 was the publication of William Shakespeare's *First Folio*" (the first printed collection of Shakespeare's plays). Davenport then announced that the class would move on and "return to our roles as attendants at the gas station of life" as he gave his first lecture on the *ABC of Acid-Base Chemistry*. J. J. Weiss, "The Question Was: What Happened in 1623?" *Medicine at Michigan*, Fall 2000, p. 20.

the desperate suffering of patients that kept the primitive practice and self-styled experts alive. Itinerant lithotomy eventually was relegated to history books and nursery rhymes as literacy, education, and growing belief in science led people to expect legitimate expertise, accurate medical information, and verifiable treatments with a fair chance for success. The idea that society should regulate professions based on reason and evidence, rather than authoritarian edicts, grew most effectively in democratic nations, unsurprisingly.

Records of genitourinary practice are sparse for colonial American times. The first published account of an elective operative procedure in the North American colonies was that of a lithotomy for bladder stone in a child of Henry Hill, a Boston distiller. The operation took place on June 24, 1720, and was mentioned in an advertisement in the *Boston News-Letter* the following month. The ad, acknowledging permission of the father, marketed Boylston's practice. Although the age of the child and anatomic route were not described, the stone was claimed to be "of considerable bigness." The surgeon, Zabdiel Boylston (1679–1766), wrote the ad himself, proudly noting the boy could hold his water afterward, and proudly concluding, referring to himself in the third person,

> This is his third operation performed in the Stone on Males and females, and all with good success: He likewise pretends to all other Operations in Surgery. Which operation the said Hill could not omit to make Publick.[10]

Boylston never attended medical school, none existing in North America until 1765, but he was a pathfinder, the first in America to remove gallstones (1710) and excise a breast tumor (1718). After he inoculated 248 people with pus from a small pox sore during an epidemic in 1721, he had to go into hiding for a time because of threats on his life.[iv]

A later successful lithotomy, described as perineal, was performed by Dr. Thomas Bond (1713–1784), a founder of America's first hospital, Pennsylvania Hospital (1751).[v]

---

iv Boylston's grandson, Dr. Zabdiel Boylston Adams, worked in conjunction with Moses Gunn of the University of Michigan during the Civil War in the Peninsula Campaign and the Second Battle of Bull Run, where they very likely interacted among the limited number of skilled physicians.

v Priority stories can be complex and nuanced. Pennsylvania Hospital, founded in 1751 by Benjamin Franklin and Thomas Bond, was the first North American hospital of any sub-stance. A medical school, the first in America, was founded in conjunction with the hos-pital in 1765. Higher education had begun earlier in Philadelphia, where a building was established in 1740 for a traveling evangelist and a charity school, although no teaching was performed there initially and it remained unused for a time. After Benjamin Franklin

Bond's lithotomy in 1756 was the first operative procedure at Pennsylvania Hospital and probably differed little in technique from lithotomies centuries earlier. Bond and his son would later play roles in developing the medical department for the Continental Army and creating its first field hospitals. Other bladder calculi experiences embellish early American medical history including Ben Franklin's flexible silver catheter invented for his stone-burdened brother, John, and presumably used later by Ben himself.

Medical skills in Boylston and Bond's time and for the next hundred years were learned during apprenticeship rather than through academic work. Dogma and experience underlay most medical practice of that era, although a body of verifiable medical knowledge had been coming together in bits and pieces through the work of Vesalius, Harvey, and many others. Prominent colonial physicians self-assembled their individual educations through patchworks of experiences. Philip Syng Physick (1768–1837), for example, graduated from the University of Pennsylvania in 1785, spent three years locally "reading medicine," two additional years in London with clinician, teacher, and innovator, John Hunter, before going to Edinburgh for yet another year to get an MD in 1792. Returning to the new United States in 1805, Physick became the first professor of surgery at Pennsylvania's medical school. Bladder stone surgery was then a significant component of general surgical practice and teaching, and Physick's lithotomy skill would later be one of his crowning achievements.[vi]

An interval of European study with a legitimate medical degree were important credentials for early leaders in American medicine, because

---

circulated a pamphlet in 1749, "Proposals Relating to the Education of Youth in Pennsylvania," an Academy of Philadelphia began teaching secondary students in the building. A Seal of the Trustees of the College of Philadelphia in 1757 shows seven stacked books on a slanted desk in rising order: *Grammatica, Rhetorica, Logica, Mathematica, Philosopica, Astronomia,* and *Theologica*. A charter for the college in 1779 created "the first" American university, actually using that term (university) and incorporating professional education of the Philadelphia medical school and colleges, then called seminaries. The medical school of the University of Pennsylvania is currently known as the Perelman School of Medicine and operates under the flag of Penn Medicine. The distinction of which institution can claim priority in higher education is discussed in a brief *Wikipedia* article "First university in the United States." The article refers to a 1911 *Encyclopaedia Britannica* paper on American universities that assigned priority historically to the University of Santo Tomas of the Philippines in 1611, then an American territory. Further confusing the issue is the blur between secondary and higher education in the seventeenth and eighteenth centuries. Nevertheless, the University of Pennsylvania can fairly claim priority as the first university, in the modern sense of the word, in Continental America.

vi In 1831, Supreme Court chief justice John Marshall, 76-years-old, came to Pennsylvania Hospital for lithotomy where Physick removed 1,000 bladder stones, allegedly, by lithotomy. Marshall, then the last living "Founding Father," lived four more years.

knowledge, education, and innovation in medicine were centered in Europe up through the mid-nineteenth century. A chapter in McCullough's book *Americans Abroad* explains the phenomenon that included significant elements of genitourinary practice.[11] John Peter Mettauer (1787–1875), a pupil of Physick and also a University of Pennsylvania graduate (1809) with European training, had an extraordinary but sparsely documented career that included great experience in lithotomies (over 400), cataract operations (800), hypospadias surgery, and, in 1838, successful closure of vesicovaginal fistula.[12] James Marion Sims (1813–1883), 10 years later, although he lacked European experience, nonetheless expanded the skills of fistula repair.[13] That work recently was thrown into controversy regarding questions of patient consent. A careful historical and ethical study of Wall concluded,

> There is no doubt that slaves in the mid-19th century American South were a "vulnerable" population who were often subjected to significant abuse by the slaveholding system. To suggest, however, that for that reason alone no attempts should have been made to cure the maladies of such enslaved women, especially when they were desperate for help and no other viable alternatives existed, seems ethically bankrupt itself. Whatever his other failings may have been, J. Marion Sims pursued this clinical goal with vigor, determination, and perseverance, and both his patients then and countless thousands of women since, benefited from his success.[14]

Contemporary medical historian, Ira Rutkow, identified the earliest American surgical textbooks.[15] Of these, the genitourinary texts began with Alexander Hodgdon Stevens (1789–1869), a Yale graduate with an MD from the University of Pennsylvania in 1819, who practiced and taught at New York Hospital. The 93-page book, *Lectures on Lithotomy*, in 1838 was America's first urology text.[vii] Stevens served as second president of the American Medical Association in 1848. Edward Dixon (1808–1880) produced a text in 1847, *A Treatise on Diseases of the Sexual System: Adapted to Popular and Professional Readings and the Exposition of Quackery* and its eighth edition in only another year reached 260 pages.

Homer Bostwick (1806–1883), another New York surgeon with a genitourinary focus, wrote two books in 1847 and 1848 with long titles.

---

vii This year was also significant for the invention of the daguerreotype by Louis-Jacques-Mandé Daguerre, which allowed formation of an image on a polished silver surface after exposure to a subject, and became a forerunner of photography after a number of process iterations. Daguerre formally publicized his invention the following year.

A Treatise on the Nature and Treatment of Seminal Diseases, Impotency, and Other Kindred Affections: With Practical Directions for the Management and Removal of the Cause Producing Them; Together with Hints to Young Men was 251 pages. *A Complete Practical Work on the Nature and Treatment of Venereal Diseases, and Other Affections of the Genito-Urinary Organs of the Male and Female* was 348 pages.[16] Bostwick discussed and illustrated anatomically-based interventions, and in his section "Mode of puncturing the bladder" he instructed that the canula must be retained, advising this operation for urinary retention from enlarged prostate but "never" in cases of "retention from stricture." The figure on the next page shows both the transurethral approach and the transrectal approach to the bladder.

Next in the Rutkow chronologic bibliography was the 1851 text of Samuel David Gross (1805–1884), *A Practical Treatise on the Disease and Injuries of the Urinary Bladder, the Prostate Gland, and the Urethra*, with 726 pages. Gross listed his position as professor of surgery at Louisville, although he was working in New York when the book was published. Similar texts followed by Alban Goldsmith (1857), William Morland (1858), Freeman Bumstead (1861), and John Gouley (1873), but one in 1874 bears special consideration: *A Practical Treatise on the Surgical Diseases of the Genito-Urinary Organs, Including Syphilis*. Its 672 pages came from William Van Buren and his younger assistant at Bellevue Hospital Medical College in New York, Edward Lawrence Keyes. This book shaped the emerging field of genitourinary surgery more than that of any others of the time. Keyes rewrote the text in 1888 with his son, who later contributed significantly to the literature on his own.

Chemical analysis and microscopy carried the inspection of urine to new levels of detail in the mid-nineteenth century and other technological paradigm shifts transformed ancient lithotomy into humane and effective genitourinary procedures, notably beginning when a young American doctor witnessed a milestone event at the Massachusetts General Hospital and reported it in a prominent journal:

> It has long been an important problem in medical science to devise some method of mitigating the pain of surgical operations. An efficient agent for this purpose has at length been discovered. A patient has been rendered completely insensible during an amputation of a thigh, regaining consciousness after a short interval. Other severe operations have been performed without knowledge of the patients. So remarkable an occurrence will, it is believed, render the following details relating to the history and character of the process, not uninteresting.

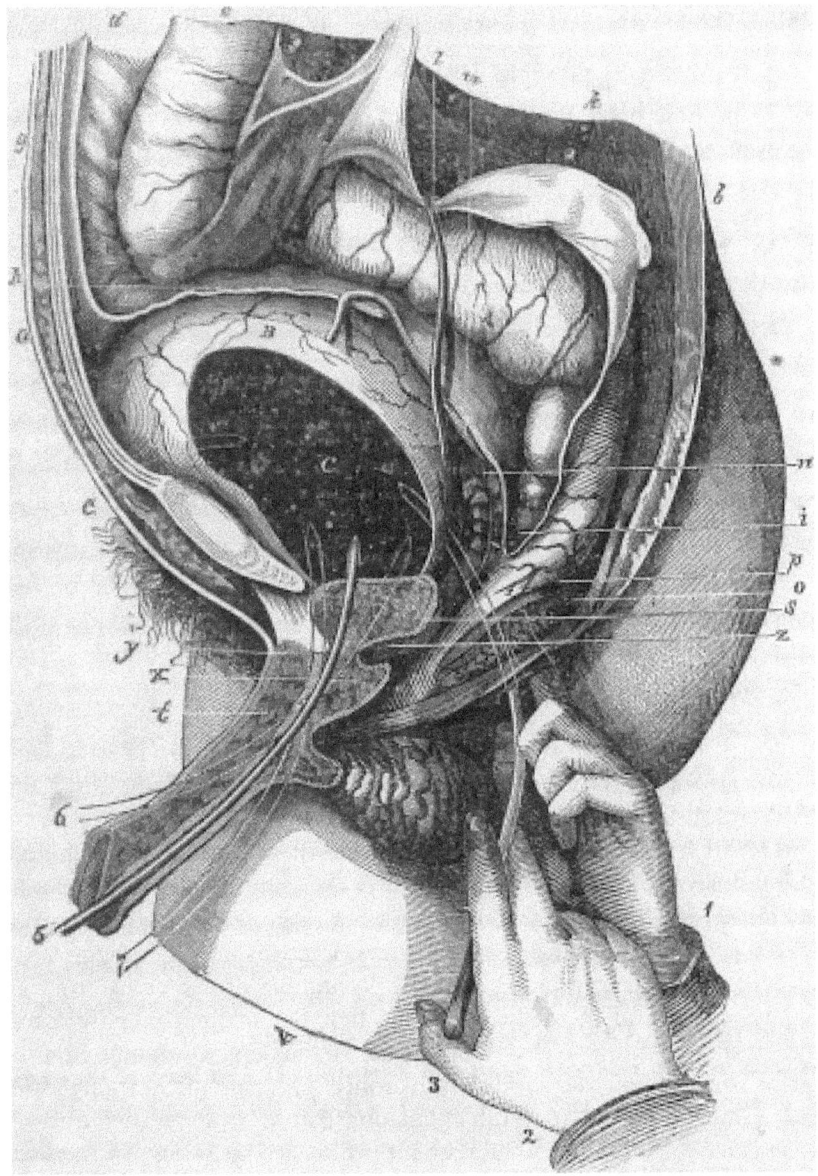

A complete practical work on the nature and treatment of venereal diseases, and other affections of the genitourinary organs of the male and female. H. Bostwick. 1848.

On the 16th of Oct., 1846, an operation was performed at this hospital upon a patient who had inhaled a preparation administered by Dr. Morton, a dentist of this city, with the alleged intention of producing insensibility to pain.[17]

Over the next half-century that young man, Henry Jacob Bigelow, would become one of the most prominent genitourinary practitioners and innovators. Oliver Wendell Holmes, another young American physician who would become no less prominent in American medicine, also witnessed the event and coined a term for the patient's insensibility, *anesthesia*. He wrote a letter to Morton on November 21, 1846:

> My Dear Sir: _ Everybody wants to have a hand in a great discovery. All I want to do is to give you a hint or two as to names, or the name, to be applied to the state produced and the agent.
>
> The state should, I think, be called "Anaesthesia." This signifies insensibility, more particularly (as used by Linnaeus and Cullen) to objects of touch. (See GOOD _ *Nosology*, p. 259.) The adjective will be "Anaesthetic." Thus we might say, the state of anaesthesia, or the anaesthetic state. The means employed would be properly called the anti-aesthetic agent.[18]

Observation, reasoning, and clinical trials of Joseph Lister brought safety in surgical care into the medical marketplace. His evidence for antiseptic surgical techniques, published in *The Lancet* and the *British Medical Journal* in 1867, was irrefutable, although acceptance was reluctant and delayed for decades in many centers.[19] Precision instruments and electrical illumination with Edison's incandescent lamp (1880) created opportunities for novel diagnostic and therapeutic cystourethroscopic interventions and elicited a new cadre of genitourinary practitioners.

Medical history, as evidenced with anesthesia, antiseptic technique, and endoscopy, is not a progressive orderly unfurling of new ideas and technology as these paragraphs suggest but rather messy collisions of old beliefs and habits against reasoned new practices and paradigms based on evidence. A transatlantic urological example of the collision of old and new is found in the story of the first documented nephrectomies and sterile technique. Gustav Simon in Heidelberg, Germany, in 1869, performed the first recorded nephrectomy. The patient, Margaret Kleb, had a long-standing ureteral cutaneous fistula and her nephrectomy was deemed a success.[20] A subsequent procedure by Simon on August 8, 1871, for renal calculus was uncovered by Peter L. Scardino. The second patient, Mary Helen (Williams) Schirm, a 31-year-old from Savannah, Georgia, had been accompanying her husband on a business trip to Germany when she had recurrence of severe left renal colic, a condition she suffered since age 18. The family consulted with Simon who declared nephrectomy necessary (an erroneous conclusion given that the lady merely had ureteral colic) and, believing the contralateral kidney normal, he removed the problematic kidney through a lumbar incision.

The procedure took 30 minutes. Anesthesia, standard of care at most major European centers at the time, was likely employed but not Lister's recent antiseptic measures, which were then only sporadically accepted in Europe. Nevertheless, the lady was well until her 21st operative day when Simon, during a routine bandage change, probed the wound to a depth of 2.5 cm with his bare finger. This was a customary habit when physicians were looking for an abscess or foreign body or perhaps if a physician was merely acting authoritatively. At that point, however, Mrs. Schirm seemed to offer no indication for Simon's deep probing. Later in the day she experienced fever and chills, followed by 10 days of sepsis and then death on September 7. The autopsy report, Scardino discovered, revealed peritonitis and pleuritis. Simon blamed the death on his finger probing and the unhygienic hospital, although Scardino suggested lack of drainage of the wound as the cause.[viii,21]

Lister's antiseptic lessons, documented so convincingly in 1867, diffused slowly throughout Europe and even more reluctantly in the United States, although one authoritative text to emphasize antisepsis and asepsis would come 22 years later from surgeon Charles de Nancrede in 1889, newly arrived in Ann Arbor.[22]

Notes

1. D. A. Bloom, E. J. McGuire, and J. Lapides, "A Brief History of Urethral Catheterization," *Journal of Urology* 151 (1994): 317–325.
2. D. A. Bloom, "Hippocrates and Urology: The First Surgical Subspecialty," *Urology* 50 (1997): 157–159.
3. D. A. Bloom, M. T. Milen, and J. C. Heininger, "Claudius Galen: From a 20th Century Genitourinary perspective," *Journal of Urology* 161 (1999): 12–19.
4. D. W. Tschanz, "The Islamic Roots of the Modern Hospital," *Aramco World* 68 (2017): 22–27.
5. D. A. Bloom, E. J. McGuire, and J. Lapides, "A Brief History of Urethral Catheterization," *Journal of Urology* 151 (1994): 317–325.

---

viii Ten years later, the death of President James Garfield in 1881 was similarly ascribed to late sepsis rather than assassin's bullet. Attending physician Willard Bliss initially probed the wound by instruments and finger hoping to find the bullet but without success. In the course of treatment, Bliss described early urinary catheterization, pus evacuation, incision and drainage, parotid abscess, probing by finger, probing by ceramic tipped Nelaton probe, and use of an "induction device" provided by Alexander Bell to locate the bullet, although again without success. Two and a half months after the assassination attempt, finger probing was repeated in the course of care, but Garfield, weakened with an 80-pound weight loss, died of sepsis, as detailed in the original paper of Bliss and the book by Candice Millard. W. Bliss, Report of the Case of President Garfield, Accompanied with a Detailed Account of the Autopsy, "The Medical Record," New York: William Wood & Company, 20 (1881): 393–402; C. Millard, *Destiny of the Republic* (New York: Doubleday, 2011).

6 G. W. Corner and W. E. Goodwin, "Benjamin Franklin's Bladder Stone," *Journal of the History of Medicine and Allied Sciences* 8 (1953): 359–377.
7 Shakespeare, 2H4 1.2.1–5.
8 F. D. Hoeniger, *Medicine and Shakespeare in the English Renaissance* (Newark: University of Delaware Press, 1992), 232.
9 J. P. Ganem and C. C. Carson, "Frère Jacques Beaulieu: From Rogue Lithotomist to Nursery Rhyme Character," *Journal of Urology* 161 (1999): 1067–1069.
10 A. S. Earle, *Surgery in America: From the Colonial Era to the Twentieth Century* 2nd ed. (New York: Praeger, 1983), 6.
11 D. McCullough, *The Greater Journey: Americans in Paris*, Ch. 4, *The Medicals* (New York: Simon and Schuster, 1911).
12 W. Bickers, "John Peter Mettauer of Virginia," *JAMA* 184 (1963): 870–871.
13 A. S. Earle, *Surgery in America: From the Colonial Era to the Twentieth Century* 2nd ed. (New York: Praeger, 1983), 226–227.
14 L. L. Wall, "The Medical Ethics of Dr. J. Marion Sims: A Fresh Look at the Historical Record." *Journal of Medical Ethics* 32, no. 6 (2006): 346–350.
15 I. M. Rutkow, *The History of Surgery in the United States, 1775–1900. Volume 1* (San Francisco, CA: Norman, 1988).
16 H. Bostwick, *A Complete Practical Work on the Nature and Treatment of Venereal Diseases: and Other Affections of the Genito-Urinary Organs of the Male and Female* (New York: Burgess, Stringer & Co., 1848).
17 H. J. Bigelow, "Insensibility during Surgical Operations Produced by Inhalation," *Boston Medical and Surgical Journal* 35, no. 16 (1846): 309–317.
18 O. W. Holmes, "Miscellany. Origin of the Term 'Anesthetic,'" *The Railway Surgeon* vol. 1, The Railway Age and Northwestern Railroader (1894–1895): 415.
19 J. Lister, "On the Antiseptic Principle in the Practice of Surgery," *British Medical Journal* 2 (1867): 246; *The Lancet* 20, no. 2299 (1867): 353–356.
20 C. P. Mathé, "Kidney Surgery," *History of Urology from American Urological Association vol. 1,* (Baltimore: The Williams & Wilkins, 1933), 296–297.
21 P. L. Scardino, "First Planned Nephrectomy for Kidney Stones," *Urology* 13 (1979): 111–112; D. A. Bloom and P. T. Scardino, "Peter Lester Scardino—A Genitourinary Surgeon in the Third Generation of the Specialty. Part 2," *Urology* 73 (2009): 944–946.
22 C. B. de Nancrede, *Lectures on the Principles of Surgery* (Philadelphia, PA: Saunders, 1889).

Medical Education, Practice, and the University of Michigan in Early America

Medical education and practice in early America had few noteworthy centers and those occasional places reflected European experience brought home by fortunate young people who had opportunities to study abroad. Philadelphia, Boston, and New York were the first major American surgical centers, but westward expansion opened new possibilities. *An Ordinance for the Government of the Territory of the United States, North-West of the River Ohio*, enacted by Congress of the Confederation of the United States on July 13, 1787, created America's first organized territory, the Northwest Territory, from lands below British North America, west of the Appalachian Mountains, north of the Ohio River, and east of the Mississippi River. The southern border later became a practical boundary between free states and the others. The *Northwest Ordinance of 1787*, as it came to be known, included a clause with a remarkably enlightened sense of government and the revised *Northwest Ordinance of 1789* of the new U.S. Congress replaced the older version with only minor changes:

> Religion, morality, and knowledge being necessary to good government and the happiness of mankind, schools and the means of education shall forever be encouraged.[1]

Notably, the word *happiness* had appeared in the second sentence of the *Declaration of Independence* 11 years earlier, as one of the three self-evident and inalienable rights of humanity. Danielle Allen's discussion of these foundational principles in her book, *Our Declaration*, should rightly precede further reading of the more parochial work immediately in front of you.[2]

New governments, cities, and infrastructure were needed to fill in the new territories and Jefferson's Louisiana Purchase in 1803 required rethinking of the meaning of "northwest." A *Congressional Act* on January 11, 1805, established the Territory of Michigan, separate from Indiana Territory, and required appointment of a governor and three judges. President Jefferson named William Hull of Massachusetts as governor and Augustus Woodward, Frederick Bates, and John Griffin, all from Virginia, as judges. Woodward and Hull arrived in Michigan Territory, on horseback, the weekend after Detroit's great fire and found their work cut out for them. Although education was not the first priority, it was not far down the list in Woodward's mind.

Woodward was an intellectual with bold ideas on epistemology and education, publishing a book in 1816 with an astonishing title for the time: *A System of Universal Science*, subtitled, *Considerations on the Divisions of Human Knowledge and on the Classification and Nomenclature of the Sciences*. The opening two sentences laid out his challenge.

> The knowledge which the human race are capable of acquiring upon this earth appears, at the first view, too multifarious to be susceptible of arrangement.
>
> On the primary approach to it, human knowledge resembles an immense structure; of which the magnitude oppresses, and the variety distracts, the mind.[3]

Woodward's ideas had a central place in the foundational document he drafted, *An act to establish the Catholepistemiad, or university of Michigania*, and that became Territorial Law on August 26, 1817, after he signed it along with Griffin and Woodbridge. The first sentences, in archaic Woodwardian terminology, laid out a university structure based on faculty and departments.

> Be it enacted by the Governor and the Judges of the Territory of Michigan, That there shall be in the said Territory a catholepistemiad, or university, denominated the Catholepistemiad, or University, of Michigania. The Catholepistemiad, or University, of Michigania shall be composed of thirteen didaxiim or professorships: first, a didaxia, or professorship, of catholepistemia, or universal science, the didactor, or professor, of which shall be president of the institution; second, a didaxia, or professorship of anthropoglossica, or literature, embracing all the epistemiim or sciences, relative to language; . . . eighth, a didaxia, or professorship, of iatrica, or medical sciences.[4]

The fragile handwritten four-page "Organic Act" was never printed, although the *Detroit Gazette* reported faculty appointments, actions of the university, and generosity of donors (called subscribers) who

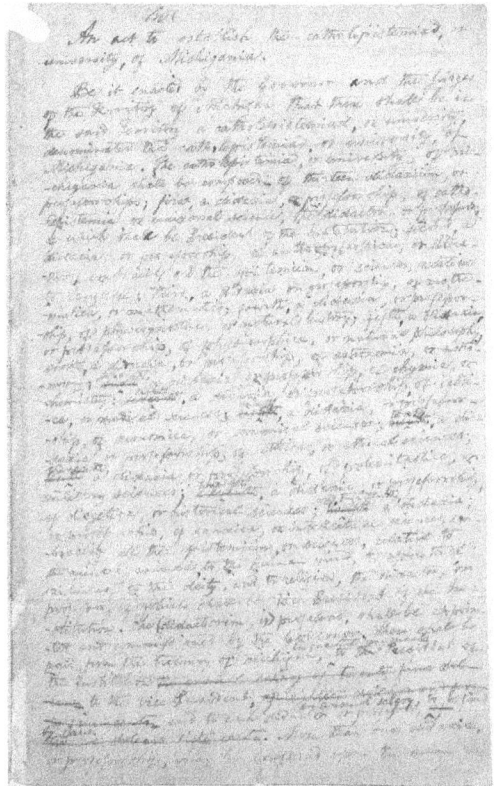

"The Organic Act." page one. Bentley Library.

contributed $3,000 within the first month. Philanthropy had a foundational role even in the first days of the university.

The 13 professorships derived from Woodward's book the previous year. The school's president, as first professor, was responsible for the entirety of the curriculum, the *Catholepistemia*. The vice president was assigned to *Ennoeica*, the intellectual sciences encompassing psychology and religion. Medical sciences, targeted as the eighth unit, *Iatrica*, would be deferred for another 30 years. The Stenecks recognized Woodward's unique vision.

> Much more than eccentric intellectualism was at work here. At a time when Eastern universities were heavy with ancient languages and literature, with religion and philosophy, and with mathematics and a nod to ancient history—the classical curriculum—Woodward had boldly emphasized science and introduced economics for the University of Michigania. He was cracking an old and powerful tradition.[5]

This university was intended as "the capstone of a statewide educational system which it would supervise." The professors were to manage the university without a supervisory board and be supported by taxation, although neither situation lasted long. Reverend John Monteith was appointed university president two weeks after the act was signed and he distributed other professorships up to, but not including, the *Iatrica* professorship. Father Gabriel Richard was named vice president, and within a few weeks the educational system established public primary schools in Detroit, Monroe, and Mackinac Island. The annual salary of the president was set at $25, the vice president $18.75, and $12.50 for professors.[i]

The only other regional colleges in the United States at the time were Transylvania University in Lexington, Kentucky, founded in 1780, and Ohio University in Athens, Ohio, founded in 1804, but neither formally anticipated a medical school as the University of Michigan had done from its start. On October 3, 1817, the university established a college in Detroit that was to have a board of trustees and visitors. Michigan's grand plan for higher education was barely reflected in its first physical iteration in Detroit, a two-story structure on Bates Street that appeared to comprise 6–12 rooms, and not at all evident in records of any students or instructional programs in its first years.

In 1821, Governor Lewis Cass and the territorial judges reorganized the University of Michigan, with a board of 20 trustees and the governor in charge of management. The *catholepistemiad* terminology and other Woodward complexities disappeared soon after their initial usage. Few details remain on classes, students, or intentions regarding the absent medical school, although complaints regarding the need to educate future Michigan doctors in Michigan reverberated over the next two decades. The Bates Street building had not delivered much in the way of actual higher education and in 1831 it was turned over to the city of Detroit as a "common school" for two years until a local taxation law allowed the city to have its own classroom buildings.

Health and disease are tied to every human era, and a cholera epidemic brought the matter home to Detroit in 1832, the city then having a population of around 3,500. Cholera reached Detroit in July via infected troops on the steamer *Henry Clay* and the disease spread quickly, claiming 34-year-old Father Gabriel Richard in September, as the epidemic was winding down. Among the estimated 200 infected people, 60–100 died. Little is recorded of any higher education activities in Detroit

---

i The purchasing power of the president's salary back then equates to around $500 now 200 years later.

around this time. With recovery from the epidemic and the university and the city having no further need for the Bates Street property, the trustees rented it to two schoolmasters for a private "high school" in 1834, but the return of cholera in the middle of July made that a short-term project. Cholera returned to Detroit again in 1849, 1854, 1866, and beyond.[6]

The fledgling University of Michigan in Detroit closed for good in 1834 with that cholera season. This year was significant to Michigan for other reasons, including the relocation in the spring of John Preston Kellogg and his family from Hadley, Massachusetts, to an area near present-day Flint. That family later included two boys who would significantly influence medical practice and health, John Harvey Kellogg (1852) and Will Keith Kellogg (1860).[ii] It was a risky time to pass through Detroit, given the cholera prevalence. One victim then, George Porter, who had been Michigan's governor since Cass left office in 1831, died of the disease on July 6, 1834, although this proved no great loss for the territory. Porter had been so ineffective in his position that territorial secretary Stevens T. Mason, who had earlier been appointed by President Andrew Jackson, was *de facto* "boy governor" for much of Porter's term. At Porter's death, Mason became territorial governor in the first days of that second cholera epidemic that lasted for eight weeks, infected over 700 people, and closed nearly all businesses in Detroit.

After recovery from that epidemic, the state sold land on the Maumee River and sequestered the funds for a new iteration of the University of Michigan. Territorial voters approved a state constitution on October 5, 1835, and elected Mason inaugural governor of the state, although statehood was delayed by U.S. Congress until a land dispute with Ohio was resolved. That dispute had escalated into the slightly bloody Toledo War in the spring and summer of 1835. Mason agreed to a compromise giving Ohio the disputed land in exchange for gaining the western two-thirds of the Upper Peninsula (Michigan already possessed the eastern third). In spite of this border controversy, sales of Michigan land were wildly popular and accounted for as much as a fifth of the federal revenue in 1836 at their peak.[7] After initial setbacks, a compromise to the border dispute was reached in December 1836, and Michigan became the Union's 26th state on January 26, 1837. Mason completed his term in 1840 and moved to New York where he died of pneumonia in 1843 at age 31. The population of Michigan at the time

---

ii Howard Markel tells this story in rich detail, and John Kellogg would attend the University of Michigan Medical School in 1873 but for only a single year in its two-year curriculum before moving to New York City where he would study under E. L. Keyes, the noted genitourinary surgeon.

of statehood was 175,000 with only 10,000 residing in Detroit. Ann Arbor, incorporated only 13 years earlier, had 2,000 people, including 11 lawyers and 9 physicians.[8]

A report to the new state legislature, resuscitating and reiterating the University of Michigan, was accepted on March 18, 1837. A conveniently formed Ann Arbor Land Company immediately offered 40 acres with a choice of one of two sites for university relocation and the offer was accepted on March 20. The university selected the flat site just east of State Street, instead of a hilly area overlooking the Huron River (that would later become the medical campus). Faculty needed to be recruited, and buildings needed to be built. A board of regents was appointed and met in June with Governor Mason as president of the board by election. Four professorships were created but the only actual appointment from that meeting was the librarian, Methodist minister Henry Colclazer. It seemed clear from the start that the Ann Arbor campus was something original and far more than a reiteration of the initial Woodward vision in Detroit. Victor Vaughan, a later dean of the Medical School, recalled, "That the original Board of Regents which was appointed by Governor Mason and began to function in 1837 had a distinct appreciation of science is shown by their first appointment to a professorship in this University."[9]

The first two professors at the university in Ann Arbor were excellent scientists and physicians as well but they performed little in the way of "professing" at the University of Michigan. Asa Gray (1810–1888), an 1831 graduate of Fairfield Medical College in New York and an avid botanist, had a brief period of medical practice apprenticeship and then found an academic path in life, moving to Manhattan as an assistant to the renowned botanist, chemist, and physician, John Torrey, at the College of Physicians and Surgeons in New York. In 1836, Gray became curator and librarian at the Lyceum of Natural History, now called the New York Academy of Sciences.[iii]

[iii] John Torrey (1796–1873) had studied and practiced medicine in New York but found teaching chemistry and studying biology more congenial, teaching the topics at West Point and later the College of Physicians and Surgeons of Columbia. He was a cofounder of the Lyceum, an important American scientific institution with democratic membership that would include two presidents, Darwin, and many other luminaries. One student of Asa Gray and Torrey at the College of Physicians and Surgeons, Charles Christopher Parry (1823–1890), would go on to a distinguished botanic career himself, identifying, among other plants, the Torrey Pine or *Pinus torreyana*, that he named for his mentor. Parry's brother would become the great-grandfather of the eminent urologist Bill Parry, head of urology at the University of Oklahoma and friend of Reed Nesbit and Jack Lapides.

Two years later, Gray was recruited to Michigan as professor of botany and zoology, arriving on July 17, 1838, as the first permanent paid professor at the newly relocated and reconstituted University of Michigan. Lacking buildings and students for teaching, the regents sent Gray to Europe to collect scientific books for the library and to outfit a vivarium. The first library acquisition was a complete copy of Audubon's *The Birds of America* at a cost of $970. Gray went on to expand the library and make connections for the new university. He met Darwin in London and they became lifelong friends. In November 1839, Gray returned to New York having acquired 3,700 books for the University of Michigan Library. The regents were impressed, but with university funds constrained they asked Gray, in April, 1840, to resign, although they covered his salary for another year. Gray never taught a class at Michigan and in 1842 he became the Fisher Professor of Natural History at Harvard, remaining in Boston until dying shortly after a stroke in 1888.

The second professor at the University of Michigan, Douglass Houghton (1809–1845), didn't last long in his job either. Born in Troy, New York, he graduated from Rensselaer School, remaining to teach chemistry and natural history, while studying medicine with a local physician and then obtaining a license to practice in 1831. He became botanist and surgeon that year on a federal expedition to explore the origin of the Mississippi River and then settled in Detroit to practice medicine, becoming state geologist in 1837. He joined Henry R. Schoolcraft (1773–1864), U.S. Indian agent and geologist, as physician-naturalist on expeditions to Lake Superior and the upper Mississippi. When Michigan became a state, Houghton organized and led the state Geological Survey and in 1839 he was named the University of Michigan's first professor of geology, minerology, and chemistry, while continuing to reside in Detroit and lead the state survey. In 1845, on a new appraisal of Lake Superior, funded by the federal government, he drowned in the lake near Eagle River along with two colleagues when their boat was capsized in a storm on October 13 and their remains were not discovered until spring the following year.

The regents, who included Schoolcraft and his friend Dr. Zina Pitcher, replaced those first two professors with men who had greater staying power. Abram Sager, another physician who was then the chief of the botanical and zoological department in the Michigan State Geological Survey, was appointed in 1842 to take Gray's place and Silas Douglas replaced Houghton in 1844. These replacements made indelible changes in the new university and its future medical school. Interestingly, three of the first four faculty at the University of Michigan were physicians.

The first university buildings in Ann Arbor, four professor's houses completed in March of 1840, were intended to contain classrooms, dormitories, living suites, library, museum, and chapel. Two were on the north side of the 40-acre site and two on the south. One on the north side became the first University Hospital in 1869. Another on the south side became the president's home. College classes in Ann Arbor began in September 1841, although it was not until 1848 when the first medical science professorships became formalized.

The medical school, initially named the Department of Medicine and Surgery, obtained its first faculty on January 19, 1848. Two of the original university faculty members of the Ann Arbor campus, Abram Sager (dean and professor of diseases of women and children) and Silas Douglas (chemistry), joined with three newcomers, Samuel Denton (medicine and pathology), Moses Gunn (anatomy and surgery), and John Adams Allen, Jr. (physiology) to comprise the inaugural medical school faculty. Classes began in the autumn of 1850, when the first medical building was completed.[iv]

Ann Arbor had a population of 28,567 in 1850, but no hospital, while Detroit was growing more quickly with 40,000 inhabitants that year and 70,000 10 years later. Detroit had hospitals well before Ann Arbor: St. Mary's (1845), the U.S. Marine Hospital (1857), and Harper Hospital (1863). Michigan's first class of medical students, 92 in number, were required to have two years of lectures (a six-month series, repeated the following year), a thesis requirement, and preceptorship before the school's five faculty members would approve their graduation. Students had no specific patient care experience beyond their preceptorships during the first 19 years of the Department of Medicine and Surgery.

In June 1850, just before the Medical Department's first class began instruction, the State of Michigan held a constitutional convention in Lansing, the new capitol. One statute that would affect the university was the public election of eight regents, one from each of the state judicial districts. This action separated the university from the state superintendent of public instruction as well as from the legislature.

> Created by the constitution, the Board of Regents of the University was as firmly founded as the legislature, the governor, or the judiciary, and was equal in its power over its designated field of state endeavor. It was a coordinate branch of state government, and unique among state universities.[10]

---

iv The Department of Medicine and Surgery was also informally called the Medical Department at the start, but the terminology became increasingly antiquated as the school grew in complexity of its disciplines. In 1915, the Board of Regents installed the term, *Medical School*.

The statute enacted April 15, 1851, remodeled the university with less specificity than the 1837 legislation, no longer enumerating specific professorships. More broadly, the act said the university should consist of at least three departments (Literary, Medical, and Law) and others according to the regents and funds available. No tuition was to be charged to Michigan residents. Later, the state Supreme Court ruled that even that stipulation for the three departments was redundant and invalid, because the regents had full authority to govern internal matters of the university and needed no specific directives. The new regents included one physician, William Upjohn of Hastings, who had been born and educated in England.

After a search process, Henry Tappan was selected president of the university and, arriving in the summer of 1852, he set about making Michigan a great American university. He promoted research along with teaching, moved students out of dormitories into the community, built a scientific curriculum modeled after West Point, and recruited remarkable teaching faculty beginning in 1854 with Corydon La Ford of Geneva Medical College and Alonzo Palmer. Ford's story enters this narrative in the next section. Palmer had graduated from the College of Physicians and Surgeons of the Western District in New York in 1839 and practiced in Tecumseh, Michigan, for the next 10 years before moving to Chicago where he dealt with the Chicago Cholera Epidemic of 1852. Coming to Ann Arbor in 1854, Palmer became professor of Materia Medica and Therapeutics as well as Diseases of Women and Children. Palmer succeeded medical school founder, Denton, who died in 1860, as leader of internal medicine. Palmer was described as one of the most enthusiastic lecturers in the school, teaching up until his death in 1887.[11]

The legislature continued to have trouble keeping hands off the university. The regents and new president Tappan resisted a directive from the legislature to appoint a professor of homeopathy, although similar pressures would return. Philanthropy again came to the aid of the university when Tappan enlarged the library with funds solicited from local citizens. He built the Detroit Observatory (1854), also using philanthropic funds. In 1855, Michigan became the second university in America to award bachelor of science degrees, these going to twin boys from Ohio. Tappan built the Chemical Laboratory Building in 1856, a fortuitous step that enhanced scientific instruction and research in the university and injected them into its medical department. The Chemical Laboratory Building proved to be a critical differentiating asset in the school's next half-century.

Notes

1 H. H. Peckham, *The Making of the University of Michigan 1817–1992.* Edited and updated by M. L. Steneck and N. H. Steneck (Ann Arbor: University of Michigan Press, 1967, 1994), p. 8.

2 D. Allen, *Our Declaration. A Reading of the Declaration of Independence in Defense of Equality* (New York: W. W. Norton, 2014).
3 A. B. Woodward, *A System of Universal Science* (Philadelphia, PA: Edward Earle, 1816).
4 H. Bernard, J. Eaton, N. H. R. Dawson, and W. T. Harris, *Report of the Commissioner of Education: Volume 1* (U.S. Government Printing Office, January 1, 1899), 601.
5 H. H. Peckham, *The Making of the University of Michigan 1817–1992.* Edited and updated by M. L. Steneck and N. H. Steneck (Ann Arbor: University of Michigan Press, 1967, 1994), 6.
6 R. Adler, *Cholera in Detroit* (Jefferson, NC: McFarland, 2014).
7 H. Markel, *The Battling Brothers of Battle Creek* (New York: Pantheon, 2017), 23.
8 H. H. Peckham, *The Making of the University of Michigan 1817–1992.* Edited and updated by M. L. Steneck and N. H. Steneck (Ann Arbor: University of Michigan Press, 1967, 1994), 15, 18.
9 V. C. Vaughan, *A Doctor's Memories* (Indianapolis: Bobbs-Merrill, 1926), 184.
10 H. H. Peckham, *The Making of the University of Michigan 1817–1992.* Edited and updated by M. L. Steneck and N. H. Steneck (Ann Arbor: University of Michigan Press, 1967, 1994), 35.
11 H. W. Davenport, *Not Just Any Medical School* (Ann Arbor: University of Michigan Press, 1999), 11.

The Department of Medicine and Surgery, Moses Gunn, and Civil War

Moses Gunn (1822–1887), one of the five founders of Michigan's Department of Medicine and Surgery, moved to Ann Arbor in 1845 after his final fall term at Geneva Medical College in New York, anticipating formation of a medical school in Michigan. Before leaving Geneva, he found a cadaver in a trunk that had been delivered by the state penitentiary to his medical college for anatomy teaching the following term. The school being closed between the terms and the trunk unclaimed outside, Gunn thought it a good idea to take it along for later teaching purposes. Gunn and his unlikely luggage took the train to Ann Arbor and in February was teaching anatomy and practicing medicine by himself. He was successful and integrated nicely into the community. Gunn was so instrumental in discussions related to Ann Arbor's future medical school that he became Michigan's first professor of surgery (and anatomy) when the school opened in 1850. That same year he married Jane Augusta Terry of Ann Arbor and they moved into a Greek Revival house they built the next year on the southeast corner of State and Ann Streets.

Gunn was a good general surgeon with particular interest in orthopaedic matters, and his operative range surely encompassed the genitourinary tract, although no record of his cases has been found. His work and that of other leading surgeons at the time was probably best reflected in the few contemporary surgical texts available to them and the most noteworthy was the two-volume *A System of Surgery* by Samuel David Gross in 1859, informed mainly by the prescientific medical knowledge of the time. Chapter 1 was titled "Irritation, Sympathy, Idiosyncrasy," Chapter 2 "Congestion," and Chapters 3 and 4 dealt with inflammation. Chapter 5, "Textural changes," had six sections: induration, transformation, hypertrophy, atrophy, contracture and obliteration, and fistula. A tiny Chapter 6 of four pages covered congenital malformations. Chapters 15, 16, and 17 in the second volume dealt with the urinary organs, male genital organs, and female genital organs, also including the breast. Therapeutic details were occasionally illustrated, such as orthopaedic dislocations.[1] Genitourinary disorders and injuries were of particular interest to Gross, his uncommonly large list of published papers includes around 150 of genitourinary relevance beginning with his second paper, *A Case of Priapism*.[2] In that three-page report, Gross, then practicing in Cincinnati, detailed his comanagement of an adult man with postcoital priapism, treated for 10 days with phlebotomy, enemas, laxatives, antimony, cold compresses, lead poultices, and flaxseed tea. On follow-up at 2.5 months, no further recurrence was noted, but as impotence was becoming evident Gross speculated that blistering therapy might have given a better result. By the mid-nineteenth century, Gross's influence on American surgical practice was profound and well-recognized, particularly in genitourinary matters. Gross wrote papers on bladder exstrophy, lithotomy, prostate diseases, urethral stricture, hermaphroditism, hernias, orchiectomy, venereology, and a number of historical profiles and obituaries. It is telling that Gross's first book, *A Practical Treatise on the Diseases and Injuries of the Urinary Bladder, the Prostate Gland, and the Urethra* in 1851 was quickly followed by a second edition in 1855, and both were published before his larger general surgery work.[3] The surgical practice and genitourinary facets that Gunn practiced and taught in mid-nineteenth-century Ann Arbor undoubtedly mirrored that described in Gross's textbooks. Furthermore, the influence of Gross as a teacher of Charles de Nancrede during their coincidence in Philadelphia extended the Gross influence in Ann Arbor beyond the first decade of the twentieth century.

Gunn believed that medical schools needed to provide clinical education in addition to classroom instruction, and medical students needed hospitals to learn how to practice medicine. Just as importantly, effective clinical teachers could only be informed by robust experiences deriving from large clinical practices and, accordingly, Gunn relocated to Detroit in 1853 to develop a large surgical practice, returning to Ann Arbor by train twice a week for academic duties. The trip lasted three hours each way, but Gunn remained a major force in the medical school and was appreciated by students, although sometimes faulted for rushing through lectures so he could catch his train home.[4] Also in 1853, the first identified African American student, Samuel Codes Watson, was admitted to the University of Michigan Medical Department. Born in South Carolina in 1832, Watson, of mixed ethnicity, passed for white while attending Michigan for a short period, without graduating for some yet unknown reason. He then received an MD from Cleveland Medical College in 1857, one of its first African American students, and later became Detroit's first elected African American city official. He was declared the city's wealthiest black property owner in 1867.[5]

Gunn's friend from medical school, Corydon L. Ford, was enticed to Ann Arbor in 1854 to take over the duties as professor of anatomy, leaving Gunn free to provide only the surgical instruction. Ford, an 1842 Geneva Medical College graduate, had remained at the school as an instructor and was teaching anatomy when Elizabeth Blackwell matriculated in 1847. It was noted that Ford had been particularly kind to that solitary woman in the class who two years later became the first woman to get a medical degree in the United States. Women medical students didn't enter the medical class at Michigan until 1871, but even that was early for most medical schools. From his start in Ann Arbor in 1854, Ford would give 600 to 700 lectures a year to the class with four daily lectures from Monday to Friday and clinical demonstrations on Saturdays during the terms from October to April. Ford lived in his office on the third floor of the Medical Building until 1865, when he married at age 52. He continued his life of education up to his end 40 years later, dying of a stroke just after completing his last lecture.

The same year as Ford's arrival, 1854, the regents dismissed one of the five founders of the medical school, John Allen, Jr., without much explanation on May 4, although Davenport suggested the dismissal was likely related to contentious national politics. The minutes of the Board of Regents were mute as to the cause for dismissal, but a local medical journal noted that Allen had "made himself obnoxious." Allen, a Democrat candidate for mayor of Ann Arbor, had supported the Kansas-Nebraska Act that would have admitted Kansas to the United States as a slave state. The prevailing sentiment in Ann Arbor and especially at the university was soundly opposed to that expansion of slavery. Alonzo Palmer, hired that same year, replaced Allen on the medical faculty. Two months after Allen's dismissal, a rally in Jackson, Michigan, of 10,000 Whigs opposed to slavery coalesced into a new Republican Party that would hold its first nominating convention two years later in Philadelphia.

With Gunn's attention turned mainly to surgical practice in Detroit and teaching in Ann Arbor, his reputation grew and in 1856 Geneva College awarded him an Honorary Masters of Arts.

Gunn and his four fellow faculty members satisfied the original mandate for the University of Michigan Medical School in populating the state with good regional physicians. William T. Bovie, Sr., one such graduate in 1858 set up practice and a farm in Augusta, Michigan, near Kalamazoo where he and his wife raised five children. One of the children, William T. Bovie, Jr., earned a bachelor's degree from UM in 1905 and a PhD in plant physiology from Harvard, remaining in Boston to work at the Harvard Cancer Commission where he invented a "bloodless scalpel" that was quickly taken up by Harvey Cushing. Bovie sold the rights to his invention for one dollar and now the device, still called "the Bovie," is routinely used in operating rooms around the world.[6]

Gunn served as dean of the Department of Medicine and Surgery for a term from 1858 to 1859. The university at the time consisted of 500 students and nine buildings, including the original four faculty homes. The Medical Department listed 143 students in 1859 and the duties as dean couldn't have been arduous given that Gunn was living and practicing medicine in Detroit, returning to Ann Arbor several times each week for his surgery lectures. Abram Sager followed him as dean, that being Sager's second term.

In 1860, university president Henry Tappan made an explicit decision to hire professors based on scholarship rather than religious affiliation, leading to criticism of the university as "godless," a charge that would return to other university leaders later in the century. In 1861, Corydon La Ford became dean of the Medical Department. The curriculum in its first two decades consisted of lectures and anatomy dissection, and students were taught ancient clinical skills of physical examination, history taking, palpation, and uroscopy, joined by auscultation invigorated by the invention of the stethoscope by René Laennec (1781–1826) in Paris in 1816. Alonzo Palmer added clinical thermometry to his practice and teaching after 1860. Pulse and respiratory rate measurement became standard parts of medical practice as the clinimetric approach expanded with the teaching of Pierre Charles Alexandre Louis (1787–1872) in Paris. There, young students from around the world, including Holmes from Boston, would come for periods of study to observe Louis on rounds introducing ideas such as medical statistics, clinical trials, and evidence-based medicine. The students formed a *Society for Medical Observation* and in 1832 a group of his American protégées including Holmes formed a branch in Boston known as the *Boston Society for Medical Improvement*.[i,7]
These ideas and numerical methods diffused slowly west to Ann Arbor.

Surgical procedures and other "clinical demonstrations" were carried out in the medical school building of 1850 in the domed (and mislabeled) "amphitheater" and these likely involved the range of interventions described by Gross, although written records are few. The Chemical

---

i William Farr, a British student of Louis, introduced epidemiological concerns to medical attention including concepts of herd immunity, dose response, death rate, and cohort effect. With William Guy and William Budd, also of the Louis bedside school, he founded the Statistical Society of London in 1834. In 1851, Holmes and George Shattuck, Jr., both students of Professor Louis, along with Shattuck's student Edward Jarvis, founded the American Statistical Society; M. Best and D. Neuhauser, "Pierre Charles Alexander Louis: Master of the Spirit of Mathematical Clinical Science," *BMJ Quality and Safety Health Care* 14, no. 6 (2005): 462–464.

Laboratory Building, built behind the medical school in 1856, and a four-story addition to the medical school building in 1864 expanded space for the growing demands of medical education including anatomy that was moved to a new room under a new dome. Medical students as well as other learners in the university took classes in materia medica, toxicology, and urine analysis in the Chemical Laboratory Building.

Materia medica derived from the ancient study of medicinal plants, exemplified in recipes of ancient Egyptian papyri as well as in the Ayurvedic *Great Trilogy* and the botanical catalog of Pedanius Dioscorides (40–90 AD) that was reproduced for many centuries. Carl Linnaeus (1707–1778) who started out as a struggling young physician in Stockholm treating venereal diseases, became a paradigm-altering botanist who expanded the field with wide-ranging discovery of new plants, binomial nomenclature, as his international disciples scoured the planet for new botanic species. Earnest healers and clever entrepreneurs brought many forms of reasonable botanical therapies as well as "snake oils" to bedsides throughout human history. Industrialization and growing understanding of chemistry added new materials to the medical armamentarium in the nineteenth century. Materia medica of the early medical curriculum at Michigan devolved into pharmacy instruction (1868) and a college of pharmacy (1876), encompassed initially within the Chemical Laboratory Building.

Silas Douglas, chemistry professor, founder of the medical school, and initiator of the Chemical Laboratory Building, brought Preston B. Rose on the faculty to teach toxicology and urine analysis. Rose, a medical school graduate from the class of 1862, became an expert toxicologist, later publishing a text, *Hand-Book of Toxicology* (1880). This was a highly relevant topic for medical students at the time, as Davenport noted,

> Poisons were everywhere. Lead was in cider and in the municipal water supply if there was one. Alum adulterated flour. Arsenic was in green wallpaper and available over the counter for a husband or wife anxious to end marital discord. In 1868–69, fifty-one medical students, well over half the class, took the course in toxicology. Preston B. Rose taught it, using his *Hand-Book of Toxicology*. He told students how to collect evidence in a case of suspected poisoning, first by careful observation of the patients and his or her surroundings and then by determining whether anyone had shown a disposition to prepare the food or medicine and to wait upon the deceased to the exclusion of others during the fatal illness. He gave explicit directions on how to conduct the post-mortem examination and how to find metals, alkaloids, or acids during subsequent chemical analysis of tissues. He concluded by describing stains made by blood

or semen. Health officials throughout Michigan regularly sent parts obtained at autopsy of suspicious cases to the Chemical Laboratory for analysis.[8]

Edgar Allen Poe's short story *The Murders in the Rue Morgue* had initiated the genre of the detective story in 1841 and the clever reasoning, Poe called "ratiocination," necessary to solve crimes. Poe's fictional detective, Monsieur C. Auguste Dupin, perhaps coincidentally endowed with the medical gaze and diagnostic acumen of Professor Louis, contributed a uroscopic reference when Dupin first described his powers of deductive reasoning to his naïve roommate, the narrator of the story:

> Perdidit antiquum litera prima sonum.
> I had told you that this was in reference to Orion, formerly written Urion; and, from certain pungencies connected with this explanation, I was aware that you could not have forgotten it. It was clear, therefore, that you would not fail to combine the two ideas of Orion and Chantilly. That you did combine them I saw by the character of the smile which passed over your lips.[9]

This genre became the *scientific crime solver meme* that continues to gather cultural momentum. Future writer Arthur Conan Doyle was barely 10 years old when Rose was teaching Ann Arbor medical students the scientific methods of forensic investigation, but only 17 years later as a 27-year-old ophthalmologist with a struggling practice, Conan Doyle recreated a sensational blend of ratiocination and scientific analysis in the intellectual superhero, Sherlock Holmes, a name that coincided with the real-life medical superhero, Oliver Wendell Holmes.[ii]

---

ii Oliver Wendell Holmes, Sr. (1809–1894) was well-known from the earliest days of his career when he observed the first public demonstration of anesthesia and shortly thereafter coined the term to describe it. He was among the most prominent of the *Americans Abroad*, who studied with Louis in Paris, as explained in David McCullough's book, and after return to Boston presented one of the first convincing hypotheses for the germ theory, as an explanation of puerperal fever. He taught first at Dartmouth Medical School and then Harvard Medical School, where he rose to the position as dean. In that role, he helped solve the Parkman murder case. George Parkman was a local physician and benefactor of the university, and George Webster was professor of chemistry at Harvard Medical School. Holmes testified for both the defense and prosecution and Webster was found guilty and hanged. Holmes dedicated his 1850 introductory lecture to the medical school class in Parkman's memory. Holmes wrote poetry and books of fiction and nonfiction, contributed to the *Atlantic Magazine*, and mingled with the literary set in Boston, including J. Elliot Cabot, James Russell Lowell, Ralph Waldo Emerson, and Henry Wadsworth Longfellow. Holmes popularized the term *Boston Brahmin* and was certainly one of them. One of his three children, Oliver Wendell Holmes, Jr., would become a Supreme Court justice. Cabot was the father of Hugh Cabot.

In 1860, the new Republican Party elected Abraham Lincoln president and the inevitable Civil War opened with a salvo of guns on Fort Sumter, April 13, 1861. News of the war unleashed broad partisan support in Ann Arbor for the Union cause and university president Henry Tappan led "a throng of students down the middle of State and Huron St. toward Court House Square."[10] Joined by Elihu Pond, editor of a local paper, the *Argus*, the crowd organized at the square, heard speeches of support for Lincoln and the Union cause, and formed a committee to consolidate military companies. One company, the Steuben Guards, had already formed a few months earlier (January 14), and a second company, the Barry Guards, was announced within a week of the Sumter hostilities. The medical school was similarly caught up in the patriotic fever, although some graduates went south to fight while others stayed north for the conflict over the next four years.

Rumors, only a week after Sumter, that Washington had been taken and President Lincoln and General Scott were prisoners of the south terrified Ann Arbor citizens, although by the next day fact-finding by the *Argus* and other papers dispelled the panic.

On May 3, 1861, a number of state militia companies including the Steuben and Barry Guards combined to form the Fifth Michigan

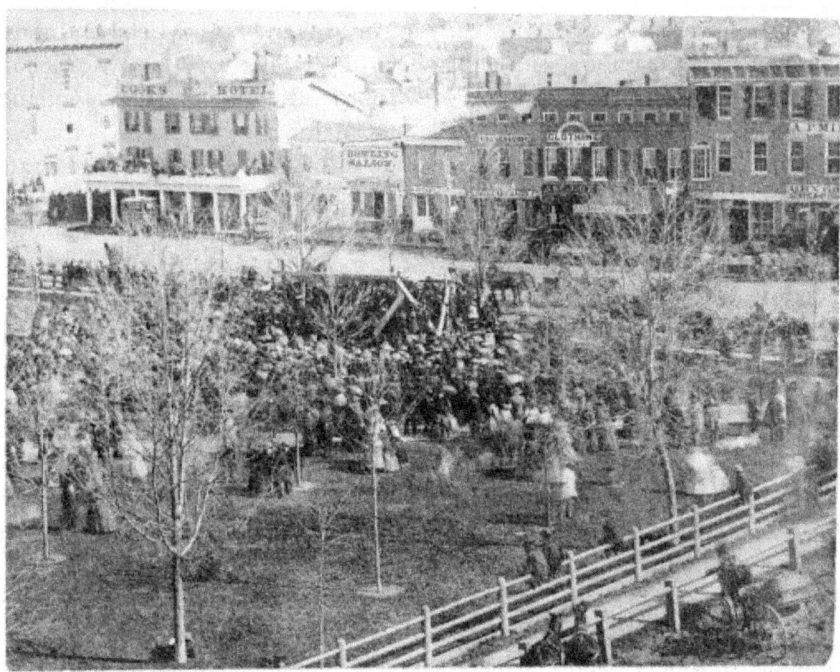

Courthouse Square, Ann Arbor, April 14, 1861. Bentley Image Bank: *BL000113*.

Volunteer Infantry, which Gunn joined in September 1861 after the First Battle of Bull Run, July 21. His medical school colleague, Alonzo Palmer had been engaged in that Bull Run action, as surgeon of the Second Michigan Infantry, but resigned in September to return to the university. That Confederate victory at Bull Run highlighted the deficits of the Union Army and indicated that the war was likely to be worse than most people had anticipated with the initial burst of patriotism. Gunn, age 39, was appointed senior regimental surgeon when the 900 enlisted men of the Fifth Michigan, ages 16 to 54, linked up with Major General George McClellan's Army of the Potomac. Confusingly, the Army of the Potomac was a name also claimed by the Confederate Army under General P. G. T. Beauregard at the First Battle of Bull Run but later changed to the Army of Northern Virginia under General Robert E. Lee. McClellan had recently returned to the army after success in the railroad industry and was praised for his expertise in "big war science," thus setting high expectations for success.[11] Although a meticulous planner, McClellan ultimately proved to be a poor general with an excess of caution and reluctance to initiate action, and he soon lost Lincoln's trust.

Gunn's duty as senior regimental surgeon involved little work and no action at first, so he took a three-week leave on December 7, 1861, returning to Michigan and Ann Arbor to deliver 50 lectures to medical students anxious to complete their medical instruction and join the war effort. Gunn returned to army duty in time for the Fifth Michigan Infantry to board steamboats in Alexandria, Virginia, with other McClellan units in mid-March enroute to Fort Monroe, Richmond, Yorktown, and eventually Williamsburg. There, the first major combat of the Peninsula Campaign occurred, involving 41,000 Union and 32,000 Confederate troops, and giving Gunn plenty of work. Among the 42 units in the Battle of Williamsburg, the Fifth Michigan (down to 500 men by then) suffered some of the heaviest losses, with 144 killed, wounded, or missing.[12] *The Fighting Fifth* remained resilient and dependable in future action, in contrast to the underperformance of McClellan and many other units. Gunn's letters to his wife documented the gruesome injuries and wretched conditions experienced by his surgical team.

Williamsburg disillusioned Gunn not only in personal hardship but also in his view of the poor administration of the Army Medical Department and the ferocity of the Confederate conviction, making him realize that the war would be long and ugly. Toward the end of May, Gunn and the Fifth Michigan fought alongside troops under Major General Erasmus Darwin Keyes, whose son Edward would join him the following year as an aide-de-camp. Twenty-five years later, Edward Keyes would become a principle founder of modern genitourinary surgery.[13] Gunn ended his military tour in July 1862 to resume practice in Detroit and teaching in Ann Arbor, newly informed by his combat experience. *The Fighting Fifth* endured the fifth highest casualty rate of all Union regiments during the war.

Gunn's clinical demonstrations back in Ann Arbor were diagnostic and surgical, using chloroform anesthesia (open drip) when necessary. Students and other observers on raised circular benches saw little more than the talkative professor and a patient, with minimal sense of close surgical details other than Gunn's narrative. Any genitourinary surgery in the early years of Michigan's Medical Department would have been performed solely by Gunn, but little evidence of these cases remains, although one example is a surgical demonstration on a man with "phymosis" [sic] for which Gunn performed a dorsal cut and sutured the incised edges. That surgical demonstration on December 5, 1866, is recounted from medical student thesis notes in Davenport's book *University of Michigan Surgeons*.

One of Gunn's students at Michigan, Mississippi native Solomon Claiborne Martin, came to the University of Michigan as an undergraduate and then studied in Germany for two years before returning to Ann Arbor to enter the medical school in 1859. Following the two years of lectures and preceptorship with Gunn and Dean Abram Sager, Martin graduated in 1861 and went south for commission as surgeon of the Wirt Adams Regiment Mississippi Volunteer Cavalry C.S.A. under General Albert Sidney. Martin then matriculated at the University of Louisiana (later Tulane University) where in 1865 he received a second MD. He practiced medicine in Port Gibson, Mississippi, and St. Louis, Missouri, where in 1892 he became professor of dermatology and hygiene at Barnes Medical College and edited the *St. Louis Medical Era*. In 1897, he began to publish the *American Journal of Dermatology and Genitourinary Diseases*. After Martin died in 1906, his two sons, S. C. Martin, Jr., and Clarence Martin, who practiced medicine together, took over management of the journal, changing the name in 1912 to *The Urologic and Cutaneous Review*, that continued in print until abrupt termination in 1952.

Attitudes about slavery and the Civil War exacerbated tensions in the university, the region, and the state. The *Detroit Free Press* had supported the southern cause, denounced abolitionists, and attacked the university and President Tappan. Ann Arbor's three newspapers separately represented three political positions, the Whigs, the Democrats, and the Republicans. Jackson, Michigan, a focal point for the rise of a new Republican Party, and Washtenaw County had voted for Lincoln. A new set of regents was parting ways with Tappan and called for his resignation after a secret meeting in June 1863. Tappan left, along with his son-in-law Professor Brünnow, the Detroit Observatory director. Tappan had met Brünnow in Berlin and recruited him to Ann Arbor as the first PhD hired by the University of Michigan.

Regent Erastus Haven became university president in October. University enrollment, having dipped at the start of the war, grew to its largest in the fall of 1863 at 871 men, with large increases in the law and medical departments as the war dragged along. The draft spared men under 20 or those who could find $300 for a substitute.[14] As the war continued, the election of 1864 evidenced growing discontent with Lincoln's management of it. Washtenaw, Wayne, and eight other counties voted for McClellan, although Lincoln still won the state. In 1864, an addition to the medical building was financed by Ann Arbor citizens. An addition to the Chemical Laboratory Building would come in 1867. That same year the legislature recommended that the university admit women, but the idea was initially dismissed.

After the war's conclusion, enrollment at the university became more national than regional, with two-thirds of students coming from other states in 1866–1867. By 1867 the Medical School enrollment reached 418. Calls for homeopathy instruction persisted but were rebuffed again by the school and regents. Davenport noted the early inclination of the university to diversity.

> Equally interesting is the fact that in 1868 two African-American students entered the university, the first of their race. Both were from Michigan, their entrance caused no headlines, and the University did not bother to record that they were African-Americans. They qualified for admission and were registered as a matter of course. One, John Summerfield Davidson stayed one year; the other Gabriel Franklin Hargo, graduated from the Law department in 1870.

The attendance of Watson in 1853 (see p. 28) qualifies that last point of Davenport.

Gunn continued efforts to move the Medical Department to Detroit but was unsuccessful. After his oldest son drowned in the Detroit River in August 1866, Gunn accepted a position of professor of surgery at Rush Medical College and moved to Chicago in 1867, to complete his career and where his younger son would get a medical degree. Gunn was widely respected throughout his academic life. He prepared for his cases carefully and built a reputation as an excellent surgeon and teacher, according to Davenport. Case reports published early in his career discussed jaw surgery, orthopaedic conditions, and hypospadias, but he published little in his later career. Gunn became a founding member and vice president of the American Surgical Association and a founding member with Keyes of the American Association of Genitourinary Surgeons, organizations that would shape American surgery and the evolving discipline of genitourinary surgery. Years later, Victor Vaughan credited Gunn as the fundamental reason that the medical school was the first professional school of the University of Michigan even though the 1837 university charter indicated that the Law School had been intended as the first professional school, an implementation that didn't happen until 1859. Vaughan offered these recollections on Gunn in his autobiography:

> One cold, snowy February day in the late forties there arrived in Ann Arbor a young man who was to become a tower of strength to both Sager and Douglas in their efforts to provide for a medical school. This newcomer in my opinion, was inferior to both Sager and Douglas, certainly to the former, in both native and acquired ability in scientific work. But he had a strong personality and a genius for organization and constructive work. While a student in a medical school at Geneva, New York, he read about the organization of the University of Michigan and the provision that a medical department would, sooner or later, be attached to this institution. Immediately on receiving his medical diploma he started out for Ann Arbor, carrying in his grip several dissecting cases and, among his grosser impedimenta, a box of suspicious shape and size and unmarked content.
>
> On arriving in Ann Arbor he hung out a shingle offering his surgical skill to the public and more discreetly he let it be known to the University students that, in his back office after a certain hour, he was prepared to initiate any of them, who might have the profession of medicine in view, into the mysteries of the structure of the human body.
>
> Personally I did not know Moses Gunn until some thirty years after his coming to Ann Arbor. However it was his custom in his later years to come to Ann Arbor on the anniversary of his first coming in the forties. On these occasions I, as his host, listened attentively to the stories of his early manhood. He told me that when he read about the prospective medical school in connection with the University of Michigan he and Corydon L. Ford were roommates at the medical school in Geneva; that they talked over the possibilities that might lie in the West; that he said to La Ford that he would come to Ann Arbor, aid in founding the school and that he would become professor of surgery and Ford should be professor of anatomy.[15]

Gunn retained affection for the Medical Department, that had formed largely on the part of his energy, returning frequently as Vaughan noted.

Over the next five years, the Surgery Department had four sequential chiefs. William Warren Greene (1831–1881), a Michigan medical graduate of 1855 and disciple of Gunn, who had returned to his native New England to teach and practice medicine, reluctantly came back to Ann

Arbor in 1867 to teach surgery in Gunn's absence but returned east the next year. Henry Lyster, Michigan medical graduate of 1860 (one of 22 graduates that year), followed as professor of surgery. Like Gunn, he had joined the Michigan volunteer infantry but remained in service until May 1865, accumulating vast experience in combat injuries, keeping detailed personal records, and making great effort to ascertain follow-up. Lyster served as professor of surgery from 1868 to 1869, later developing his practice in Detroit and having an important role in founding the State Board of Health. Alpheus Benning Crosby was the next surgery professor (1869–1871) and as a good friend of President Angell he was a willing partner in the inclusion of the first women in the medical classes. As a Civil War surgeon Crosby was an early adapter of wound irrigation and carbolic acid, which significantly reduced his rate of infections. Crosby also maintained simultaneous practices and appointments at medical schools in Vermont, New Hampshire, and on Long Island, likely during the summer quiescence of the medical school in Ann Arbor. Theodore McGraw followed from 1871 to 1872. A Detroit native he graduated from UM in 1859, obtained a medical degree from the College of Physicians and Surgeons in New York, served in the Civil War, and then returned to Ann Arbor as lecturer in surgery for one unhappy year before returning to practice in Detroit, operating at Harper and St. Mary's hospitals. His later career was distinguished as a surgeon, teacher, and innovator. He was the first serious surgical investigator in Ann Arbor with extensive canine experimental work.

Donald Maclean came next and he lasted from 1872 to 1889. Born in Ontario in 1839, he graduated in medicine from the University of Edinburgh, serving as an assistant to the famed surgeon James Syme, as had Joseph Lister. Maclean then, in 1864, became professor of surgery at Queen's University in Kingston, Ontario, moving to the Michigan surgery chair in 1872. Maclean lived and practiced in Detroit and lobbied strongly but unsuccessfully to move the clinical teaching to Detroit. He operated extensively in southeastern Michigan, specializing in removal of ovarian cysts, and published his cases.[16] Losing the battle to relocate the Ann Arbor medical school, Maclean left the university in the aftermath of a contentious location debate in 1889 and continued his Detroit practice. In 1894, he became AMA president. He died in 1903 and the inaugural *Medical Portrait* in the *Detroit Medical Journal* six years later depicted him very favorably as "perhaps in his day the best known surgeon Michigan ever had," concluding that under his teacher Syme, Maclean

> ... became himself one of the most brilliant operators of his day. He was possessed of a most winning and striking personality and was greatly beloved by his pupils. Many of the best surgeons in the west

today acknowledge with pride and affection the debt they owe to their great teacher and friend, Donald Maclean.[17]

Gunn's influence lingered long after he had left Ann Arbor largely through the work of his trainees but so too persisted the unresolved tension between the academic mission in Ann Arbor and the lure of hospital-based practice in Detroit, even long after Maclean's departure.

Notes

1 S. D. Gross, *A System of Surgery* (Philadelphia: Blanchard and Lea, 1859).
2 S. D. Gross, "A Case of Priapism," *Western Medical Gazette* 2 (1834): 14–16.
3 S. D. Gross, *A Practical Treatise on the Diseases and Injuries of the Urinary Bladder, the Prostate Gland, and the Urethra* (Philadelphia, PA: Blanchard and Lea, 1851).
4 H. W. Davenport, *University of Michigan Surgeons, 1850–1970. Who They Were and What They Did* (Ann Arbor: Historical Center for the Health Sciences, University of Michigan, 1993), 7–8.
5 Michigan's Story: The History of Race at U-M / The Firsts - Online Exhibits. https://www.lib.umich.edu/online-exhibits/exhibits/show/history-of-race-at-um/diversity-in-student-life/the-firsts.
6 J. L. O'Connor, D. A. Bloom, and T. William, "Bovie and Electrosurgery," *Surgery* 119 (1996): 390–396.
7 D. A. Bloom, J. Wan, and H. P. Koo, "Barometers & Bladders: A Primer on Pressures," *Journal of Urology* 163 (2000): 697–704; M. Karamanou, A. Karakatsani, I. Tomos, and G. P. C. A. Androutsos, "Louis (1787–1872): Introducing Medical Statistics in Pneumonology," *American Journal of Respiratory and Critical Care Medicine* 182 (2010): 1569–1570.
8 H. W. Davenport, *Not Just Any Medical School* (Ann Arbor: University of Michigan Press, 1999), 4–6.
9 E. A. Poe, "The Murders in the Rue Morgue" *Graham's Magazine*, April 1841.
10 L. Duff, "Ann Arbor Yesterdays," *Ann Arbor News*, April 17, 1961.
11 Wikipedia, George B. McClellan.
12 T. E. Sebrell, II, "The 'Fighting Fifth': The Fifth Michigan Infantry Regiment in the Civil War's Peninsula Campaign," *Michigan Historical Review* 35 (2009): 27.
13 E. S. Smith, E. D. Vaughan, E. S. Belt, and D. A. Bloom, "Edward Lawrence Keyes: A Pivotal Early Specialist in Modern Genitourinary Surgery," *Urology* 62 (2003): 968.
14 H. H. Peckham, *The Making of the University of Michigan 1817–1992*. Edited and updated by M. L. Steneck and N. H. Steneck (Ann Arbor: University of Michigan Press, 1967, 1994), 64.
15 V. C. Vaughan, *A Doctor's Memories* (Indianapolis: Bobbs-Merrill Company, 1926),187–189.
16 D. A. Maclean, "Tabular Statement of the Surgical Work Done in the Department of Medicine and Surgery of the University of Michigan during the School Year 1881 and 1882," *Physician and Surgeon* 5 (1883): 385–396.
17 Medical Portraits I—Dr. Donald Maclean, 1839–1903. *Detroit Medical Journal* 9, no. 1 (1909): 18.

A Medical School Hospital and Scientific Curriculum

Michigan's medical school, late in its second decade, recognized the need to incorporate clinical education in the curriculum with proximity to a hospital and in 1869, two years after Gunn's exit, it created its first University Hospital in one of the original professor's houses on North University Avenue. This was an unprecedented solution to the problem that had distressed Gunn, although that first iteration of a University Hospital was basically just a 20-bed dormitory for patients undergoing surgery or demonstrations in the medical school. With a medical building, a chemical laboratory, and a hospital in 1869, Michigan was soon to become a noteworthy American medical school.[i]

Scientific inquiry and advancing technology were producing something new in human history around this time—a verifiable understanding of health, disease, and therapy. No better example in 1869 was the finding of Paul Langerhans, a medical student in Berlin, of cellular clumps in normal pancreatic tissue that he was investigating under the microscope for his thesis. He called the clumps islets or insula and those beta cells later proved to be the source of insulin. The rapid changes in medical knowledge in the wake of the Civil War quickly spilled over into the worlds of medical education, research, and care.[ii]

---

i Successive hospital iterations in 1876 with a 60-bed pavilion-style hospital and the Catherine Street Hospital in 1892 aimed to match state-of-the art hospitals for their times but fell short.

ii Langerhans had already (two years earlier) discovered epidermal dendritic cells as a student in the laboratory of German pathologist Rudolf Virchow (1821–1902). Twenty years later, Oscar Minkowski (1858–1931) and Joseph von Mering (1849–1908) removed a pancreas from a dog and found abnormally large amounts of sugar in the dog's urine. Fast forward to the 1923 Nobel Prize in Medicine to Frederick Banting (1891–1941) and J. J. R. Macleod (1876–1935). Credit was acknowledged by Banting to Charles Best (1899–1978) and by Macleod to James Collip (1892–1965) for their roles

As the university grew after the Civil War, President Haven needed help from the state legislature. A millage (one-twentieth of a mill on every dollar of property tax) was granted with the caveat that a professor of homeopathy be added to the Medical Department. The regents refused, although offered to help create a School of Homeopathy in any community other than Ann Arbor, even offering a building and endowment for such a university branch. The counteroffer was not accepted and no millage funding came to the university at the time. Homeopathy pressures continued to be applied to the University of Michigan and President Haven again appealed to the state legislature for funding in 1869.

> Courageously, he told the legislature that the University had never in its Medical Department taught any exclusive theory of medicine (which homeopathy was) and should not do so. Further he remarked that the Board of Regents had always enjoyed full freedom to decide which course should be taught, just as they appointed professors they deemed best. A vital constitutional question was at stake, aside from scientific policy, about whether the legislature could dictate University courses through acts of appropriation.[1]

A compromise was reached whereby the university got a yearly appropriation, but no millage, yet without the homeopathy stipulation. Still, the homeopathic question would return. President Haven resigned that spring of 1869 without revealing at first his intention to move to the presidency of Northwestern University.[iii]

Henry Frieze took Haven's place, *pro tem* for two years presiding over the initial admission of women to the university in 1870. The Medical Department followed in 1871, with separate lectures for women but ended that segregation after a year. Surgery and its genitourinary component were taught by the succession of Surgery Department chiefs mentioned earlier who, although not distinguished for their genitourinary skills on the national scene, were competent teachers and practitioners, according to Davenport and other accounts. Gunn's charge that a medical school needed a hospital in tandem was not completely deflected by the small Ann Arbor University Hospital during the next two decades, and a number of his successors continued to lobby to move the medical school to Detroit.

---

in the discovery of insulin. Both laureates shared their awards with the collaborators. By 1922, diabetic patients were being successfully treated with insulin.

iii The drift of Michigan presidents and provosts to presidencies of private peer universities over the next 150 years may be partially attributable to the complexities of publicly elected governance.

James Angell came to Ann Arbor as university president in 1871 for a career that would last 38 years and he ultimately put the relocation pressures to rest. Faculty salaries were low when Angell began his presidency and Michigan's best teachers were being plundered by peer institutions. The regents had refused Dean Sager's request to extend the six-month lecture terms of the Medical Department to nine months, on the grounds of additional cost. The Michigan legislature had continued to pressure the university for homeopathic inclusion in the medical school curriculum, but the regents resisted and were supported by the state Supreme Court, until the legislature made an appropriation contingent on deployment of a complete homeopathic school, separate from the medical school. Thus, compelled by Lansing in 1873, the regents agreed to attach an independent school of homeopathy to the university, provided the state fund its faculty. The next year the state provided $6,000 for two homeopath positions and, on the advice of the Homeopathic Society, the regents appointed Samuel Jones from the Homeopathic Medical College of Pennsylvania to teach materia medica and therapeutics as well as John Morgan from Hahnemann College of Philadelphia to teach theory and practice of medicine. The first class of Michigan's Homeopathic College had 24 students in 1875 and enrollment soon grew to as many as 125 compared to Medical and Surgical Department enrollment of 370 students in 1874–1875. Students were allowed to take classes and courses with the Medical Department.[iv]

The University of Michigan Homeopathic School was never fully independent, rather dependent on the medical school for fundamental scientific instruction and laboratory work. Vaughan noted that the homeopathic students were relatively small in number and lived and worked among the other students with "but little friction."[2] However, as the Medical School increased its requirements, the Homeopathic School did not keep pace and disparity grew in quality of students. Vaughan sensed that Medical School professors came to expect less of the homeopaths in terms of academics. Over time, homeopathic courses and departments

---

iv Homeopathy was a system of medical practice created by German physician Samuel Hahnemann (1755–1843), who was dissatisfied with medical practice of his time, that included treatments such as phlebotomy and other harmful practices with little therapeutic benefit. He gave up his village practice around 1784 to become a medical writer and translator, publishing his idea that "like cures like" in 1796 and coining the term *homeopathy* in 1807. A student of his, Hans Birch Gram, brought the homeopathic idea to North America in 1825 and a homeopathic medical school opened in Philadelphia in 1835. The movement gained public support, but encountered professional resistance, notably with the 90 page essay *Homoeopathy and Its Kindred Delusions* by Oliver Wendell Holmes in 1842. [O. W. Holmes. Homeopathy and its Kindred Delusions; Two Lectures. William D. Ticknor 1842 Boston.] An American Institute of Homeopathy formed in 1844.

strained the university budget, homeopathic enrollment dwindled in the twentieth century, and the college was closed in 1922 under Dean Hugh Cabot, merging resources back into the Medical School.

W. Henry Fitzbutler (1842–1901) came into the Michigan story in the early years of the first hospital. The son, of an enslaved African-American who worked as a coachman and a mother who was an indentured servant from England who fled the American South by Underground Railroad to Amherstburg, Canada, in the early 1840s, Henry grew up in Canada and graduated from Detroit Medical College in 1869 and then from the medical school at the University of Michigan in 1872. He was the first recognized African American student at both schools. He moved to Louisville, Kentucky, where he lobbied the state legislature for a medical school that would not exclude applicants because of color. Fitzbutler was successful in his lobbying, the school opened in 1888, its first graduate was a woman, and he served as dean and the majority owner of Louisville National Medical College for the rest of his life. The school added a hospital in 1896. In 2002, the University of Michigan organized the Fitzbutler Jones Society to honor both Fitzbutler and Sophia Bethena Jones (1857–1932), who in 1885 was the first African American woman to graduate from the medical school. She became a faculty member at Spelman College where she organized the nursing training program.[3]

In 1874, President Angell persuaded the legislature to remove the $15,000 ceiling on the one-twentieth mill tax, thereby doubling the university income. He also instituted annual student dues that year of $10 to $20. While Angell "worked to cultivate Tappan's educational vision," he also steered the university fully into the new secular world of science, open inquiry, and new ways of thinking without expectation of a single religious flavor. Blouin, in the quote below, described Angell's remarkable leadership:

> Politically, it was essential that Angell accommodate the university to the religious culture of the time, and he did truly believe that moral discipline was a proper goal for education. . . . In these discussions [i.e. concerning religious framing of truth-seeking, ethics both sectarian and nonsectarian, and science], Angell found a remarkable middle ground, accepting an importance for moral issues but remaining staunchly open to the authority of new ideas and to those who expressed them.[4]

In this middle ground, the university and its medical school underwent the major reputational transformation that Blouin detailed, going from the minor to the major leagues of higher education. For the medical school, the principle driver of that transformation was a young man who came north from Missouri for postgraduate study in chemistry in 1874. Coincidentally, another young man, who would also become a major force in American health care and worldwide culture, left Ann Arbor's small medical school that year. Victor Vaughan was the one who came, and stayed as will be noted shortly, while John Kellogg was the student who left.

The Kellogg story, well-detailed in Howard Markel's book, tells how John Kellogg, sponsored by Ellen and James White of the Seventh Day Adventist Church in Battle Creek, entered the two-year program of the Medical Department at the University of Michigan in the fall term of 1873 but became dissatisfied with the six-month lecture terms and lack of clinical experience. Furthermore, Markel found that as a late registrant to the school, Kellogg's assigned seat for the lectures, number 336, was too far from the lecturers and any patients to foster adequate comprehension.[5] The new University Hospital in Ann Arbor was hardly comparable to the busy metropolitan hospitals in large cities and several faculty, including Gunn's replacement Donald Maclean, shared discontent over the lack of proximity to a large city and its hospitals and advised some students to complete their education in major urban settings. After the winter term of 1874, Kellogg decided not to return to Ann Arbor for the second year of medical school but to begin medical school anew in New York City at Bellevue Hospital Medical College. The Whites reluctantly lent Kellogg $1,000 to start the fall term at Bellevue. This was the equivalent of $22,500 in 2019 currency.[6]

At Bellevue, Kellogg was taught and influenced by William Van Buren and Edward Lawrence Keyes, early genitourinary surgeons and concomitant venereology experts, the latter topic of greater interest to the morally self-righteous student from Battle Creek than the former. Coincidentally, 1874 was a big year for Keyes and Van Buren with their new urology textbook, *Genito-Urinary Diseases and Systems*, that solidified the conceptual basis for the practice of genitourinary surgery of the time. As the knowledge base, technology, and surgical repertoire expanded, new editions came out in 1888 and 1895. Comparison of the tables of contents in the textbook of Gross in 1851 with that of Keyes and Van Buren in 1874 shows steady replacement of dogma and opinion with observation, experience, and science. Keyes, and later his son, became major players in the evolution of the field, although in 1874 there was only modest recognition of this new arena in the Michigan medical curriculum.

In 1875, the state of Michigan gave the University of Michigan $3,000 for a Dental Department and appropriated $8,000 for a new hospital building contingent on a contribution from the city of Ann Arbor of $4,000. As a result, twin pavilion-style buildings, each 30 × 114 feet, were built from the back of the original faculty house, opening in 1877 with room for 150 patients:

> When built it was understood that this hospital would become so badly infected within ten years that it would be necessary to burn it. . . . It served as a hospital until 1890 and for at least twenty years more as a class and laboratory room.[7]

The Homeopathic College shared the hospital until 1879 when another faculty house on North University was converted for the homeopaths.

Bolstered by new funds from the millage and student fees, the regents granted the Medical Department request, that had been refused six years earlier, to extend the six-month instructional terms to nine months, benefitting the Homeopathic Medical College as well.[8] Under Angell's watch, the two-year MD program lengthened to three in October 1877. The following year, 1878, faculty salaries were cut because of economic depression: professors dropped from $2,500 to $2,200 that year and President Angell went from $4,500 to $3,750. In 1880, the medical curriculum was extended to four years and that year Angell was appointed by President Rutherford Hayes as minister to China to negotiate a new immigration treaty, a contentious issue given national concern over usurpation of jobs in the delicate economy. During Angell's two years away, Dean Frieze returned to the office of university president. The university and the Medical and Surgical Department made impressive gains under Angell from 1871 through 1909, a time period matched by the rise of the specialty of genitourinary surgery and its transition to the terminology of urology.

A problem that blew up in the chemical laboratory early in Angell's term had lasting consequences. Preston Rose, a young instructor and graduate of the medical school, was teaching under the aegis of Professor Douglas. Rose, although a popular teacher, wasn't destined to become a forensic celebrity, like Poe's detective or the later Sherlock Holmes, but his chemical analysis teaching lured students. His urinalysis class enrolled 55 in 1866, 41 in 1869, and 143 in 1871, utilizing George Harley's text, *The Urine and Its Derangements*.[v]

Rose was promoted to assistant professor of physiological chemistry in 1875, perhaps the first academic title of its sort, further evidence of the expansion of science into health care in the nineteenth century.

---

v Harley (1829–1896), a great English physiologist, had dictated the book during a period of personal visual difficulty and it was published in 1872, reprinted in America, and also translated into French and Italian.

An $800 discrepancy in the accounting of student fees led Douglas to fire Rose in October 1875, and the dispute reached the state legislature. A state committee began to investigate in 1877, but the matter and the money in question escalated. The committee found Rose responsible for $497 of the discrepancy, while Douglas was held responsible for $4,477. The regents accordingly dismissed Douglas, an astonishing action considering that he was one of the original medical school faculty members. The regents tried to collect the funds, suing both Douglas and Rose for the discrepancy that had grown to $5,671. The court held Rose liable for $4,624 and Douglas for $1,047. Two new regents joined the board in January 1878, further splitting the regents bitterly over the issue and the matter reached the Michigan Supreme Court in 1881. Philanthropy saved the day, in terms of the financial dispute, when Rice Beal, owner and editor of the *Ann Arbor Courier*, and a Rose supporter, persuaded the regents to accept a gift of a huge natural history collection he owned.[vi] The Rose-Douglas affair was the most serious controversy faced by President Angell during his otherwise excellent 38 years in office and the effects lingered for decades, in spite of the ultimate financial settlement.[9]

The immediate teaching void in 1875 was solved when a new PhD in chemistry, Victor Vaughan, was asked to teach Rose's course on physiology and class on urinalysis.[10]

Notes

1 H. H. Peckham, *The Making of the University of Michigan 1817–1992*. Edited and updated by M. L. Steneck and N. H. Steneck (Ann Arbor: University of Michigan Press, 1967, 1994), 66.
2 V. C. Vaughan, *A Doctor's Memories* (Indianapolis: The Bobbs-Merrill Company, 1926), 104.
3 University of Louisville School of Medicine website; *Medicine at Michigan*, Fall 2002; http://www.medicineatmichigan.org/sites/default/files/archives/fitzjones.pdf.
4 F. X. Blouin, Jr., "The Components of Reputation: Pragmatism, Science, and the Transformation of the University of Michigan, 1852–1900," *Michigan Historical Review* 43, no. 1 (Spring 2017), 13–14.
5 H. Markel, *The Kelloggs: The Battling Brothers of Battle Creek* (New York: Pantheon, 2017), 49.

vi Joseph Steere, a UM graduate and then assistant professor of paleontology in 1876, collected "an immense number of butterflies, bird skins, tropical woods, insects, fish, shells, fossils, and rocks" on a worldwide trip in 1870 backed by Beal. In June 1878, the regents bought half the collection at the price of their claim against Rose (then $4,624), while the other half was gifted to the university. Douglas and the court were paid $3,650. The only winners in this ugly matter were the lawyers, accountants, and expert witnesses who received more than $8,000. H. H. Peckham, *The Making of the University of Michigan 1817–1992*. Edited and updated by M. L. Steneck and N. H. Steneck (Ann Arbor: University of Michigan Press, 1967, 1994), 82–83.

6 H. Markel, *The Kelloggs: The Battling Brothers of Battle Creek* (New York: Pantheon, 2017), 51.
7 V. C. Vaughan, *A Doctor's Memories* (Indianapolis: Bobbs-Merrill Company, 1926), 203.
8 H. H. Peckham, *The Making of the University of Michigan 1817–1992*. Edited and updated by M. L. Steneck and N. H. Steneck (Ann Arbor: University of Michigan Press, 1967, 1994), 86.
9 H. H. Peckham, *The Making of the University of Michigan 1817–1992*. Edited and updated by M. L. Steneck and N. H. Steneck (Ann Arbor: University of Michigan Press, 1967, 1994), 82–83.
10 H. W. Davenport, *Not Just Any Medical School* (Ann Arbor: University of Michigan Press, 1999), 6.

Victor Vaughan's Time

Victor Vaughan was born on October 27, 1851, on a family farm in Mount Airy, Missouri, northwest of Columbia. His autobiography recounts a pleasant boyhood in Missouri in spite of the Civil War. Attending Central College in Fayette, Missouri, for one year and then Mount Pleasant College, in Huntsville, he became enamored with chemistry, after he discovered a locked room that turned out to harbor a long-neglected chemistry laboratory. Barker's *Chemistry* and *Qualitative Analysis* by Silas Douglas and Albert B. Prescott, from Michigan's chemical laboratory, made inspirational impressions on Vaughan.[1]

After graduating with a BS in 1872, Vaughan remained at Mt. Pleasant to teach Latin and chemistry, leaving abruptly in February 1874 when the school president halved the salaries of teachers in order to add to the school buildings. In his autobiography, Vaughan wrote that he "found it necessary to look outside my native state for university training" later writing, "Michigan was the great state university," and "my final decision was made when I learned that there was a large and well-equipped chemical laboratory." Vaughan also at the time was well aware of great Michigan intellects including James Craig Watson (Ann Arbor Observatory director after Brünnow left and discoverer of 23 asteroids beginning in 1863), Thomas M. Cooley (Law School dean), Henry Frieze (Latin professor and former university president), Louis Fasquelle (professor of Italian and French), and President Angell, among others. Things were happening at the University of Michigan, and Vaughan was anxious to partake of the intellectual excitement. As Vaughan went north to Ann Arbor, John Kellogg left the medical school to go east.

In September 1874, Vaughan and a friend from Mt. Pleasant who intended to enter Michigan's pharmacy school traveled by the Wabash Railroad through Toledo and Detroit to Ann Arbor.

My companion and I spent a forenoon in youthful admiration of the beautiful homes on Fort Street, Lafayette, Woodward, Jefferson, Avenues and other thoroughfares in Detroit. Our bucolic eyes had never realized that earth could be so fair. Certainly in the seventies and eighties Detroit in the early fall was one of the most fascinating of cities. A wider observation led me to the belief that there was only one other city and that was Cleveland which could favorably compare with it. It was an intoxication of the imagination to visit either.[i]

After alighting from the train at Ann Arbor in the late afternoon and entering the disreputable station of that time, and especially after dining at the 'Cook House' we, boy-like, cursed the lack of wisdom which led the early authorities to select Ann Arbor instead of Detroit as the seat of the University. This opinion was strengthened by a night of attempts at sleeping and a scanty breakfast at the famous hostelry named above.[2]

Fortunately, things got better for Vaughan, who remained in Ann Arbor undeterred to study chemistry under Douglas, coauthor of the book that had inspired young Vaughan to come north.

Hidden away behind the medical building was the chemical laboratory, then the largest and best equipped chemical laboratory in the United States, and with but one in the world to compare with it—the laboratory of Fresenius at Wiesbaden.[3]

Two years later, Vaughan completed three theses to obtain one of the first two PhD degrees given by the University of Michigan, the other going to William H. Smith in biology. Before receiving his degree, however, an unexpected teaching opportunity occurred with the Rose-Douglas controversy and Vaughan took over Rose's class in January 1876.

Vaughan needed to win over the medical students with his first lecture in physiological chemistry, later recalling that Rose "held a medical degree and was deservedly popular in both classroom and laboratory." As a new instructor, Vaughan had not even matriculated as a medical student. Strategically, he immersed himself deeply in a novel topic and

---

i Nearly a half-century later, when Vaughan wrote A *Doctor's Memories* in 1926, conditions had changed because the next sentences that followed his bucolic recollections of Detroit neighborhoods were quite different: "Now, I drive miles to avoid penetrating them. 'The banners of industry,' in the form of great volumes of smoke, now shut out the sunlight which at the time kissed their pavements and played 'hide and seek' on their beautifully wooded lawns."

then gave the first of many lecture hours on "the structure and function of the kidney." The students were enthusiastic and sang "He is a jolly good fellow" at the end of the first class. Vaughan took medical student teaching seriously, planning to join the class himself soon. He complained that the medical school had only two microscopes available for the students "and these were well nigh worthless." President Angell responded by authorizing Vaughan to spend a few hundred dollars on better equipment, and after a trip to the Centennial Exposition at Philadelphia in September 1876, Vaughan returned with six English Crouch microscopes. A year later, he purchased six Zentmayer microscopes, with additional funds from the president.

Vaughan and his fellow PhD Smith entered the medical school in the fall of 1876, in the last years of the two-year curriculum and in parallel with the new homeopathic students. In 1878, Vaughan collected an MD and continued to teach physiological chemistry throughout much of his impactful career at Michigan and his international celebrity until retirement in 1921. Vaughan's lecture notes were printed, revised, and sold to students for many years. The 1879 edition was 315 pages, according to Davenport, with 160 pages on urine composition including Vaughan's observations on his personal diurnal variance. He detailed physiology and pathology of the constituents of urine and detection of drugs.[4] As for the Douglas-Rose financial dispute that launched his career as a medical educator, Vaughan recalled, "Knowing both men as I did I have never thought that either stole a dollar."[5]

The expanded medical curriculum of three years in 1877 reflected a verifiable scientific knowledge base far different from the dogmatic duplicate lecture series of the first decade of the school. The first-year students had classes on descriptive anatomy, comparative embryology, histology and microscopy, physiology, chemistry (general, organic, and physiologic), botany, bacteriology, and sanitary science. Second-year topics were physiology, materia medica and therapeutics, pathology, physical diagnosis, medical jurisprudence, practice of medicine, systemic surgery, obstetrics, physiology and pathology of menstruation, and diseases of women and children, in addition to 12 weeks of afternoons dedicated to urinalysis in the chemical laboratory. Optional courses in the second year included laboratory work in physiology, electrotherapeutics, advanced histology, pathological chemistry, and an extended course in analysis and toxicology. The third-year classes included the practice of medicine, systemic surgery, clinical medicine, clinical surgery, surgical anatomy, minor surgery, obstetrics, clinical gynecology and children's diseases, ophthalmology and otology, laryngology, diseases of the skin, eye and ear clinic, with optional classes of an extended course in clinical surgery and a course in clinical ophthalmology. The curriculum was heavily lecture-based with 473 lectures in year one, 516 in year two, and 653 in the third. A four-year curriculum began optionally in 1880.[6]

Surgery, from 1872 to 1889 under Edinburgh-educated Donald Maclean, who insisted on clean technique, was wide-ranging in anatomic terrain, including genitourinary problems such as the management of traumatic urethral stricture with early catheterization.[7] Like his earlier predecessor, Gunn, Maclean lived and practiced in Detroit and advocated relocation of the Ann Arbor medical school. Maclean was a committed medical educator and a versatile surgeon, and among the many students he taught over 17 years two are especially notable. The 1883 graduate, William Mayo (three-year program) would have a profound influence over American health care and medical education. In the fall of 1883, Vaughan with six other university faculty members (in astronomy, two in chemistry, engineering, geology, physiology) formed a Scientific Club and invited 12 other faculty members for monthly dinners and discussions related to science in its broadest sense of "methodologic observation and reasoning to create new knowledge." At another place and another time this might have been called a "Natural History Club," but the "science" terminology was pre-ordained even into the fabric of the University of Michigan with the vision of Augustus Woodward in 1816. The Scientific Club continues to meet 136 years later.[8]

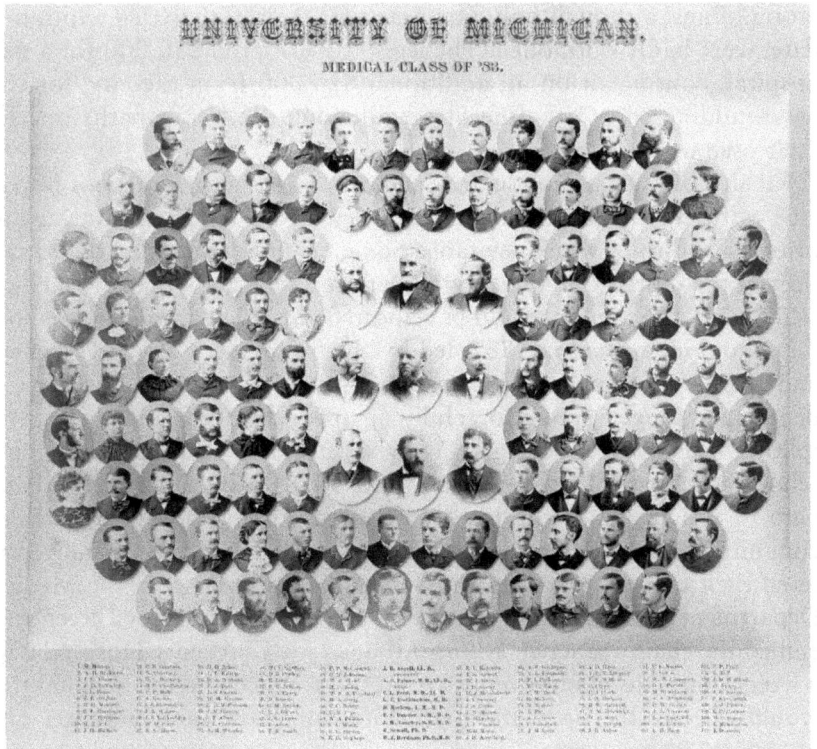

Class of 1883 picture. Mayo second row from bottom, eighth from left.

An 1884 graduate, Herman Webster Mudgett, became one of the most despicable sociopaths in American medicine, whose disturbing story is well told by Erik Larson in *Devil in the White City*. Mudgett moved to Chicago after medical school and inexplicably changed his name to Dr. Henry Howard Holmes and began (or possibly resumed) a career of serial murder until the law caught up with him and he was executed by hanging in Philadelphia, 12 years after graduation from medical school.[9]

Ford resigned as dean of the Medical Department in 1885 and was replaced by Vaughan. The Vaughan era of three decades would bring the University of Michigan Medical School into the top tier of American medical education. Angell took another leave from the university presidency in 1887 to serve with the national Fishery Commission to negotiate U.S. fishing rights off Newfoundland, Nova Scotia, and New Brunswick.[10] Rising property values in 1888 inflated the university's one-twentieth mill tax yield and the faculty salary cuts, from 10 years earlier, were restored, with Angell's pay raised to $5,000. A new hygiene and physics lab was built, and the chemical building enlarged, again. Vaughan's attention was somewhat diverted with his role on the State Board of Health and by this time the pavilion hospital buildings, although only one year past their anticipated expiration date, were badly outmoded. The legislature offered $50,000 for a new hospital, contingent on an additional $25,000 from the city, for two new buildings on Catherine Street allowing the homeopaths one for their own use.[11]

Faculty physicians conducted medical and surgical practices in parallel with their educational duties, so tensions between clinical and instructional roles were inevitable. Some faculty maintained their practices in the more populous city of Detroit and argued that the medical school and its hospital should be relocated there. The campaign to move the school intensified in 1887, led by chief of surgery Donald Maclean and George Frothingham, professor of ophthalmology. University president James Angell spoke forcefully against relocation and the regents followed his advice, voting in 1889 on a policy to keep the medical school and hospital in Ann Arbor and asking Maclean and Frothingham to resign. Given the history of intermittent tenures and divided commitments of the five surgery chiefs after Gunn, who usually centered their clinical practices and personal lives in Detroit, the Medical Department offered a fulltime model for the next surgery director, to embed the chair's practice in Ann Arbor at the University Hospital with a fixed salary based on revenues from the practice and the hospital that would obviate the need and permission for extramural practice. This model enticed Charles de Nancrede from Philadelphia, a rising figure in American surgery and surgical education, to Ann Arbor in 1889. This was also a notable year for the medical school and university in many other ways, including the death of Henry Frieze that December. Frieze was one of the university's most valuable "utility players" as a nationally known intellect, a respected educator, a valued colleague, and twice-serving acting president.

The enrollment for entire University of Michigan graduating class in 1890 was 2,153, making Michigan the largest university in the country, exceeded three years later by Harvard. Michigan's professors were among the nation's most gifted teachers and writers. Their work and textbooks in math, chemistry, education, law, astronomy, and languages created a new generation of knowledge that branded the University of Michigan as a place of deep expertise, similar to the branding that had attracted a young Victor Vaughan from rural Missouri a generation earlier.[12] President Angell recognized the power of a large and successful alumni cohort and reported that the number of degree-bearing university alumni that year was 10,700.[13] In 1891, the state added an additional $25,000 to complete the two hospital buildings and Joshua Waterman offered $20,000 for a gymnasium, early evidence of a growing interest in collegiate-level athletics. In 1891, Michigan's University Hospital had its first "house physician"[14] and by 1899, the hospital had as many as six interns, aided by senior medical students acting as interns. Alice Hamilton in the 1892–1893 term was one of those students, who received free room and board for their service.[ii]

The remarkable partnership of the State of Michigan and City of Ann Arbor culminated in an overdue new University Hospital on Catherine Street in 1892. The state legislature provided for two buildings, one for the Department of Medicine and Surgery, as the medical school was still known, and another for a Homeopathic Department. The medical school's University Hospital occupied the eastern building with open wards containing three rows of beds, a five-bed obstetrical ward, and

---

ii Alice Hamilton (1889-1970) would become a leading expert in occupational health. She was born in New York City and raised in Indiana where she was home schooled and matriculated at the University of Michigan Medical School in 1891. After internships at Northwestern Hospital for Women and Children and studies in Leipzig Germany and Johns Hopkins, she returned to the faculty at Northwestern. In 1908 she was appointed to the Illinois Commission of Occupational Diseases and in 1911 to the United States Department of Labor. In 1919 she joined Harvard Medical School as its first woman on the faculty. *Alice Hamilton Exploring the Dangerous Trades: The Autobiography of Alice Hamilton MD*, Northwestern University Press, 1943. Reprinted 1985.

twelve single rooms for seriously ill patients. No classrooms or laboratories were provided. Patients were prepared for surgery in a bathroom and the surgical theater was a small pit beneath semi-circular benches. The architectural firm obviously had little hospital experience.[15]

Instructors, laboratories, and classrooms for the new disciplines of physiology, pharmacology, and pathology were squeezed into the old curriculum and the medical school physical plant just as the rest of the university was similarly accommodating to new instructional topics of the later nineteenth century, such as engineering and physics. A multidisciplinary building was planned, but budgetary reality excluded engineering, so the new building was dedicated to hygiene and physics, with space for Vaughan's programs including chemistry, physiology, and bacteriology. It wasn't until 1903 when a new medical building opened and the medical programs moved into it that physics was left all to itself.

Homeopathic issues continued to pester the University of Michigan toward the end of the nineteenth century. In 1894, the American Institute of Homeopathy demanded resignation of Michigan's dean Henry Lorenz Obetz, who was accused of advocating consolidation of the two medical schools. The homeopathic faculty supported this complaint. Regent and Detroit physician Herman Kiefer investigated, found the charge untrue, and blasted the homeopathic institute for interference in university affairs. Nonetheless, the homeopathic dean resigned and the regents fired the rest of the homeopathic faculty. The homeopathic lobby then persuaded the Michigan legislature to compel the university to move the Homeopathic Medical College to Detroit. The Board of Regents refused and the dispute worked its way to the Michigan Supreme Court in 1896, which (again) defended the autonomy of the university. The same guarantee of autonomy was made in subsequent state constitutions of 1908 and 1963.

A new homeopathic dean, W. B. Hinsdale, appointed in 1895, recruited new homeopathic faculty, but student enrollment continued to dwindle, given that homeopathic theory was becoming further irrelevant in the context of the rapidly evolving scientific basis of medical knowledge. A chemistry fellowship, funded this same year by Parke-Davis in Detroit, was an indication of growing university partnerships with industry. Another landmark event that year was the medical school's first endowed professorship, $100,000, given by Dr. Elizabeth Bates of Port Chester, New York, who had no connection with the university other than her admiration for Michigan's early open door to women for medical education. Just as philanthropy fueled the start of the University of Michigan in Ann Arbor, the novel gift of Bates at the *fin de siècle* to establish a professorship was followed by many others over the next century creating a strong professoriate that made the university a leader among the best of its peers.

The final decade of the nineteenth century oddly brought new sectarian ideas to health care, namely chiropractic and osteopathic philosophies. These new paradigms of health care, based on personal and idiosyncratic ideas of individual practitioners rather than verifiable knowledge based on scientific method, would have been more logical 50 years earlier, when homeopathy, mesmerism, magnetic therapy, phrenology, water cures, and other medical memes were popular. "Regular medicine," the so-called orthodoxy of the earlier nineteenth century, in fact had little of a verifiable or scientific basis behind it to counter the proliferating sectarian medical ideas of those earlier times. The American Medical Association was formed in 1847 largely for purpose of distinguishing "regular practitioners," who had trained in the orthodoxy of their time, from sectarian programs of instruction. The robust and verifiable scientific basis for medicine, including germ theory, biochemistry, physiology, pharmacology, organ basis of disease, and so forth had not existed in the early nineteenth century to counterbalance those sects. It is ironic that new personal medical ideologies would gain traction in spite of the accruing scientific knowledge base at the end of the century.

Osteopathy was based on the belief that most disease emanates from impaired blood flow to a part of the body and can be corrected by osteopathic manipulation therapy. Andrew Taylor Still (1828–1917), a physician trained largely by his father and Civil War experience as a *de facto* surgeon, developed this idea after he lost his wife and four children to diseases that conventional medical practice could not repair. Still also had a remarkable career, as an anti-slavery state legislator in Kansas for a time, before he created the American School of Osteopathy in Kansas City, Missouri, in 1892.

Chiropractic medicine came from Daniel David Palmer (1845–1913), a Canadian who came south for various careers including teaching beekeeping, shopkeeper, and practice as a magnetic healer. After some instruction in osteopathic medicine, he hypothesized that disease came from impaired nerve supply that could be improved by spinal manipulation, proposing his ideas in 1895, calling it "a science of healing without drugs."[16] He established the Palmer College of Chiropractic in Davenport, Iowa, in 1897.

By this time, Victor Vaughan and the University of Michigan Medical School were at the center of American medical orthodoxy. Vaughan had arrived in Ann Arbor in 1874 as a young man with a mission to learn chemistry, obtained one of Michigan's first two PhDs and then became one of its last two-year MDs, steadily rising to become dean of the Medical Department in 1885. The medical curriculum went from a rudimentary set of lectures barely adding up to 12 months over two years to a four-year graduated mix of lectures, laboratories, and clinical experiences based largely on science delivered in nine-month terms. The medical students diversified during Vaughan's time. Vaughan grew up amidst the Civil War, had important leadership positions in the Spanish-American War, and national roles during World War I. He took the University of Michigan Medical School from a small regional medical school to become one of the noteworthy medical centers of the world by the start of the twentieth century, and even with all that, his work was hardly completed as the new century began.

Notes

1 H. W. Davenport, *Victor Vaughan: Statesman and Scientist* (Ann Arbor: University of Michigan, 1996).
2 V. C. Vaughan, *A Doctor's Memories* (Indianapolis: Bobbs-Merrill Company, 1926), 87–89.
3 V. C. Vaughan, *A Doctor's Memories* (Indianapolis: Bobbs-Merrill Company, 1926), 91.
4 H. W. Davenport, *Not Just Any Medical School* (Ann Arbor: University of Michigan Press, 1999), 6.
5 V. C. Vaughan, *A Doctor's Memories* (Indianapolis: Bobbs-Merrill, 1926), 103.
6 H. W. Davenport, *Not Just Any Medical School* (Ann Arbor: University of Michigan Press, 1999), 17.
7 H. W. Davenport, *University of Michigan Surgeons 1850-1970 Who They Were and What They Did* (Ann Arbor, MI: Historical Center for the Health Sciences, University of Michigan, 1993), 34.
8 P.c. Bob Bartlett.
9 E. Larson, *Devil in the White City* (New York: Knopf Doubleday, 2004).
10 *Harpers Weekly*, Volume XXXI, October 15, 1887, The Fisheries Commission p. 739, Personal p. 743.
11 H. H. Peckham, *The Making of the University of Michigan 1817–1992*. Edited and updated by M. L. Steneck and N. H. Steneck (Ann Arbor: University of Michigan Press, 1967, 1994), 94.
12 H. W. Davenport, *Not Just Any Medical School* (Ann Arbor: University of Michigan Press, 1999), 94.
13 H. W. Davenport, *Not Just Any Medical School* (Ann Arbor: University of Michigan Press, 1999), 96.
14 H. W. Davenport, *Not Just Any Medical School* (Ann Arbor: University of Michigan Press, 1999), 130.
15 H. W. Davenport, *Not Just Any Medical School* (Ann Arbor: University of Michigan Press, 1999), 29.
16 E. Ernst, "Chiropractic: A Critical Evaluation," *Journal of Pain and Symptom Management* 35 (2008): 544–62.

PART II

A New Medical Subspecialty in North America and Ann Arbor

Origin Claims for Genitourinary Surgery in North America

The distinct practice of genitourinary surgery gained little traction throughout most of the 25 centuries following Hippocrates beyond the recognition that bladder stones required special skills and practitioners. In the late seventeenth century in Europe scientific thought and products of industrialization began to expand the conceptual basis and technology of medical practice, spilling over to lithotomy slowly. Colonial and post-colonial America lagged behind, where early leading medical practitioners, subservient to European medical sophistication, undertook periods of observation and study across the Atlantic, returning with new skills and knowledge. Nevertheless, genitourinary practice in terms of knowledge base and procedures had changed little even by the early nineteenth century when the University of Michigan formed initially in Detroit in 1817 or 21 years later when it moved to Ann Arbor. Lithotomy and simpler genitourinary interventions were not much different than they had been in Hippocratic times. Ancient uroscopy, bladder catheterization, preputial interventions, and horrific lithotomy were still the main skills of the trade along with empiric amelioration of venereal disease in spite of improved anatomic understanding and technology in the mid-nineteenth century. Urologic care then reflected the condition of health care in general, and in those early days at this university, medical practice in its entirety had not substantially improved in its preceding two millennia, a verifiable conceptual basis for medical practice and precision technology only assembling later in the nineteenth century.

The attempted practice of immunization that nearly caused the death of Boston lithotomist Zabdiel Boylston in 1721 (see p. 9) wasn't widely embraced until long after its proven demonstration by Edward Jenner (1749–1823) in 1798 and even now is contentious in some places. Germ theory, introduced conceptually by Oliver Wendell Holmes in the 1843 talk to the *Boston Society for Medical Improvement*, didn't deploy in clinical practice until Joseph Lister's conclusive published evidence more than 20 years later and even then, diffused only slowly over the next 20 years. General anesthesia, in contrast, spread rapidly across the Atlantic within a month after its initial public demonstration in Boston in 1846. Microscopy verified the organ basis of many diseases and investigations in biochemistry, physiology, and pharmacology opened up relevant new fields in the second half of the nineteenth century as medical ideologies such as mesmerism, homeopathy, hydrotherapy, and phrenology were replaced by scientific epistemology. Yet, with Darwinian persistence, old medical ideologies reentered clinical marketplaces and new therapeutic fantasies emerged. Public and professional discontent with prevailing medical orthodoxy made simpler explanations for disease and remedy attractive and opened the way for the chiropractic and osteopathic paradigms of the 1890s. Politically purposed scientific ideologies, such as eugenics and Lysenkoism, in the next century, would continue to corrupt marketplaces, academia, and nations.[i]

Genitourinary surgery is not an ideology but an enduring facet of health care, and urology is its twentieth-century neologism. A pedantic competition developed for the distinction as the "birthplace of American urology" and *The History of Urology*, a book commissioned by the American Urological Association (AUA) in 1933, claimed seven locations important to the origin of American urology: Baltimore, Boston, Chicago, the "Middle West,"

---

i Trofim Lysenko (1898–1976), Russian biologist, rejected Mendelian genetics and proposed a theory of environmentally acquired inheritance. His experimental results showing improved crop yields (unverified by others) convinced Joseph Stalin to embrace Lysenkoism nationally. Soviet scientists who opposed the idea were dismissed from their posts, if not killed as "enemies of the state"; S. Fitzpatrick, *Stalin's Peasants: Resistance and Survival in the Russian Village after Collectivization* (Oxford: Oxford University Press, 1994), 4–5. Forced collectivization and famine followed in the 1930s, but Lysenko's political power consolidated and in 1940 he became director of the Institute of Genetics of the USSR Academy of Sciences. In 1948, scientific dissent from Lysenko's theory was outlawed. After Stalin died in 1953, Nikita Khrushev retained Lysenko in his post, but scientific opposition resurfaced and Lysenko's agricultural influence declined. In 1964, Andrei Sakharov (1921–1989), physicist, architect for the Soviet thermonuclear bomb (RDS-37), later Soviet dissident, and Nobel Peace Prize recipient (1975), denounced Lysenko to the Russian Academy of Sciences in 1964 saying, "He is responsible for the shameful backwardness of Soviet biology and of genetics in particular, for the dissemination of pseudo-scientific views, for adventurism, for the degrading of learning, and for the defamation, firing, arrest, even death, of many genuine scientists"; L. Norman, N. L. Qing, and J. L. Yuan, "Biography of Andrei Sakharov, Dissent Period," *The Seevak Website Competition*; B. M. Cohen, "The Descent of Lysenko," *Journal of Heredity*, 56 (1965): 229–233; B. M. Cohen, "The Demise of Lysenko," *Journal of Heredity*, 68 (1977): 57. Lysenko died in Moscow in 1976 and the daily national newspaper accorded him only brief mention. His politically enforced pseudo-science had tragic consequences for millions of people in Soviet Russia, yet the effects of environment on Mendelian and other proven and verified genetic functions, suspected by countless scientists from Lamarck, if not earlier, is now the field of epigenetics.

New York, Philadelphia, and the "West Coast." Many of those claims describe names, personalities, and some "firsts" of medical practice but mainly detail the final decades of the nineteenth century and first two decades of the twentieth. Michigan's part in the American medical story was well underway in those years, although Michigan didn't contribute then to the developing story of genitourinary surgery, as urology was known in that time. While it is neither essential nor possible to identify a single time and place where American urology appeared *de novo* and replicated itself, it is useful to explore its multiple roots and early sites of practice. Baltimore, Boston, Indiana, New York, Philadelphia, and two medical organizations are the principle contenders for the "origin" status of American genitourinary surgery.

After Edison's incandescent bulb of 1880 merged with the cystoscope of Max Nitze, the new technology demanded a new skillset that opened and consolidated genitourinary surgical practice in clinical workplaces around the world. Before that time, isolated operative procedures, clever instrument innovations, random genitourinary clinics, and sporadic academic appointments were insufficient to create a new free standing specialty of surgery. The cystoscope was the critical factor that allowed unimagined diagnostic and novel therapeutic possibilities to evolve, thereby requiring a new breed of specialists.

Baltimore

Baltimore came first among the chapters in *The History of Urology* origin examination due to alphabetical order and because Johns Hopkins Hospital, after 1889, was the focal point for the modern surgical residency training system and later the first full-range urological institute to fulfill the tripartite mission of clinical care, education, and research in one geographic place. The name, Hugh Young (1870–1945), is central to the story of urology and its place in Baltimore, detailed in Jewett's biographic sketch and Young's autobiography.[1] Young created the first formal urologic training program and was a surgical innovator with few peers. His conservative perineal prostatectomy in 1903 for benign disease and radical cure of prostate cancer in 1905 were surgical tour de forces that set new standards for the time.[2]

Gynecologist Howard Kelly (1858–1943), one of the "Big Four" physicians to inaugurate Johns Hopkins Hospital and a senior contemporary of Young, improved the cystoscope design and integrated it into his practice. Kelly became an expert in ureteral catheterization in both sexes, writing,

> As previously stated in a brief preliminary note, published in the ANNALS OF SURGERY, January, 1898, I have insisted from the very first, when I began my work of inspecting the female bladder and catheterizing the ureters through an open speculum, that there was no reason why the same methods should not be applied, with a few changes

and slightly increased difficulties, to the male sex. Although I have repeatedly dwelt upon this in conversations with friends and during my cystoscopic demonstrations in women, I have not yet been able to induce any one to take up the matter and to thoroughly investigate it.

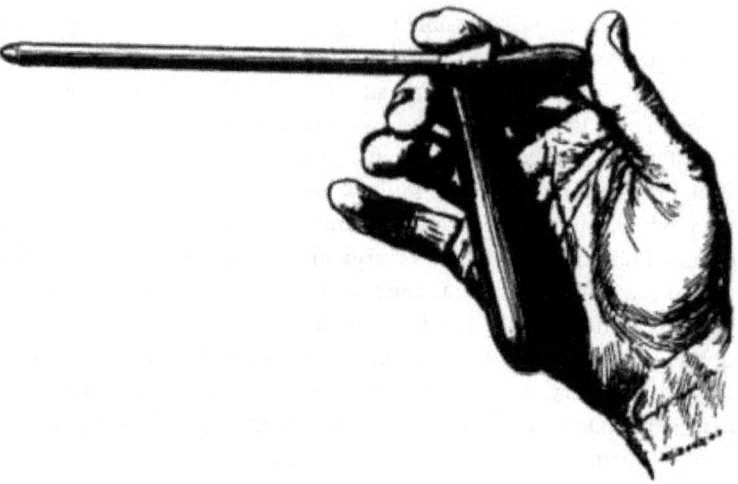

FIG. 1.—Showing male cystoscope reduced to a little less than one-half size; it is held gently poised between index and middle fingers, and during its introduction the thumb keeps the obturator in place.

Figure from Kelly's paper on cystoscopy and ureteral catheterization, 1898.

Kelly then tells how, on November 18, 1893, he commissioned construction of a device he described as a speculum "eight millimeters in diameter, eighteen centimeters long" and later used it in the genitourinary clinic at Johns Hopkins on a patient under the care of Hugh Young (figure from the paper above).[3]

Kelly, a renowned gynecological surgeon and devout Episcopalian, held prayer meetings before his operative procedures. He was also an avid naturalist and collector finding room at home, in addition to his wife and nine children, for a library of over 10,000 books. H. L. Mencken (1880–1956), cultural critic, journalist, and "sage of Baltimore," commented on the "Big Four" founders of Johns Hopkins Medical School with a somewhat negative view of Kelly and William H. Welch (1850–1934), one of the other founders.[4] Welch was a particular friend of Victor Vaughan in Ann Arbor and the two were among the most prominent American medical leaders and educators of their time.[ii]

---

ii Later in his life Kelly developed a curious Michigan connection, being named Honorary Curator of Reptiles and Amphibians in the Museum of Zoology at the University of Michigan,

Young took up Kelly's challenge. The Brady Institute, opened in 1915, gave Young space and resources for his work, and the institute itself would have a formative role in modern urology. Young became a preeminent urologist, educator, and innovator for much of the first half of the twentieth century. Diamond Jim Brady also produced another great Brady Institute at New York Hospital, after he died in 1917. The placement of the permanent office of the AUA in 1952 was yet another fortunate coincidence for Baltimore and urology.[5]

Philadelphia

This claim could begin on December 8, 1752, when Benjamin Franklin of that city wrote a letter, with details of a flexible silver catheter he designed, to his older brother John, a sufferer of bladder stone. American urologic technology possibly began with this device. Thirty years later, when Benjamin himself was suffering from stone, it is likely that he used his own invention.[6]

Philip Syng Physick (1768–1837), considered by many as the first "father of American surgery," had a career at Pennsylvania Hospital that was also a genuine starting point for Colonial American genitourinary surgery. Physick graduated from the University of Pennsylvania in 1785, studied medicine under a regional mentor and then spent 1790–1792 in Europe, working in London as house surgeon at St. George's Hospital and assistant to John Hunter, and next obtaining an MD from the University of Edinburgh. Back in Philadelphia in practice at Pennsylvania Hospital he became distinguished for innovations in urethral surgery. His successful lithotomy in 1831 on Chief Justice John Marshall was a career highlight (see p. 10n).[7] John Syng Dorsey (1783–1818), nephew of Physick, also studied with Hunter as well as with Alexis Boyer in Paris, another European authority in genitourinary surgery. Dorsey returned to Philadelphia in 1803 with skills in diagnostic uroscopy, catheterization, urethral sounding, lithotomy including pediatric bladder stone management, and urethral stricture therapy. His *Dictionary of Practical Surgery* in 1810 and *Elements of Surgery* in 1813, were important early American contributions to surgery and its genitourinary aspects including topics such as upper tract stones, imperforate anus, vaginal anomalies, and spina bifida.[8] Philadelphia was also the eventual home and primary career site for S. D. Gross, author of *A Practical Treatise* in 1851, which surely bolsters that city's claim in the origin story (see p. 27–28).

---

where he gifted his library, paintings, and other gifts to the herbarium in 1928; B. Kanouse, "Doctor Howard Atwood Kelly," *Mycologia* 35, no. 4 (1943): 383–384. (See pp. 221–5.)

Boston

Three names encapsulate this claim as a birthplace of American urology: Henry Jacob Bigelow (1818–1890), the Massachusetts General Hospital, and Harvard Medical School. Bigelow was entitled to all three labels and his name came to national attention in 1846 as a 27-year-old observer of the first public demonstrations of general anesthesia described earlier (see p. 14).[9] Bigelow's genitourinary interests began with a paper in 1849 on "Employment of a New Agent in the Treatment of Stricture of the Urethra" and he reached international acclaim with his paradigm-changing litholopaxy publication in 1878 in the *American Journal of Medical Sciences*.[10]

Bigelow's students, Arthur Tracy Cabot (1852–1912) and Francis S. Watson (1853–1942), had similar great impact in genitourinary surgery, and Cabot's younger cousin Hugh Cabot followed as a major leader in urology, as the field was rebranded, and had a fundamental part of the Michigan Urology story.[11] Watson's influence on the specialty has been underrated in the historical record. He was credited with the first median perineal prostatectomy in modern times (1889) and a paper in 1905 captured a sense of the new scientifically based performance art of twentieth-century surgery: "Some anatomical points connected with the performance of prostatectomy with remarks upon the operative treatment of prostatic hypertrophy."[12] Watson's two-volume textbook in 1908, assisted by John H. Cunningham, Jr., *Diseases and Surgery of the Genito-Urinary System* was dedicated to Edward L. Keyes, "surgeon, author, teacher, and master in his field of the profession." Watson didn't use the Guiteras *urology* neologism in his book, although *urology* subsequently became the textbook term of choice in the twentieth century.[13] Watson and Cunningham wrote the entire text themselves. Watson was becoming a senior authority in the developing field, later writing the "Historical Sketch of Genito-Urinary Surgery in America" for the first chapter of Hugh Cabot's 1918 textbook, *Modern Urology*. The sketch included profiles of Samuel David Gross, Henry J. Bigelow, Edward Keyes, Arthur Cabot, John Bryson, and Samuel Alexander. Also, included in the chapter was a sketch of Watson himself by Edward L. Keyes, Jr.:

> at the request of the editor of this work, who desires to include its subject in this chapter: "Among the circle of men who have maintained the high standard of urology in Boston during the past forty years, Dr. Francis S. Watson is unique."[14]

The "Middle West"

The "Middle West," with Indiana in particular, was a contestant for the birthplace competition according to William Wishard, albeit with a heavy

New York influence. Born in Greenwood, Indiana, in 1854, Wishard had a long and influential career and as author of the scholarly *Preface to the AUA History of Urology* in 1933, he had the privilege of including his region. Like Solomon Martin who obtained two medical degrees (University of Michigan, 1861, and University of Louisiana, 1865) a decade or so earlier (see p. 35), Wishard undertook two medical school courses, completing one in 1874 at Indiana and another in 1876 at Miami Medical College (later Cincinnati University), then entered general practice. In 1879, he was persuaded to become superintendent of Indianapolis City Hospital, which had run down sadly since its military function during the Civil War. His job was viewed as "somewhat odious" at the time, according to Wishard's son in a later obituary.[15]

The hospital was then described as more of an "asylum for destitute and dying poor."[16] Wishard had a better vision and turned the decrepit hospital around after raising $60,000 to upgrade it, adding three buildings, and creating a nursing school, all the time performing his daily clinical work. He began to develop particular interest in genitourinary surgery, influenced by the Van Buren and Keyes text of 1873. Attending an autopsy of a man who had died a week after catheterization for urinary retention, Wishard discovered a hypertrophied ("almost pedunculated") middle lobe and believed that its removal earlier might have spared the man's life. Wishard determined to learn more about genitourinary surgery, although his father, a distinguished regional physician and volunteer surgeon during the Civil War, disapproved of the son's genitourinary interest.

Wishard later recollected how his career developed, in the following quote in which he, himself, was "the writer" during a conversation with the professor of general surgery in 1886, who

> intimated to the writer that there would probably be an early vacancy in the chair of gynecology and abdominal surgery, in which the writer had already been assisting, and inquired if he would like to have an associate position in that department with assurance of promotion. The writer expressed his appreciation and stated that he did not wish to continue teaching in that department, and in reply to further inquiry indicated his intention of limiting himself to surgical urology. The surgeon seemed greatly surprised and replied, "That is a minor department of general surgery. I will be glad to get rid of it and have a special chair established, but why do you prefer such work? You will be nothing but a respectable venerealist."[17]

Wishard resigned from City Hospital on January 1, 1887, to spend the next several months in New York at the Polyclinic Medical School observing emerging leaders of the field, Eugene Fuller (1858–1930),

Frederic R. Sturgis (1845–1919), and E. L. Keyes (1843–1924) in their pathfinding genitourinary surgical practices. He returned to Indianapolis later in 1887 even more committed to the field and founded the Department of Genitourinary Surgery at the Medical College of Indiana, the first American academic department of genitourinary surgery, and served as its chief for 49 years. That department has also been the site of the longest continuous academic practice of what is now called *urology*. Note that Wishard's recollection, in 1933, used the Guiteras' neologism, *urology*, which replaced *genitourinary surgery* after 1902.

In his new academic and clinical capacity, Wishard in 1889 performed Indiana's second recorded nephrectomy. (L. H. Dunning, in South Bend, did the first in 1887.)[18] Wishard was an innovator in prostatic surgery and his soft-nosed rubber catheter was widely used until Foley's balloon improvement in 1935. Wishard became AUA president in 1904 and was still active nearly 30 years later when the AUA turned to him for the preface to its 1933 *History of Urology*.[19] Wishard's successors, Homer Hamer and Henry Mertz, also became national leaders of the first rank.

The "Middle West" should, by all geographic rights, include Chicago, although that city rated its own chapter by Herman Kretschmer in *The History of the AUA*, with profiles of important individuals and clinics but no strong evidence for foundational originality in the field. Ann Arbor, until well into the twentieth century, having only opened its medical school at mid-nineteenth century offered nothing at the cutting edge of genitourinary care, education, or research, but that status would change.

New York City

New York may be the best contender for birthplace of American genitourinary surgery. Edward Loughborough Keyes (1873–1949), son of the founding figure of organizational modern genitourinary surgery and an important presence in the field himself, made the New York case in this hyperbolic sentence: "On Friday, March 2, 1849, Dr. William H. Van Buren, surgeon to Bellevue Hospital and son-in-law of Alexander Mott, the greatest surgeon New York had ever known, opened the new amphitheater at Bellevue Hospital by performing the operation of perineal lithotomy at a public clinic."[iii,20]

Overstatement aside, this was a landmark event. Other times and places might qualify for historical priority of lithotomy in America, the operating room was not technically "an amphitheater," and proof is elusive that

---

iii Keyes listed his name for a chapter in the 1933 AUA *History of Urology* as "E. L. Keyes, Jr.," although his middle name Loughborough, his mother's maiden surname, differed from his father, Edward Lawrence Keyes.

Mott was "the greatest" in New York up to 1849. It can be assumed that general anesthesia was employed, and that fact alone represented the most noteworthy improvement of lithotomy since Hippocratic times. It is also significant that the ancient operative procedure of lithotomy happened to be the operation selected for that first surgical demonstration in Bellevue Hospital's new operating room. The term *urology*, as has been noted, didn't exist in Van Buren's time and the full range of genitourinary surgery had yet to be determined, inasmuch as venereology initially dominated much of the clinical attention of the emerging subspecialty. Nonetheless, Van Buren (1819–1883) was the first identifiable American genitourinary surgeon with a career of practice, innovation, and teaching in the field that became twentieth-century urology, and in 1851 he became its first North American academician, as clinical professor of genitourinary diseases at New York University. While this wasn't then a distinct academic department, it was the first formal genitourinary academic title in America and afforded Van Buren opportunity to develop uncommon expertise in the new arena. Transferring to Bellevue Hospital Medical College, when Freeman Bumstead (1844–1879) resigned from its clinic of syphilology, Van Buren became professor of the principles of surgery and professor of genitourinary diseases.

Van Buren's early assistant, John W. S. Gouley (1832–1920), became a well-known "clinical urethral specialist" and split with Van Buren over which of them invented a certain catheter. Gouley left Bellevue for the Medical Department of the University of the City of New York, as professor of clinical surgery and genitourinary surgery and in 1873 he published an influential book of 368 pages, *Diseases of the Urinary Organs Including Stricture of the Urethra, Affections of the Prostate and Stone in the Bladder*. This book mentions an endoscope invented by Fisher in Boston in 1824, among other early devices, although Ira Rutkow doubts Gouley used any of them.[21] Cystourethroscopy was primitive until the merger of the endoscope of Max Nitze and the incandescent bulb of Thomas Edison in 1880. The actual question of the invention of the disputed tunneled catheter, whether by Van Buren or Gouley, is unresolved and irrelevant except for the fact of fracturing their collaboration. Gouley was unusually cantankerous, later noted to have been excluded from membership in an important emerging organization of his peers due to his temperament.[22]

Van Buren's textbook, published the year after Gouley's, was aided by another assistant, Edward Lawrence Keyes, then a professor of dermatology and adjunct professor of surgery at Bellevue Hospital. *A Practical Treatise on the Surgical Diseases of the Genito-Urinary Organs Including Syphilis*, was 672 pages, nearly double that of the Gouley text.

Fessenden Nott Otis (1825–1900), another noteworthy New York genitourinary surgeon, wrote *Stricture of the Male Urethra, Its Radical Cure* in 1878. A graduate of Union College (1849) with an MD from

New York Medical College (1852), Otis practiced in New York City and in 1871 became professor of genitourinary and venereal diseases at the College of Physicians and Surgeons.[iv]

A second edition by Otis came out in 1880 and other books by him followed in 1883 and 1888. Otis is credited with the first use of local anesthesia in urology.[23] With Van Buren near the end of his career, Keyes carried on their collaboration in *The Venereal Diseases, Including Strictures of the Male Urethra* in 1880, dedicating the text to his teacher. Keyes made a remarkable comment in the preface to the book:[v]

> Finally I have raised my voice, for what it may be worth, in protest against the views of the new school in urethral pathology, which seems to claim that every natural undulation in the diseases of the pendulous urethra is a stricture fit for cutting, and that all the ills of the genitourinary passages may be accounted for by the existence of these undulations, and, usually, made to disappear when the latter are cut.[24]

The book included a number of woodcuts, made from photographs taken by Dr. G. H. Fox of New York, such as the "Otis Urethrameter," used to calibrate strictures (on next page).

The New York origin case includes other important genitourinary names, particularly Eugene Fuller and Reinhold Wappler. Eugene Fuller (1858–1930) became the principle pioneer of suprapubic prostatectomy in North America. Fuller had come to New York from Boston as the younger Keyes recalled,

> Eugene Fuller who came from Harvard with an excellent boxing record, was associated with Keyes from 1885–1895, and during this period published the most strikingly original work that New York urology has produced.[25]

---

iv King's College, founded in New York in 1754, contained a medical school in 1767 that was the second medical school of the original 13 colonies, although it claims to have been the first to give the degree of Doctor of Medicine, which went to Robert Tucker in 1770. Samuel Bard and John Jones cofounded its teaching hospital in 1771 and, after the Revolutionary War, King's College renamed itself Columbia College. In 1807, the College of Physicians and Surgeons (P&S) was established by charter and in 1814 its faculty merged with that of Columbia College. In 1884, William Vanderbilt donated land for P&S at what is now Columbus and Amsterdam Avenues. Presbyterian Hospital formally partnered with Columbia and P&S in 1911, and the school admitted its first women in 1917. The Arnold Gold Foundation began its first White Coat Ceremony at P&S in 1993 and after a gift of $250 million, the medical school changed its name to the Columbia University Roy and Diana Vagelos College of Physicians and Surgeons, as announced in 2017 at its 250th anniversary by university president Lee Bollinger, former president of the University of Michigan.

v Rutkow deserves credit for identifying this passage, as none of the present authors read the entire 348 pages of the Keyes text of 1880.

Otis Urethrameter, 1880.

The boxing coincidence with Ramon Guiteras, who shortly followed Fuller in New York, is curious but Fuller left the sport behind for urological innovation, albeit with some academic jousting. Fuller's report, "Six successful and successive cases" in 1895, of suprapubic prostatectomy was challenged across the Atlantic by Sir Peter Freyer in London with "a clinical lecture on total extirpation of the prostate for radical cure of enlargement of that organ with four successful cases" in 1901. New York and London vied for priority in suprapubic prostatectomy for benign prostatic hypertrophy until an editorial in the *British Medical Journal* in 1907 laid the matter to rest in favor of priority going to Fuller.[26]

Reinhold Wappler (1870–1933) emigrated from Germany in 1890 and worked in New York City as an instrument maker. Until then the electroendoscopic instruments of Maximilian Nitze (1848–1906) were the only cystoscopes available throughout America, but they were delicate and repair was problematic. New York urologist Ferdinand Valentine convinced Wappler to repair them, and soon Buerger, Young, and Keyes became involved in designing better and more durable urological instrumentation. Wappler's first patent, an electrical muscle stimulator in 1896, formed the basis for the Wappler Electric Controller Company, founded the following year. The American Cystoscope Makers Inc. (ACMI), established in 1908, produced the first American cystoscopes and became closely entwined with Wappler Electric.[vi,27]

Organizations

It could be argued that genitourinary surgery came of life in professional societies, and New York City was the origin of urology's first two, although the story begins with another organization, the American Surgical Association (ASA) that formed in 1880 to legitimize surgeons and create a forum for their socialization, an essential part of the development of any specialty. Moses Gunn was an early member. His successor at Michigan, Charles de Nancrede, recalled that Gunn would comment freely at ASA meetings, sometimes with biting criticism.[28] No organization at the time specifically represented genitourinary surgeons and in 1886 Claudius Mastin, a general surgeon in Mobile, Alabama, and ASA member, proposed a triennial congress of several different surgical societies, acknowledging the diversification of surgery. He contacted Edward Keyes in New York City, "the best known genitourinary specialist," and asked that he create a new surgical society of that cadre of surgeons. Keyes, in turn, contacted two dozen

> surgeons known especially for Genito-Urinary work—or at least who have done good service in that field. . . . gentlemen especially known in relation to syphilitic practice, teaching or research.[29]

Twenty expressed interest and 10 attended an organizational meeting at Keyes's home in Manhattan on October 16, 1886. These included Arthur Tracy Cabot, F. N. Otis, and Roswell Park. Gunn, formerly of Ann Arbor and currently in Chicago, was also invited but didn't come to the organizational meeting. An invitation also had been sent to Henry Bigelow of Boston, who didn't respond. Keyes and his guests thus initiated the American Association of Genito-Urinary Surgeons (AAGUS), urology's first professional organization, and held a first scientific meeting in Lakewood, New Jersey, in May 1887. The meeting records noted that "on motion, Dr. Moses Gunn, of Chicago, was declared an original member of the Association," although there is no evidence that he attended at Lakewood, presented a paper, or was active in any subsequent meetings. Eleven members presented papers and the proceedings appeared in the *Journal of Cutaneous and Genito-Urinary Diseases* in

---

vi The NY Academy of Medicine established the Ferdinand C. Valentine Fellowship Award for Research in the Field of Urology in 1963; "The Ferdinand C. Valentine Award," *Journal of Urology* 108, no. 1 (1972): 180. The award first went to Charles Huggins and later, in 1976, to his one time room-mate at UM Reed Nesbit.

July 1887. In addition to A. T. Cabot, Keyes, and Gunn, the 22 original members included Roswell Park and Samuel W. Gross (one of the two sons of Samuel David Gross).[30] The *History of the American Association of Genito-Urinary Surgeons 1886–1982*, by Harry Spence, lists 11 presenters at that first meeting and Cabot, third on the program, discussed two topics: "The case for hysterectomy for the relief of pyelitis from obstruction" and "prostatectomy for obstruction—2 cases."[31] Keyes presented "Suprapubic cystotomy for vesical tumor and large calculus."

The second meeting, held in Washington, DC, featured a paper by Samuel W. Gross regarding masturbation and urethral stricture and another paper by Arthur Cabot called *A case of bowel ending in the urethra of a child four weeks old: relief by operation*.[32] Keyes gave a paper on nephrectomy for pyonephrosis followed by death from renal failure. The author had appropriately catheterized the contralateral kidney and assumed that the presence of urine from it was evidence of normal function, more precise proof of renal function lacking at the time. The remaining kidney was "cirrhotic" on autopsy.[33] These papers indicate the growing range of scientifically informed genitourinary practice as the nineteenth century was concluding. The AAGUS excluded J. W. S. Gouley (see p. 67) for his incivility, behavior well-known to his contemporaries. Ramon Guiteras was elected to membership in 1895 at the Niagara Falls meeting and gave his first paper to the AAGUS at its Washington, DC, meeting in 1900, the topic being "Deformities of the Prostate." Arthur Cabot continued to be a robust member of the society and his presentation record reflects the inclusive range of genitourinary surgery as it transitioned into modern urology. Arthur's nephew and protégée, Hugh Cabot, was elected at the 1907 meeting and also contributed to the organization although not to the same degree in terms of presentations or organizational influence (see table below).

Table 1. Papers presented at AAGUS from 1887 through 1911 by Arthur Tracy Cabot and Hugh Cabot.

Dr. Arthur T. Cabot	
Year	Title
1887	Case of hysterectomy for the relief of pyelitis from obstruction. Prostatectomy for obstruction. Two cases, by Dr. A. T. Cabot.
1888	Case of bowel ending in the urethra of a child four weeks old; relief by operation, by Dr. Arthur T. Cabot.
1889	A case of scirrhus of the bladder, with specimen, by Dr. Arthur T. Cabot.
1890	A case of cystitis, with the formation of a thick epidermal sheet in the bladder, by Dr. A. T. Cabot.
1890	A case of cyst of the kidney, apparently cured by a single aspiration, by Dr. A. T. Cabot.

Year	Title
1890	A case of extrophy to the bladder, with photographs, by Dr. A. T. Cabot.
1891	Observations upon the surgery of the ureter, by Dr. A. T. Cabot.
1892	A case of sacculated bladder, with autopsy, by Dr. A. T. Cabot.
1893	A case of calculus pyelitis with complete suppression of urine for seven days; relieved by operation, by Dr. A. T. Cabot.
1895	A case of cancer of the urethra, by Dr. A. T. Cabot.
1898	Cases of recurrence of stone in the bladder, by Dr. A. T. Cabot.
1898	Personal experience in the operative treatment of prostatic obstruction, by Dr. A. T. Cabot.
1900	Some observations upon hydronephrosis, by Dr. A. T. Cabot.
1903	Specimen of strangulated testis, from torsion of the cord, by Dr. A. T. Cabot.
1903	Report of a case of calculus anuria, by Dr. A. T. Cabot.
1906	A note on the cyst of the prostate, by Dr. A. T. Cabot.
1907	Modern operations for the complete removal of the prostate, by Dr. A. T. Cabot.
1907	Spontaneous fracture of stones, by Dr. A. T. Cabot.
1909	Specimens from a trans-peritoneal cystotomy for cancer; no sign of recurrence at the end of one year, by Dr. A. T. Cabot.

Dr. Hugh Cabot

Year	Title
1907	The value of palliative operation for cancer of the bladder, by Dr. Hugh Cabot.
1908	Varicose veins of a papilla of the kidney, a cause of persistent hematuria, by Dr. Hugh Cabot.
1909	Treatment of stricture of the bulbar portion of the urethra by resection partial or complete, by Dr. Hugh Cabot.
1909	Some observations upon total extirpation of the bladder for cancer, by Dr. Hugh Cabot.
1910	The diagnosis of stone in the pelvic portion of the ureter; a preliminary report in certain limitations of radiographic diagnosis and a suggested remedy, by Dr. Hugh Cabot and W. J. Dodd (by invitation).
1910	Value of vaccines in the treatment of infections of the urinary tract, by Dr. Hugh Cabot.
1911	Phenolsulphonephthalein as a test of renal function, by Dr. Hugh Cabot (paper prepared by Dr. Hugh Cabot and Dr. Edward L. Young, Jr.).

The American Urological Association (AUA) was the second major organization of the specialty and it also formed in New York City, although initially with a different name in 1902. Oddly, the New York chapter in the 1933 AUA *History of Urology*, written by Keyes's son, Edward Loughborough Keyes, omits any direct mention of the name of the AUA founder, Ramon Guiteras, a highly influential genitourinary specialist in New York and originator of the *urology* neologism. The younger Keyes concluded his chapter with a curious comment that alluded to Guiteras: "the genial smile of the man who had once knocked down John L. Sullivan was to help make him the founder of the American Urological Association." Guiteras was, like Fuller, a competent amateur boxer (see p. 89).[34]

A third association of urologists formed internationally, and Watson described the origin of that group in his introductory chapter for Hugh Cabot's 1918 textbook:

> In 1907 a few distinguished French surgeons took steps for the organization of an international body of urologists and in 1908 there came into existence l'Association Internationale d'Urologic. The most renowned specialist of his time, Professor Felix Guyon, was its first president. The officers of the first congress, which met in September 30–October 3, 1908, in Paris were: President, Professor J. Alberran. Vice Presidents: Professor Karl Posner of Berlin; Dr. F. S. Watson of Boston, Secretaire-général Dr. E. Desnos, of Paris, Tresorier-général Dr. O. Pasteau of Paris. A committee composed of Drs. F. S. Watson of Boston (chairman), John Vanderpoel of New York (secretary and delegate), and Hugh H. Young of Baltimore, manages the affairs of the American branch of the international organization.[35]

Watson's chapter in 1918 offered a remarkable summary of the "More important steps of progress in genito-urinary surgery in the last forty years":

1. The revolutionary method of litholapaxy
2. All the knowledge of nature and treatment of vesical tumors
3. Radical surgical treatment of hypertrophied prostate
4. Cystoscopy and the knowledge it secures
5. Ureteral catheter and study of renal functional capacity
6. Tests to determine renal function
7. Radiography knowledge of stones and conditions of renal pelvis and ureter
8. Numerous surgical procedures and contrivances

"Each and all of these have resulted in a great saving of human life and sparing of human suffering."

This list indicates the quantum leap in knowledge and skills from the pediatric cystolithotomy reported by Zabdiel Boylston in 1720, and Alexander Stevens book, *Lectures on Lithotomy* in 1838. That first American genitourinary procedure was most likely closer in technique to Galen and Frère Jacques than to that of Watson and his contemporaries of the 20th century. Similarly, that first American urology textbook recapitulated ancient teachings rather than modern clinical science.

Origin claims for any field are foolish exercises if taken too seriously, but they can be useful constructs to understand the emergence of branches of medicine. The origin of modern urology in North America was multifocal, as observations, ideas, and skills were consolidated, shared, and tested. New learners over generations criticized, verified, debunked, and built upon the knowledge of their teachers, adding new discoveries and incorporating new technology until a coherent new field became established. The explanations for new areas of inquiry and practice in health care are ultimately social, because if an area is to persist and grow its knowledge and skills must be useful, verifiable, and freely taught. This happens best in societies that embrace freedom to inquire, share, criticize, innovate, and test ideas and technology. These freedoms are the crux of universities, science, and liberal democracy. Although the University of Michigan was a late comer to modern genitourinary surgery and the earliest years of urology, the twentieth-century iteration, the Ann Arbor campus soon became a powerful epicenter, largely through Hugh Cabot, but that path had begun with Moses Gunn.

Notes

1. H. J. Jewett, "Hugh Hampton Young: A Biographical Sketch," *Urological Survey* 21 (1971): 69–77; H. H. Young, *A Surgeon's Autobiography* (New York: Harcourt, Brace, 1940).
2. H. H. Young, "Conservative Perineal Prostatectomy," *JAMA* 41 (1903): 999–1009; H. H. Young, "The Early Diagnosis and Radical Cure of Carcinoma of the Prostate," *Johns Hopkins Hospital Bulletin* 16 (1905): 315–321.
3. H. A. Kelly, "Cystoscopy and Catheterization of the Ureters in the Male," *Annals of Surgery* 27 (1898): 475–486.
4. C. S. Roberts, "H. L. Mencken and the Four Doctors: Osler, Halsted, Welch, and Kelly," *Proceedings (Baylor) University Medical Center* 23, no. 4 (Oct 2010): 377–388.
5. C. E. Cox, T. Lee, C. Miksanek, and D. A. Bloom, "Evolution of Surgical Professional Organizations: A Case Study of Thomas Moore, Graceland, and the American Urological Association," *Urology* 107 (2017): 82.
6. G. W. Corner and W. E. Goodwin, "Benjamin Franklin's Bladder Stone," *Journal of the History of Medicine and Allied Sciences* 8 (1953): 359–377.

7   L. Herman, "Philadelphia's Contribution to the Development of Urology in America," *History of Urology vol. 1* (Baltimore, MD: Williams and Wilkins, 1933), 92–94.
8   M. T. Milen, N. W. Thompson, and D. A. Bloom, "John Syng Dorsey and Postcolonial Genitourinary Surgery," *Urology* 59, no. 4 (2002): 626–630.
9   H. J. Bigelow, "Insensibility During Surgical Operations Produced by Inhalation," *Boston Medical and Surgical Journal* 35 (1846) 16: 309–317.
10 R. M. Hodges, O. W. Holmes, H. Lee, D. W. Cheever, H. Derby, R. H. Fitz, A. T. Cabot, "The Memorial Meeting of the Boston Society for Medical Improvement," *Boston Medical and Surgical Journal* 123 (1890): 505; T. Dwight, "The Claim That the Merit of Introducing Ether Belongs to the Late Dr. Henry J. Bigelow," *Boston Medical and Surgical Journal* 123 (1890): 553.
11 R. F. O'Neil, "Early History of Urology in Boston," *History of Urology vol. 1* (Baltimore, MD: Williams and Wilkins, 1933), 27–29.
12 F. S. Watson, "Some Anatomical Points Connected with the Performance of Prostatectomy with Remarks upon the Operative Treatment of Prostatic Hypertrophy," *Annals of Surgery* 41 (1905): 507–519.
13 F. S. Watson, J. H. Cunningham, Jr., *Diseases and Surgery of the Genito-Urinary System* (Philadelphia; New York: Lea & Febiger, 1909).
14 H. Cabot, *Modern Urology in Original Contributions by American Authors*, vol. 1 (Philadelphia, PA; New York: Lea & Febiger, 1918), 32.
15 http://urology.iupui.edu/history/img/pdfs/Wishard/Wishard%20obituary%201941.pdf.
16 R. A. Mannion, "William Henry Wishard (1816–1913): The Urologist's Father or a Physician of the Old School," *Journal of the Indiana State Medical Association* 70 (April 1977): 186–188.
17 W. N. Wishard, "Preface," *History of Urology vol. 1* (Baltimore, MD: Williams and Wilkins 1933), viii–ix.
18 H. G. Hamer, "Early History of Urology in the Middle West," *History of Urology vol. 1* (Baltimore, MD: Williams and Wilkins, 1933), 67.
19 W. N. Wishard, Jr., and W. N. Niles Wishard, Sr., "Urologist, Educator, Administrator, Medical Statesman, Church and Family Man," *Urological Survey* 19, no. 3 (1968): 113–121.
20 E. L. Keyes, Jr., "Early History of Urology in New York," *History of Urology vol. 1* (Baltimore, MD: Williams and Wilkins, 1933).
21 I. M. Rutkow, *The History of Surgery in the United States 1775–1900*, vol. 1 (San Francisco, CA: Norman, 1988), 339.
22 E. L. Keyes, Jr., "Early History of Urology in New York," *History of Urology vol. 1* (Baltimore, MD: Williams and Wilkins, 1933), 72–73.
23 I. M. Rutkow, *The History of Surgery in the United States 1775–1900*, vol. 1 (San Francisco, CA: Norman, 1988), 342.
24 I. M. Rutkow, *The History of Surgery in the United States 1775–1900*, vol. 1 (San Francisco, CA: Norman, 1988), 343–344.
25 E. L. Keyes, Jr., "Early History of Urology in New York," *History of Urology vol. 1* (Baltimore, MD: Williams and Wilkins, 1933), 80.
26 E. Fuller, "Six Successful and Successive Cases of Prostatectomy," *Journal of Cutaneous and Genito-Urinary Diseases* 13 (1895): 229–234; P. Freyer, "A Clinical Lecture on Total Extirpation of the Prostate for Radical Cure of Enlargement of That Organ with Four Successful Cases," *BMJ* 2 (1901): 125–129; Anonymous, "Regarding the Controversy," *BMJ* 1 (1907): 551.
27 M. A. Reuter and H. J. Reuter, *Reinhold H. Wappler and the American Cystoscope Makers, Inc.* (Stuttgart, Germany: Max Nitze Museum for Medical Endoscopy, 1966).

28 M. M. Ravitch, "A Century of Surgery: The History of the American Surgical Association" (Philadelphia: J. B. Lippincott, 1981).
29 H. M. Spence, *A History of the American Association of Genito-Urinary Surgeons 1886-1982*, (Dallas: 1982), 6.
30 E. B. Smith, E. D. Vaughan, E. S. Belt, and D. A. Bloom, "Edward Lawrence Keyes: A pivotal early specialist in modern genitourinary surgery," *Urology* 62 (2003): 968–972.
31 H. M. Spence, *A History of the American Association of Genito-Urinary Surgeons 1886–1982* (Dallas, 1982), 39.
32 H. M. Spence, *A History of the American Association of Genito-Urinary Surgeons 1886–1982* (Dallas, 1982), 9.
33 E. L. Keyes, Jr., "Early History of Urology in New York," *History of Urology* vol. 1 (Baltimore, MD: Williams and Wilkins, 1933), 80.
34 G. M. Crane and D. A. Bloom, "Ramon Guiteras: Founder of the American Urological Association, Surgeon, Sportsman, and Statesman," *Journal of Urology* 184 (2010): 447–452.
35 H. Cabot, *Modern Urology in Original Contributions by American* Authors, vol. 1 (Philadelphia; New York: Lea & Febiger, 1918), 20.

The Bumpy Path to Charles de Nancrede and the Fulltime Salary Model

After Moses Gunn left Ann Arbor for Rush Medical College in Chicago in 1867, Ann Arbor had a succession of surgery chiefs, noted earlier, but none so influential over the next 32 years. William Warren Greene (1831–1881), Henry Lyster (1837–1894), Alpheus Crosby (1832–1877), Theodore McGraw (1839–1921), and Donald Maclean (1839–1903) were all principally clinical surgeons, although Maclean lasted the longest as surgery chief, from 1872 to 1889. Born in Ontario, he trained in Edinburgh with the legendary surgeon and educator James Syme and brought new European ideas including Joseph Lister's carbolic acid method to Ann Arbor in 1877, although Maclean soon abandoned it, citing deaths from "carbolic acid poisoning" and preferring "perfect cleanliness." Records are sparse, but he operated on 326 patients in the 1881–1882 academic year and the cases included bladder fistula, perineal tumor, bladder stone (treated by left lateral lithotomy), varicocele ("radical operation, cure"), and gonorrhea, among orthopaedic, gynecologic, dental surgery, cutaneous procedures, cleft lip, and eye procedures.[1]

Just as his predecessors, Maclean lived and practiced in Detroit, arguing forcefully to move clinical teaching to the larger city and its hospitals. His main ally in this fight was George Frothingham, professor of ophthalmology. Ann Arbor's rudimentary first two hospitals had not fully satisfied the need for a clinical milieu to match classroom medical education. Faculty member Victor Vaughan had initially favored relocation, particularly after his son set up practice in Detroit, but changed his opinion as dean when the issue heated up in the late 1880s and aligned with university president James Angell who had become a focal point of the relocation pressure. Vaughan and Angell convinced the regents that clinical teaching should remain in Ann Arbor with the medical school, as Vaughan later recalled, with some selective memory in his autobiography:

> I never believed in the removal of the Medical School, or even its clinical teaching, to Detroit. It was on this rock that I broke with two of the best friends I ever had, Frothingham and Maclean. But I did believe that the Medical School could utilize the clinical facilities of the large city to the benefit of its students, and to that of the profession and the people.[2]

Vaughan's idea for clinical collaborations in Detroit, however, was never pursued, mainly due to faculty disinterest. A new hospital, to replace "the small and expendable pavilion hospital," was an obvious necessity and collaborative state and city funding was arranged. On June 24, 1889, the regents voted,

> That in the opinion of this Board Professors Maclean and Frothingham have placed themselves in such antagonism to the policy adopted by this board. . . . that they should no longer continue their connection with the University.[3]

The role of Victor Vaughan in the story of the University of Michigan Medical School, seen again in this example, was pivotal and is told in multiple sources including his autobiography and notably in the work of Horace Davenport.[4] After medical school dean Alonzo Palmer died in 1887, the medical faculty elected Corydon La Ford dean. Ford was time-tested and at that time the oldest faculty member. Wisely, he trusted Vaughan to act as *de facto* dean and when Ford resigned in 1891 the regents named Vaughan to replace him. Vaughan recalled,

> When Dean Palmer died in 1887, Doctor Ford nominally became dean but practically turned over that function to me. My relation to Doctor Ford and his family had been most intimate for many years. I was his family physician, the family consisting of himself, his very intelligent wife, and two adopted daughters. I had all along urged advancement in the requirements for admission to the school and lengthening the course to four years. Good naturedly Doctor Ford had replied to my plan: "Have your way, but I will look forward to the time when I shall begin the opening lecture, which I will give as long as I live, with *My dear sir*, since there will be only one student on the benches."[5]

Vaughan did have his way and annual sessions were extended from six to nine months over two years in 1877, a third year was added in 1880, and a fourth in 1890, with no decrease in matriculation, as Ford had speculated. Ford, however, did fulfill his promise, dying immediately after his last lecture. Vaughan took office at an opportune time.

> About the time I made dean (1891) there were seven chairs in our school to fill. This was in a way and in some particulars a most fortunate occurrence. It is seldom that a new dean has opportunity to select a Faculty to suit his own ideas, but it brought upon me my greatest strain as dean. I was determined to have men of general culture and of productive scholarship and none others. I knew full well if I could fill all the chairs with men possessed of these qualifications the success of the School would be assured and the task of the dean would be easy.[6]

Vaughan, already hard at work for several years as *dean de facto*, was the reason for the vague phrase, "About the time I made dean" in his autobiography. Vaughan's new recruits were Charles de Nancrede (1847–1921) in surgery in 1889, George Dock (1860–1951) in medicine in 1891, Paul Freer (1862–1912) in chemistry in 1889, James McMurrich (1859–1939) in anatomy in 1894, John Abel (1857–1938) in pharmacology in 1890, and Flemming Carrow (1853–1932) in ophthalmology in 1889. Arthur Cushny (1866–1926) followed Abel in 1893 who left for the new medical school in Baltimore.

Abel's chair of pharmacology became the nation's first. Abel (1857–1938) was a Michigan graduate (1883), then working in Europe where he isolated epinephrine from the adrenal medulla. Abel stayed only until 1893 when Johns Hopkins recruited him to its new medical school, where he collaborated on an early form of a renal dialysis device, along with one other Michigan faculty member (William Howell) and two other Michigan graduates (Henry Hurd and Franklin Mall). Vaughan was proud to point out that those four Michigan men comprised half of the new medical faculty at Johns Hopkins.[7]

Frederick George Novy (1864–1957) would deploy Vaughan's intellectual legacy more than any other of his trainees or faculty hires. Born and raised in Chicago, Novy came to the University of Michigan and achieved a chemistry BS in 1886 and stayed for a master's degree in 1887 with a thesis called "Cocaine and its derivatives," published as a monograph the same year, listing his title as assistant in organic chemistry.[i]

---

i The short text, while not a riveting page turner, begins with a historical introduction: "The startling accounts given by the Early European travelers in South America of the wonderful effects produced by coca leaves, have led at quite an early period to their chemical examination." He then discussed the three related alkaloids ecgonine, benzoylecgonine, and cocaine, the last being "the alkaloid of coca leaves." For each, he described

While teaching bacteriology as an instructor, Novy qualified for a PhD with a thesis in 1880 on "The toxic products of the bacillus of hog cholera." He obtained an MD from the University of Michigan in 1891 and followed the footsteps of his teacher and dean Victor Vaughan as assistant professor of hygiene and physiological chemistry. Visiting key European centers in 1894 and 1897, he brought a high level of expertise back to Ann Arbor and became an international expert in medical basic sciences, particularly microbiology. Novy became full professor in 1904 and first chair of the Department of Bacteriology at the University of Michigan. He was one of the earliest modern physician-scientists. He worked on trypanosomes and spirochetes, including laboratory culture techniques, he studied anaerobes, researched the tubercle bacillus, and investigated the 1900 bubonic outbreak in San Francisco. Novy became Vaughan's educational, investigational, and (to a great extent) administrative successor and had a major role in the upcoming transformative years of Hugh Cabot, Vaughan's actual successor as dean.

George Dock, said to be the best clinical pathologist in the country, was a major recruitment of Vaughan in 1891 and his resignation in 1908 over Vaughan's inability to provide a student laboratory was ameliorated when the dean replaced him with Albion Walter Hewlett.[ii,8]

Vaughan's autobiography tells his version of his recruitments, although the larger narrative is not quite so simple. After the threat to relocate the medical school to Detroit was averted and the regents dismissed Maclean and Frothingham, a committee of three regents was created to oversee Vaughan's recruitments. With Vaughan they visited Boston, New York, and Philadelphia where they met de Nancrede and were impressed.[9] The full-time employment model was the essential element to solve the persistent tension between private practice and the academic mission. de Nancrede had served under Samuel David Gross at Jefferson and remained in Philadelphia with appointments at three state-of-the-art hospitals, although he had no academic appointment. By age 42 when he came to Ann Arbor, de Nancrede was skilled in the full gamut of general surgery including brain surgery, cataract extraction, abdominal exploration, orthopaedic procedures, and genitourinary operations. He was

---

preparation, properties, salts, reaction, physiological action, synthesis, and chemical constitution, providing greater chemistry details for cocaine itself. The last chapters covered homologues of cocaine and doubtful alkaloids; G. F. Novy, *Cocaine and Its Derivatives* (Geo. S. Davies, Detroit, 1887).

ii The Dock influence in Ann Arbor and nationally was large and has been recounted well. H. W. Davenport, *Doctor Dock*, (New Brunswick and London: Rutgers University Press, 1987). Hewlett in turn resigned in 1916 to become professor of medicine at Stanford, where years later his son with a friend named David Packard developed a great company in a garage.

an early adapter of new ideas, being the first in his region to perform appendectomy and recognize the diagnostic value of McBurney's point, a controversial idea at the time. He embraced Listerism, in spite of the negative stance of his teacher, Gross. de Nancrede recommended Listerian principles in a talk to the American Surgical Association in 1882, later becoming president of the organization. de Nancrede's influential textbook, *Essentials of Anatomy and Manual for Practical Dissection* in 1888 endured through seven editions until 1911 and he published *Lectures on the Principles of Surgery* in 1889, one of the first American textbooks on antiseptic technique, with a second edition in 1905. de Nancrede was recalled as an effective surgeon, astute clinician, and excellent teacher.[10]

The full-time job at the University of Michigan brought de Nancrede from Philadelphia with his wife and nine children in 1889. Michigan's remarkable decision to attract a full-time surgery professor with an ample salary that made a separate private practice unnecessary was irresistible, although the pavilion hospital was primitive by Philadelphia standards and the town of Ann Arbor must have seemed rustic. Arriving in Ann Arbor, de Nancrede found little in the way of clinical resources and had to obtain his own instruments, however, he was free to teach, write, investigate, and care for patients as he liked, and he recognized that newer facilities were coming on line. An anatomical laboratory building, just completed in 1889, freed up space in the medical building and served anatomic dissection purposes up to 1903. The small surgical practice de Nancrede developed in Ann Arbor reflected his commitment to an academic life of teaching and investigating. Over most of the next two decades, the Surgery Department remained mainly his one-man show, with gradual emergence of a few partial specialists in gynecology, neurosurgery, and genitourinary surgery by the early 1900s.

The Ann Arbor Surgery Department was in turmoil when de Nancrede arrived, in part because of the recent Detroit relocation controversy. His first clinical ally was Cyrenus Darling, who had graduated from the medical school in 1881, during the three-year curriculum phase, and then entered local general practice. Darling maintained close ties to the school, teaching anatomy and physical diagnosis. Soon after arrival, de Nancrede began a mandatory surgical laboratory for fourth-year students, to teach aseptic and antiseptic technique, anesthetize dogs, operate on cadavers, and perform intestinal anastomoses. Darling became the teacher, and de Nancrede was proud enough of the course to describe it at the American Surgical Association (ASA) national meeting in 1894. An annual summer course was announced at the same time, to teach practitioners new developments in medicine and developed into a robust continuing medical education program over more than 20 years with Darling covering the surgical part. de Nancrede encouraged Darling's interest in dental surgery and in 1892 Darling became a lecturer in oral pathology and surgery in the Dental Department, and Darling had a turn as dental dean from 1903 to 1907. Teaming up with another oral surgeon, Darling accumulated a large experience in repair of cleft lip and palate.

The medical school had 14 faculty, half preclinical and half clinical, with de Nancrede as the sole surgeon in 1891, when a new hospital opened.[11] This was the third sequentially for the university and it was placed on Catherine Street, nearly a half mile from the central campus, because President Angell wanted it separate from the rest of the university.[12] This 400-bed facility aligned with the determination of the regents, President Angell, and Dean Victor Vaughan to dispel any notion of relocation. The new hospital was imperfect as it soon became evident but was a major upgrade for patients, faculty, and medical students. It had two nearly identical buildings, one for the practice of the Homeopathic Department and the other, to the west, for "regular medicine" of the Medical Department. (Interestingly, similar awkward language distinctions persist today with the opposing terms, *osteopathic* and *allopathic* medicine.) Davenport noted,

> The hospital had been designed by architects with very little experience in hospital construction, and it had no classrooms or laboratories. de Nancrede operated before the class in a pit from which rose a semicircular array of wooden benches. He probably had about a hundred beds for his patients.[12]

A roentgenological laboratory was later established and administered by de Nancrede. Anesthesia was delivered by open drip ether until the 1900s when closed circuit systems were implemented. The Homeopathic Department moved out of its building on Catherine Street in 1901 to a new facility on North University leaving space for the Departments of Internal Medicine, Neurology, and Dermatology in what was then called the West Ward. University Hospital became the East Ward for the Department of Surgery and its specialties. The outdated original medical school building of 1850, with its 1865 addition, was replaced by a new medical building in 1903.

de Nancrede, although an authoritative figure in the world of surgical practice and academia, was not a part of the emerging genitourinary intelligentsia. Nevertheless, as disciple of Gross and an accomplished general surgeon, his repertoire included genitourinary procedures for trauma, bladder stone, and kidney problems. He embraced the new technology of the Crookes tube to locate foreign bodies as well as stones in the urinary tract, noting that some stones were radiolucent and required endoscopic confirmation. He was a bold yet cautious surgeon, using anterior approaches for nephrectomy, so he could be certain that each patient had a second kidney. He was reluctant to undertake exploratory laparotomy and did not favor palliative surgical procedures.[13] Over the next two decades, de Nancrede parsed out facets of his general surgical practice and teaching in gynecology, oral surgery (Darling), genitourinary surgery (Darling and Loree), and in 1911 to the first full-time anesthesiologist, Allen Richardson.

The Spanish-American War, a prelude to the twentieth century, tugged at the patriotic strings of de Nancrede and Vaughan who both volunteered in 1898. The combat experience of de Nancrede was mainly in a diversionary operation at the Battle of Las Guasimas on June 23, 1898, near Santiago, Cuba, where 9,644 infantrymen, three field guns, and 800 irregulars of the U.S. Army and the Republic of Cuba faced 1,500 infantry and two field guns of the Kingdom of Spain. It was a decisive U.S. victory although with 27 dead and 52 wounded on the American side, while the Spanish had 7 dead and 14 wounded. The American side included the 1st U.S. Volunteer Cavalry, known as the Rough Riders, under Leonard Wood and the 10th U.S. Regular Cavalry, called the Buffalo Soldiers. Wood, before becoming U.S. Army general, army chief of staff, military governor of Cuba, and governor general of the Philippines, started out as an army surgeon with an MD from Harvard Medical School.[iii] Vaughan briefly came under fire and had a turn taking care of the wounded, until yellow fever took him down, nearly at the cost of his life. He later was assigned to a commission, along with Drs. Walter Reed and Edward Shakespeare to study infectious diseases, and it was Vaughan who completed the report, outliving his two colleagues. During service both in Cuba and with the commission, Vaughan developed friendships with colleagues at Johns Hopkins, Harvard, Penn, and other elite medical faculty that continued well beyond that war and extended their influence not only into military medicine and science but also bringing revolutionary change to American medicine, education, and public health. Welch in Baltimore and Vaughan in Ann Arbor were at the pinnacle of this elite group.[14]

The combat injuries de Nancrede managed were equivalent to a few weeks of experience in a major urban trauma center today, but they gave him newfound authority on ballistic injuries of that time. He offered this new expertise in talks at the American Surgical Association (of which he was president in 1909) and elsewhere as well as in papers over the rest of

---

iii Later as a general, Leonard Wood would send advice to Michigan students urging them to finish their college work before enlistment in World War I.

his career. He remained proud of his short military duty and was recalled proudly wearing his broad-brimmed campaign hat when traveling to work at University Hospital years later. His personal provenance seemed to inspire him around that time and a newspaper clipping from the *Ann Arbor Gazette* February 6, 1906, tells that the professor petitioned the probate court in Ann Arbor and paid the county $3 to change his surname to that of his grandfather Paul J. G. de Nancrede:

> Dr. Nancrede states in his petition that there is a desire in the family, of which he is the oldest living male representative, for reasons of sentiment that the name be changed to the original and that the petition is not sought with any fraudulent intent.[15]

Thus, Nancrede became de Nancrede. When World War I broke out 11 years later, he bitterly resented the fact that Victor Vaughan, then on the Executive Committee of the General Medical Board in Washington, DC, vetoed active duty for the 70-year-old professor.

In counterpoint to de Nancrede's recollection of Gunn's sharp commentaries at the ASA, years later at the same organization Ravitch mentioned de Nancrede's habits of discussion: "Nancrede's four pages of discussion on this subject, on which 'I have nothing especially new to offer' bore witness to the accuracy of his statement."[iv,16] de Nancrede's accomplishments as an educator, author, proponent of asepsis, and gunshot wounds expertise took him to the highest levels of American surgery. His writings later in his career were mainly contributions to general surgery textbooks.

Darling was the first Michigan surgeon to hone genitourinary skills within a larger general surgical practice and his student Ira Dean Loree would become the first to have a professorial title as a genitourinary surgeon. Darling had many other interests including orofacial surgery, dentistry, and administration, whereas Loree more exclusively expanded into genitourinary surgery. When St. Joseph Mercy Hospital opened a few streets away from University Hospital, the clinical faculty who lacked the full-time salary of de Nancrede found a receptive facility for their private practices. Darling, a founder of the Catholic hospital, became its first chief of staff. The hospital was initially a converted house on the southwest corner of State and Kingsley (still standing) and it received its first patients on December 19, 1911. In 1914, a new facility opened on North Ingalls, across the street from the University Hospital, with six operating rooms

---

iv Because it was later in his life when de Nancrede added "de" to his last name, the literature offers both versions. This text adheres to the later version that de Nancrede preferred from 1906 to the end of his life.

and "accessory rooms" for anesthesia, instruments, orthopaedic plaster, cystoscopy, library, doctors' offices, nurses, utilities, sterile supplies, and waiting rooms. The two larger operating rooms included glassed-off viewing stands that accommodated 25 doctors and 25 students.[17]

In November of 1914, de Nancrede's academic effort was reduced due to personal illness and Cyrenus Darling was placed in charge of the surgical department. Loree then became associate professor of genitourinary surgery and, by dropping the "clinical" part of his title, presumably gave up his private practice.[18] Darling's effectiveness as a leader was diminished by his interim status, having been told by Dean Vaughan that he was not good enough to be chosen as permanent director of the department.[19] In 1917, de Nancrede retired completely and he died in 1921, with *The University Encyclopedic Survey* commenting, "leaving, as do most physicians, little tangible evidence of the great service he rendered to humanity."

Notes

1 H. W. Davenport, *University of Michigan Surgeons 1850-1970 Who They Were and What They Did* (Ann Arbor, MI: Historical Center for the Health Sciences, University of Michigan, 1993), 34.
2 V. C. Vaughan, *A Doctor's Memories* (Indianapolis: The Bobbs-Merrill Company, 1926), 228.
3 H. W. Davenport, *University of Michigan Surgeons 1850-1970 Who They Were and What They Did* (Ann Arbor, MI: Historical Center for the Health Sciences, University of Michigan, 1993), 37.
4 H. W. Davenport, *"Victor Vaughan: Statesman and Scientist* (Ann Arbor: Historical Center for the Health Sciences, University of Michigan, 1996).
5 V. C. Vaughan, *A Doctor's Memories* (Indianapolis: The Bobbs-Merrill Company, 1926), 213.
6 V. C. Vaughan, *A Doctor's Memories* (Indianapolis: The Bobbs-Merrill Company, 1926), 217–218.
7 V. C. Vaughan, *A Doctor's Memories* (Indianapolis: The Bobbs-Merrill Company, 1926), 223–224.
8 H. W. Davenport, *Victor Vaughan: Statesman and Scientist* (Ann Arbor: Historical Center for the Health Sciences, University of Michigan, 1996), 20–21.
9 H. W. Davenport, *Victor Vaughan: Statesman and Scientist* (Ann Arbor: Historical Center for the Health Sciences, University of Michigan, 1993), 18.
10 D. A. Bloom, G. Uznis, and D. A. Campbell, Jr., "Charles B. G. de Nancrede: Academic Surgeon at the fin de siècle," *World Journal of Surgery* 22 (1998) 11: 1175–1181.
11 H. W. Davenport, *Fifty Years of Medicine at The University of Michigan 1891–1941* (Ann Arbor: The University of Michigan Medical School, 1986), Table in p. 10.
12 H. W. Davenport, *University of Michigan Surgeons 1850-1970 Who They Were and What They Did* (Ann Arbor, MI: Historical Center for the Health Sciences, University of Michigan, 1993), 46.
13 H. W. Davenport, *University of Michigan Surgeons 1850–1970 Who They Were and What They Did* (Ann Arbor, MI: Historical Center for the Health Sciences, University of Michigan, 1993), 47–48.

14 J. M. Barry, *The Great Influenza* (New York: Viking Penguin Books, 2005), 86.
15 *Ann Arbor Gazette*, "He Changes His Name," February 6, 1906.
16 H. W. Davenport, *Fifty Years of Medicine at The University of Michigan 1891–1941* (Ann Arbor, The University of Michigan Medical School, 1986), 301; M. W. Ravitch, *A Century of Surgery, 1880–1980* (Philadelphia, PA: J. B. Lippincott, 1981).
17 Bentley Historical Library, University of Michigan, Undated St. Joseph's magazine clipping, Burton files; also reference to Ann Arbor News article.
18 H. W. Davenport, *University of Michigan Surgeons 1850–1970 Who They Were and What They Did* (Ann Arbor, MI: Historical Center for the Health Sciences, University of Michigan, 1993), 56.
19 H. W. Davenport, *University of Michigan Surgeons 1850–1970 Who They Were and What They Did* (Ann Arbor, MI: Historical Center for the Health Sciences, University of Michigan, 1993), 53.

Challenges and Changes in a New Century

Fin de siècle is a phrase that encompasses the transition from one century into the next, usually involving the 20 years that straddle the New Year's Eve between centuries. Common sense might view that celebration on December 31, 1899, although technically it was after New Year's Eve, December 31, 1900, when the nineteenth century concluded and the twentieth century began on January 1, 1901. That actual moment, or even the actual year, is irrelevant to understanding this particular story of the roots of genitourinary surgery at the University of Michigan, and the broader perspective of the *fin de siècle* concept is more useful. Either way, the emergent twentieth century brought new terminology with *urology* replacing genitourinary surgery, *Medical School* replacing the Department of Medicine and Surgery in Ann Arbor, new technology such as the *X-ray* and *radiology*, and new concepts of *graduate medical education* and *medical specialty boards*.

The vagueness of the *fin de siècle* is also convenient to understanding the paradigm shifts in medical education, science, and practice of the twentieth century. The comparison with the UM Medical School at its beginning 50 years earlier is stark. The two-year six-month lecture terms in 1850 had become a graduated four-year curriculum with embedded laboratory experience and clinical practice in a hospital by 1900. Ancient dogmatic topics such as *materia medica* and *inflammation* had shifted into verifiable concepts of biochemistry, physiology, organ-based pathology, microscopic histology, and pharmacology that informed clinical practice, and subspecialties were emerging in medicine. Internships and residency programs were forming.

Other factors and forces brought changes to science, education, and health care, locally and nationally. Near Ann Arbor, in Midland, Michigan, Herbert Dow (1866–1930) started a company to extract bromine from brine in 1890 and the following year he figured out how to do the extraction with electrolysis, thus inventing the Dow process. Roentgen's X-ray in 1896 became more than a tool, launching a distinct specialty itself, variously called roentgenology, radiology, and diagnostic imaging over the next century as well as becoming an intrinsic part of modern urology. Medical research moved from the periphery to a central position in medical education and practice as the century progressed. In 1901, John D. Rockefeller established 10 fellowships for advanced medical research of which Michigan received two, and this was a prelude to massive private and public financing of research and education that followed in the century. The University of Michigan was becoming a major force in American education, although it had yet to become a national leader in clinical care, much less urology.

President Angell noted in 1903 that students on campus came from all states and territories except Alaska. A new medical building of stone had been completed adjacent to the old wood structure. A larger medical campus was assembling beginning with a bequest to University Hospital that year from the widow of Alonzo Palmer for a children's ward in honor of her husband and a psychopathic ward was under construction funded by a special state appropriation. The Pasteur Institute established a unit for rabies care in the UM Medical Department, in response to a local epidemic, and 23 persons bitten by rabid animals were treated in the first six months.[1]

When Angell resigned in 1905, regent Herman Kiefer assumed the role as the medical school's guardian in that period of leadership uncertainty as the university continued to grow.[2] Dr. and Mrs. Walter Nichols in 1906 gave 30 acres for a botanical garden, that continues to bedazzle visitors, adjacent to today's Mott Children's and Women's Hospital. The Michigan Union opened in 1907 on State Street and alumni raised over a hundred thousand dollars for a war memorial building across the street. The regents added another $50,000, flush from a recent millage increase, and accordingly Alumni Hall was dedicated in 1910, quickly bringing its main use to the university as an art museum. These and many other factors transformed the University of Michigan Ann Arbor campus as the new century unfolded.

At the start of the twentieth century, genitourinary surgery was split between venereology practice (heavily admixed with dermatology) and the genitourinary anatomic terrain navigated by general surgeons. The Nitze-Edison technology marriage in 1880 had created new opportunities for expertise and was further amplified by X-ray, precision instruments, and endoscopic electrical therapy. The domain of general surgery expanded in the *fin de siècle* beyond the capacity of any single individual to master all the emerging surgical subspecialties of ophthalmology, orthopaedics, and otolaryngology as well as genitourinary surgery. A talented cadre of surgeons was enlarging the scope of genitourinary surgery internationally with Enrico Bottini's operation for benign prostatic hyperplasia, inversion of the tunica vaginalis for hydrocele by Robert Green, relief of bladder neck contracture by Charles Chetwood, hypospadias repair by Charlie Mayo, exstrophy closure by Friedrich Trendelenburg, perineal prostatectomy by Hugh Young, and suprapubic prostatectomy of Eugene Fuller and Terence Millin.

One of these new specialists, Ramon Guiteras, began to use a new word, *urology*, combining the Greek terms for urine (uro) and study (logy). *Urology* seemed to catch on, even if semantically it didn't quite hit the mark of accuracy. Guiteras, no doubt, intended the word to capture the idea of the study and practice of the urinary and genital tracts.[i,3]

Guiteras, a prominent New York surgeon with interest and skills in genitourinary surgery, had assembled a team of similarly oriented surgeons at the New York Postgraduate Hospital. He left something to posterity beyond the new word—a new organization. Following work one day in 1900, Guiteras took his colleagues to an East Side tavern, the Frei Robber, known for homemade wine and limburger cheese. He claimed the pungent cheese kept other patrons strategically away from the clinical shoptalk and amidst the fruitful conversation, the group named itself the New York Genitourinary Society and continued to meet socially with that slight increase in organizational formality. Two years later, assembling at the home of Guiteras in February, the group renamed itself the American Urological Association, an intentional stretch, considering that they all were New Yorkers. They held a "first convention" in June 1902 at Saratoga Springs. Membership expanded and the following year a second convention was held in New Orleans and a third in 1904 in Atlantic City, with 34 members in the convention photograph. In 1905, when the group met in Portland, Oregon, it had truly become a national organization.

In 1904, the American Medical Association (AMA) formed a Council on Medical Education in response to a growing call from within the medical profession and externally from public voices to reform medical education. The 50-year evolution of the rudimentary medical curriculum in Ann Arbor, with a duplicate six-month course of lectures for students with meager preliminary academic credentials in 1850, to a four-year graduated curriculum with laboratories and clinical experience for qualified students, had not been widely mirrored throughout the country, even

---

i The 1908 two-volume text of Watson and Cunningham from Boston, *Genito-Urinary Diseases*, didn't pick up on the new terminology, but others that followed, starting with that of Guiteras in 1912, would use the more compact word, *urology*. The term was repeated in 1918 by Hugh Cabot, by then an internationally famed Boston surgeon, in his text *Modern Urology*.

by 1900. The council inspected 162 schools and produced a confidential report in 1907 that had little effect in improving standards. The AMA gave the report to the Carnegie Foundation but insisted that the report stay confidential, whereupon the Foundation commissioned a young PhD, Abraham Flexner, to do another survey. Flexner, a former Johns Hopkins student, began by conversations with William Welch (1850–1934) and Franklin Mall (1862–1917), later reporting, "The rest of my study of medical education was little more than an amplification of what I had learned during my initial visit to Baltimore."[4] Welch and his friend Victor Vaughan were then at the top of the academic medical establishment and Mall was an acolyte of both men.

Welch, born in Norfolk, Connecticut, received an MD at Columbia College of Physicians and Surgeons in 1875, studied in Germany with Rudolf Virchow among others, and in 1877 opened a laboratory at Bellevue Medical College before moving to Baltimore as a founding member of Johns Hopkins Medical School. Mall, of Belle Plaine, Iowa, had been drawn to Michigan's medical school by three professors, Corydon La Ford, Victor Vaughan, and Henry Sewall, graduating in the class of 1883 with William Mayo. After further study in Germany until 1886, Mall went to Baltimore to train in pathology under Welch and ultimately became the first professor of anatomy at the new Johns Hopkins School of Medicine in 1893. Mall became a strong advocate for reform of medical education and the full-time model of clinical faculty salaries. Mall, Vaughan, and Welch were the best of the classically educated physicians in the *fin de siècle* transition of American medicine and leading advocates for change in medical education, but national inertia was strong.

Flexner's report in 1910 to the Carnegie Foundation for the Advancement of Teaching, *Medical Education in the United States and Canada*, changed medical education throughout North America. At the end of his book, he concluded that 120 of the 150 plus medical schools of North America should be closed. The first half of the book discussed the history of medical education and its current status. The second half provided detailed descriptions of schools in each state and each province of the United States and Canada.[5] Commercial medical schools received poor reviews and most of them disappeared in the wake of Flexner's book.

Flexner had visited Ann Arbor in 1909 and inspected its two medical schools: (a) the University of Michigan Department of Medicine and Surgery (now the Medical School), organized in 1850 and described as an "integral part of the university," and (b) the University of Michigan Homeopathic College, organized in 1875 and described as an "organic department of the university." Flexner noted each school had its own hospital, no bed count was offered for the former, but the Homeopathic

Hospital was listed for 100 beds. The medical school (formally known then as the Department of Medicine and Surgery) required two years of college "including sciences, strictly enforced," while the Homeopathic College required only a four-year high school education. Enumerating the teaching staff for the Medical School, Flexner noted,

> 63, of whom 22 are professors. The laboratory work is wholly in charge of full-time instructors; but assistants adequate in number are lacking. The clinical teachers are salaried and owe their first duty to the school.

Regarding the teaching staff of the Homeopathic College, Flexner reported that of the 26 faculty more than half (15) were professors. The instate percentages for the Medical School and the Homeopathic College students were 45 percent and 38 percent. Flexner had no intrinsic bias against the homeopathic schools; he himself continued to see a homeopathic physician for his personal health.[6]

The Homeopathic College, initially forced upon the university unconstitutionally by the Michigan State Legislature reflected the inevitable tension between government and education; that is, the public regulation of (medical) education through legislative purse strings and the free inquiry implicit in education and science are irreconcilable. Whether a society is monarchy or plutocracy, faith-based or nonsectarian, socialistic or capitalistic, democracy or corpocracy, authoritarian or libertarian, tension necessarily always remains between universities and the rest of society.

This last point is too important to relegate to a footnote: *The University* or *The Academy* is the only free-standing institution that exists for the "tomorrow" of humanity, representing education of tomorrow's citizens, builders, teachers, leaders, and thinkers. The purpose of the university, *writ large*, is to educate society and in doing so refine and discover knowledge. Evolving over the course of more than a millennium, *The University* has become a *Multiversity* of education, investigation, criticism, health care, technology innovation, policy formulation, public commentary, leadership training, and many other public goods that vary across institutions. The three strands that Margaret and Nicholas Steneck described in their update to Howard Peckham's *The Making of the University of Michigan 1817–1992* have become a giant coaxial cable thickening as it courses through generations.[7]

While it is often said, and always hoped, that "the arc of the moral universe is long, but it bends toward justice," regressions happen along the way. So, it was that after women first came to the medical school class in 1871, they comprised 25 percent of the class when Vaughan became dean in 1891, but by 1910 only 2 percent. Since 2000, however, the male–female ratio has seesawed around 50 percent. Possibly, before the next century, the gender reporting will become more than a binary choice.[ii,8]

The University of Michigan Medical School entered the twentieth century as a far more complex iteration of an academic medical center than at its start in 1850 when medical education was the sole basis for its existence. The Chemical Laboratory Building in 1856 introduced the service of research (chemical analysis, toxicology, and urinalysis) to medical education, clinical practice, and scientific discovery. A more complete linkage of medical education to clinical practice came with the first University Hospital in 1869 and by its third iteration in 1891 the triple mission of an academic medical center was fully in place, although uncertainty in mission balance played out in such disputes as relocating the Medical School, compensation of clinical faculty, and criteria for academic promotion. Mission balance continued to confuse faculty and perplex leadership through the next century and into the present one, but history and ethics bring clarity to the matter: the University of Michigan Medical School began with an *educational mission* of training the next generation of physicians, *research* followed quickly to bring science (chemistry, at first) into education as well as to public service, and *clinical care* was recognized as the necessary milieu for medical education and research. Nonetheless, it was not widely accepted throughout university leadership or within the faculty that among the three parts of the conjoined mission, clinical care is the moral epicenter, trumping any other part of the mission at any moment. Clinical care, now an activity requiring complex intellectual teams, is the financial engine that currently underpins the other missions. Any great academic medical center in the twenty-first century must be first and foremost a state-of-the-art health care system that not only delivers excellent and efficient patient-centric service but also studies and improves systems of care and technologies in addition to its traditional scholarly and clinical disciplines. Clinical care is the epicenter and most essential deliverable of academic medical centers.

---

ii The phrase, "Let us realize the arc of the moral universe is long, but it bends toward justice," was employed by Dr. Martin Luther King in 1958 in *The Gospel Messenger*, noting it to be a known aphorism, and he used it again in 1964 for a baccalaureate sermon at Wesleyan University Commencement exercises. The phrase has a deep history, traceable to 1853 and "A Collection of Ten Sermons of Religion" by Theodore Parker, Unitarian minister, American transcendentalist, and abolitionist. A book in 1918, *Readings from Great Authors*, quoted Parker. A columnist in the *Cleveland Plain Dealer* reiterated the phrase but omitted the word "moral" in 1932. The phrase has been since repeated on many occasions such as in a 1940 New Year version by Rabbi Jacob Kohn in Los Angeles: "Our faith is kept alive by the knowledge, founded on long experience, that the arc of history is long and bends toward justice." President Obama used the phrase and credited Dr. King in 2009.

Notes

1. H. H. Peckham, *The Making of the University of Michigan 1817–1992*. Edited and updated by M. L. Steneck and N. H. Steneck (Ann Arbor: University of Michigan Press, 1967, 1994), 113.
2. H. H. Peckham, *The Making of the University of Michigan 1817–1992*. Edited and updated by M. L. Steneck and N. H. Steneck (Ann Arbor: University of Michigan Press, 1967, 1994), 123.
3. G. M. Crane and D. A. Bloom, Ramon Guiteras: Founder of the American Urological Association, Surgeon, Sportsman and Statesman. *Journal of Urology* 184 (2010): 447–452.
4. K. M. Ludmerer, *Learning to Heal*, (Baltimore and London: The Johns Hopkins University Press, 1996), 172; J. M. Barry, *The Great Influenza*, (New York: Penguin Group, 2005), 83–84.
5. A. Flexner, *Medical Education in the United States and Canada* (New York City: The Carnegie Foundation for the Advancement of Teaching, 1910), Bulletin no. 4, 243–244.
6. J. M. Barry, *The Great Influenza*, (New York: Penguin Group, 2005), 86.
7. H. H. Peckham, *The Making of the University of Michigan 1817–1992*. Edited and updated by M. L. Steneck and N. H. Steneck (Ann Arbor: University of Michigan Press, 1967, 1994).
8. H. W. Davenport, *Not Just Any Medical School* (Ann Arbor: University of Michigan Press, 1999), 31.

Cyrenus Darling and Ira Dean Loree

During the de Nancrede era, Cyrenus Darling (1856–1933) and Ira Dean Loree (1869–1936) performed the genitourinary clinical work and teaching of the University of Michigan Medical School and its hospital. Darling was born on a farm to a family that neither expected or encouraged higher education, but a local minister directed the young Cyrenus to college. Living as a student in the home of a Dr. William F. Breakey (UMMS 1859), Darling found further encouragement to advance his education. After a leg fracture and treatment at no cost by a kind local physician, Darling was inspired to attend Michigan's Medical School and graduated in 1881. He opened a small town practice, where he was described as a "born doctor" who embraced the full range of surgery at the time, including dentistry and genitourinary surgery.

When de Nancrede arrived in Ann Arbor in 1889, Darling learned of the need for an assistant to the professor and took the part-time job. Enjoying teaching more than writing, Darling became a bedrock of the surgical department. His 81-page memoir gives insight into his career, although lack of dates makes it difficult to reconstruct a chronology.[1] Darling was known to be particularly circumspect regarding patient confidentiality. He took interest in university politics, Ann Arbor government (serving as mayor, 1894–1895), the state medical society, and state legislation regarding medical practice. Darling had a summer home in northern Michigan where a neighbor and fellow physician, Dr. Clarence Edmonds Hemingway, would vacation from the Chicago area. The neighbor's son, Ernest, likely fished at some of the same streams as Darling.

Darling developed genitourinary expertise during his career at Michigan and became skilled in cystoscopy in its earliest days. In June 1902, the regents noted his appointment as lecturer on genitourinary and minor surgery at a salary of $500.[2] Darling's main career impact, however, was in oral surgery and he teamed up with Chalmers Lyons (UM Dentistry,

1898) to operate upon as many as 200 children with cleft lip or palate in some years. Lyons trained Michigan's first oral surgery intern in 1917 and developed an excellent residency training program.[i]

Darling served as dental school dean from 1903 to 1904. His contribution to the medical literature was small and he was described by Fredrick Coller as "a strong local rather than a national figure."[3] As had a number of other clinical faculty, Darling operated his own private hospital for a time, in a building he built on Fifth Avenue. He sold it in 1915 and began construction of a brick "fireproof" structure that became office space in 1917 for him and Dr. Charles Washburne at a new location on 213–293 East Liberty, later known as the Zwerdling-Darling Block. Osias Zwerdling was a ladies' tailor and furrier who built the adjacent building.[4]

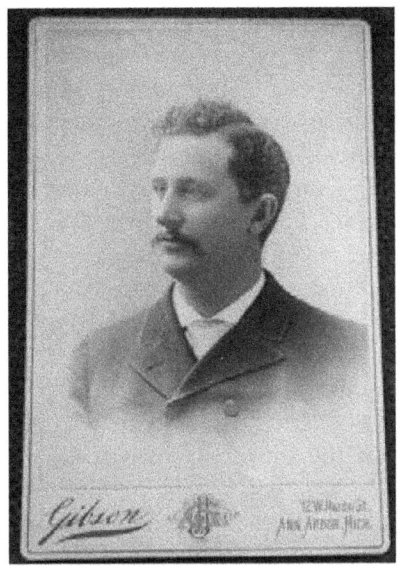

Gibson Studio photograph of Darling as a young faculty member.

The other genitourinary specialist, Ira Dean Loree, was an 1891 UMMS graduate. He went into private practice locally and ran for political office as a county commissioner in 1897 but was disqualified on a technicality. He joined the de Nancrede faculty in 1901 as a Fourth Assistant in Surgery, appointed without pay according to the June meeting of the Board of Regents.[5] A year later, the regents gave Darling an appointment as lecturer on oral surgery at a salary of $500 and Loree was named demonstrator of oral surgery at a salary of $200. Presumably, for Darling and Loree, these oral surgery salaries were additional to their genitourinary and minor surgery positions. Loree assisted Darling with oral surgery and on Saturday mornings with genitourinary procedures in the University Hospital. In 1903, Loree was advanced over two more senior assistants

---

i Chalmers Lyons (1874–1935) was a respected teacher as well as clinician and a study/alumni club was founded in 1927 as the C. J. Lyons Club, later becoming the Chalmers J. Lyons Academy of Oral and Maxillofacial Surgery. One of the founding members, Reed O. Dingman, would become chief of the plastic surgery section of the Surgery Department at Michigan. The academy continues to meet. A Chalmers J. Lyons Memorial Lecture and medal were established in his honor.

to first assistant in surgery "in the place of Dr. Willard H. Hutchins, at the same salary $200" and Darling was reappointed lecturer on genitourinary and minor surgery.[6] Loree continued to serve in 1902–1903 as a demonstrator in oral surgery, displaying the versatility of surgeons of his time. In 1904, the regents reappointed Darling as lecturer on genitourinary and minor surgery and demonstrator of surgery "without change in salary, $500," while increasing Loree's salary as first assistant in surgery at $400.[7] In 1905, Loree was named lecturer in genitourinary surgery and became clinical associate professor of genitourinary surgery in 1907, while maintaining an additional private practice.

Those genitourinary titles, the first at Michigan, indicated that Darling and Loree had taken ownership of genitourinary practice at the university. Loree's professorship in 1907 of genitourinary surgery was the first for the University of Michigan. It was reported in the *Detroit Medical Journal* that Loree was one of two leaders in a discussion of "certain phases of the treatment of syphilis" at the 35th semiannual meeting of the Northern Tri-State Medical Association on January 12, 1909. The issue also noted, "Dr. Dean Loree has established his office in the Glazier building where he will devote his attention to general surgery, with especial reference to surgery of the genito-urinary tract." That particular issue of the journal carried other news relevant to the University of Michigan, no surprise given that Victor Vaughan, Jr., was associate editor. An obituary of Donald Maclean noted the death earlier in the month in Detroit and another notice titled "Dr. Hewlett succeeds Dr. Dock" offered an encapsulation of Hewlett's promising career.[8]

Loree's clinical range included prostatectomy for benign disease, reporting results in a 1916 paper with R. W. Kraft, who had worked with Loree since medical student days.[9] Loree's genitourinary service grew, documenting 3,304 outpatient visits in the first six months of 1917, but complaints and demands from him resulted in a contentious relationship with Dean Vaughan, who nonetheless helped bolster resources. In October 1917, the *Regents Proceedings* recorded that Drs. Darling and Sawyer intervened to give Loree further support in the form of "One Demonstrator or Assistant at $900, One Assistant at $400, One Interne without Salary, Fifteen Beds, and Instruments $125."[10] The 1918 April meeting discussed the cystoscope situation at the hospital:

> *Gentlemen—*
> At a meeting at your Executive Committee held March 14, 1918, Dr. Loree at the Department of Genito-Urinary Surgery strongly urged permission to use approximately $350 out of salaries saved in that Department for the purchase of an operating cystoscope, at a cost of about $225, and a diagnostic cystoscope, at a cost of $125.

There is only one diagnostic cystoscope in the Surgery Department, and when this is out of commission, as in fact it was at the time of our annual meeting when it was in New York for repairs, the diagnostic work of the Department and the interests of the patients suffer.

Likely, the cystoscope repair was performed in Wappler's shop (see p. 69–70).[11] Darling and Loree, the first genitourinary specialists at the University of Michigan over the initial two decades of the twenty-first century, held on to the old terminology rather than *urology*. Loree's title in 1907 and Darling's attention to oral surgery and dentistry provided Loree opportunity to become Ann Arbor's primary urologic clinician and teacher, although Loree never achieved much recognition on the national scene.

Vaughan was unwilling to appoint Darling as head of the Surgery Department for a number of reasons, as de Nancrede faded away, preferring an individual with greater academic stage presence. Vaughan, on the center stage of international health care himself, certainly knew or knew of the major surgical talents in North America and beyond, but he was unable to entice anyone to Ann Arbor until 1919. The full-time model, although offering a reasonable living wage by academic standards for the de Nancrede recruitment in 1889, had fallen far enough below the marketplace incomes for most surgeons with the desired *stage presence* over the ensuing 30 years. It was a lucky break for Vaughan to find Hugh Cabot interested in the job, and he quickly accepted the position, although salary issues persisted even after Cabot's start in September, 1919.

Darling was insulted when mistakenly not included for Cabot's welcoming reception. Out of pique, Darling refused to attend the dinner in honor of himself and de Nancrede. A long letter of apology with some remonstrance from Vaughan was the final straw and Darling withdrew from the medical school.[12] The September meeting of the Board of Regents noted:

> Regent Sawyer presented a letter of resignation from Dr. C. G. Darling as professor of surgery to be effective when his successor should take up his duties. On motion of Regent Sawyer, Dr. Darling's resignation was accepted with deep appreciation of the value of his long and devoted services to the Medical School and to the university. At this point the Board took a recess for lunch.

Darling moved his practice entirely to St. Joe's, the hospital he was instrumental in building in 1911 and that had quickly become an excellent surgical resource for Ann Arbor. No record has been found of his thoughts regarding the Cabot interlude at Michigan, but Darling remained respected by university leaders to the end of his days. Darling retained his appointment as professor of dental surgery until resignation in November, 1926, when he was named Professor Emeritus of Dental Surgery.

Loree, like Darling, was unwilling to embrace the new chief and resigned on March 9, 1920, moving his practice entirely to St. Joes. Loree's final reference in the *Regents' Proceedings* came in a special meeting on June 1920:

> Dean Vaughan transmitted the resignation of Dr. Ira D. Loree as Associate Professor of Genito-Urinary Surgery, effective as of June 30, 1920. On motion of Regent Sawyer, the resignation of Professor Loree was accepted with regret.[13]

With Michigan's first two genitourinary surgeons gone, Cabot was suddenly the sole remaining expert in that field, although he preferred to call himself a urologist rather than the older term. In addition to being chief of surgery, other leadership duties would quickly accrue, no doubt taxing his clinical capacity and even though Ann Arbor had the two other valued specialists only a short distance away there is no evidence that Cabot called for their help in teaching or staffing the university cases.

Upon Darling's death in 1933, President Ruthven called him "one of the greatest figures in the history of the university." Novy, Lyons, and

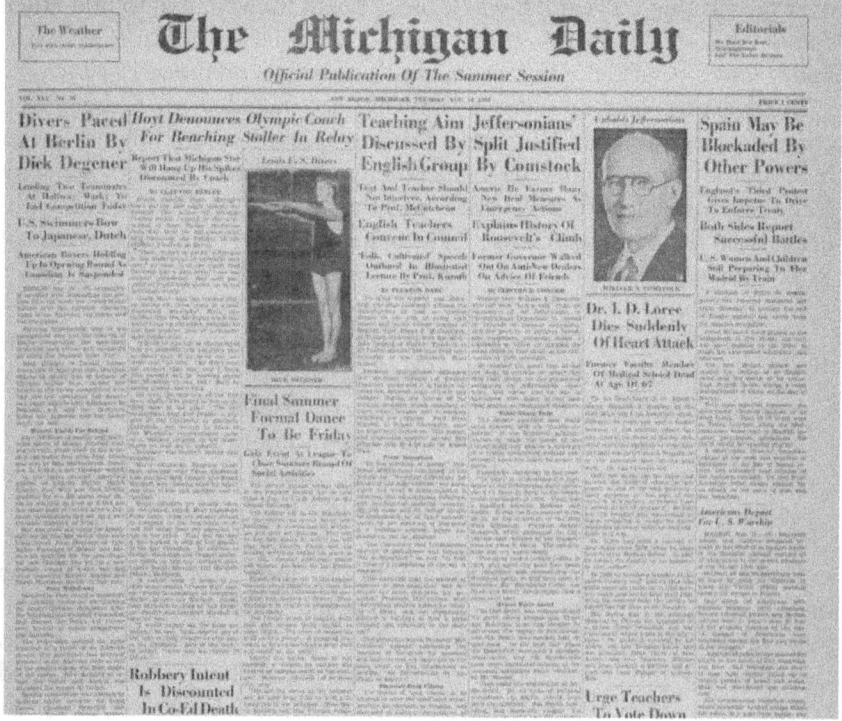

Dr. I. D. Loree dies suddenly of heart attack. *Michigan Daily*, August 11, 1936.

Wolaver wrote Darling's memorial note and an obituary was recorded in the *New York Times*. Loree continued his respected work at St. Joes until he died at home in Barton Hills in 1936 of a myocardial infarction at age 67. An obituary was carried in the *Michigan Daily*. (See previous page.)

Darling and Loree contributed good service to the University of Michigan and were the foundational genitourinary specialists. They were appreciated by colleagues and the Ann Arbor community, but their loss from the university was reluctantly accepted as collateral damage of the recruitment of Michigan's first celebrity urologist.

Notes

1 Bentley Historical Library, University of Michigan, B-161-D call #93183 Aa1.
2 University of Michigan Board of Regents, June 1902.
3 H. W. Davenport. *University of Michigan Surgeons 1850–1970 Who They Were and What They Did* (Ann Arbor, MI, Historical Center for the Health Sciences, University of Michigan, 1993), 53.
4 Ann Arbor District Library, Zwerdling-Darling Block, 1915.
5 University of Michigan Board of Regents, June 1901, 669.
6 University of Michigan Board of Regents, June 1903, 209.
7 University of Michigan Board of Regents, June 1904, 373.
8 H. M. Rich and V. Vaughan, "Dr. Hewlett Succeeds Dr. Dock," *Detroit Medical Journal* 9, no. 1 (1909): 18, 21, 30, 1909.
9 I. D. Loree and R. W. Kraft, "Results after Prostatectomy," *The Journal of the Michigan State Medical Society* 15 (1916): 435–436.
10 University of Michigan Board of Regents, October 1917, 36.
11 University of Michigan Board of Regents, April 1918, 198.
12 H. W. Davenport, *Fifty Years of Medicine at The University of Michigan 1891–1941* (Ann Arbor: The University of Michigan Medical School, 1986), 300.
13 University of Michigan Board of Regents, June 1920, 952.

The Post-Flexnerian Decade and Hugh Cabot

The University of Michigan, approaching its centennial in the decade after Flexner's report of 1910, was internationally respected for its faculty, prodigious alumni, favored textbooks, and landmark research accomplishments. The medical school, although rising in reputation, had sparse iconic names, and Victor Vaughan was the predominant one. The Surgery Department could boast historically of Moses Gunn and Charles de Nancrede, but these reflected the previous century. Few other names in surgery were prominent outside the region and none were present in the emerging realm of urology. Michigan's genitourinary clinic had been competent under Loree with an occasional national publication but little engagement in the new frontiers of the field, much less leadership in the emerging national organizations.

Overall enrollment at the University of Michigan in 1910 was 5,339, making it the third national university in size, after Columbia and Chicago, while Harvard was fourth. (Within a few years, Harvard and California would jump ahead of Michigan.) The highly successful presidency of James Angell that had begun in 1871 was running out of steam. He felt he was losing his suitability for the job and tried to resign in 1905, but the regents refused to accept resignation then, although they did so in 1909. Law dean Harry B. Hutchins was named acting president for the term of a year, during which the regents considered external candidates including Woodrow Wilson, president at Princeton. Lacking any more attractive alternatives willing to consider the job, the regents offered Hutchins the presidency in 1910 for three years. Hutchins, age 63, insisted on a five-year term, although later at the regents' request he would stay for a second term into 1920.

In 1910, the AUA elected Hugh Cabot president. The organization had been growing rapidly and at its eighth year then had 320 active and 16 honorary members. Cabot's presidential address the following year at the Chicago convention was "Is Urology entitled to be regarded as a specialty?" Clearly, the Guiteras neologism was widely embraced. Cabot, in Boston, was successfully following the path of his older cousin Arthur Tracy Cabot and emerged as one of the leaders in urology. Cabot's rhetorical question reflected daily tension in workplaces between general surgeons and genitourinary specialists, still often dismissed as "clap doctors." General surgeons resisted the loss of turf to a new cadre of skilled genitourinary surgeons like Cabot who were claiming the new clinical territory. Anesthesia, antisepsis, analgesia, and modern technology with electrical illumination, X-rays, cystoscopes, and precision instruments allowed this new iteration of lithotomists to differentiate themselves from their predecessors of Hippocratic times.

Franklin H. Martin, a prominent general surgeon in Chicago, had created the journal *Surgery, Gynecology and Obstetrics (SG&O)* in 1905 for surgeons to share and test ideas and methods. This surgical socialization expanded in 1910 to the *Clinical Congresses of Surgeons of North America*, organized sequentially by *SG&O* in large surgical centers for continuing education of practicing surgeons. After advertising the first congress in *SG&O*, the staff estimated an attendance of 200 participants, but the 10-day event in Chicago attracted 1,300 physicians, evidence of an unanticipated appetite for continuing medical education in the new century of subspecialty health care.[1] The American College of Surgeons (ACS), an educational fellowship of surgeons, formed in 1912 as an outgrowth of the clinical congresses and would have a strong relationship over the next century not only with urology and the American Urological Association but also with the University of Michigan.[i]

As good as the University of Michigan Medical School looked to Flexner in 1909, its hospital deteriorated in the post-Flexnerian decade, as Vaughan's extramural responsibilities distracted him from the deanship in Ann Arbor. Vaughan was a leader at the Michigan Board of Health, the National Board of Medical Examiners, and the AMA, in 1913–1914

---

i One early member of the ACS, Ernest Amory Codman (1869–1940), a product of Harvard Medical School and the Massachusetts General Hospital, initiated the first morbidity and mortality conferences to formalize the sense of responsibility of surgeons for their clinical outcomes. He extended this to what he called "the end-result idea." Codman built a hospital around this concept and published a book at his expense called *A Study in Hospital Efficiency* in 1916. His hospital closed in 1917, when Codman and his team went to Halifax as volunteers after the catastrophic explosion, but it never reopened. Codman's outspoken ideas made him a pariah in Boston and American surgery, and his concepts were largely neglected until resurrection by Avedis Donabedian of Michigan in 1988, at a speech at Harvard; A. Donabedian, "The End Results of Health Care: Ernest Codman's Contribution to Quality Assessment and Beyond," *Milbank Quarterly* 67, no. 2 (1989): 233–256.

serving as its president. Additional work as founding editor in 1915 of the *Journal of Laboratory and Clinical Medicine*, along with numerous other responsibilities, including expert witness testimony nationally against quackery, stretched his attention so widely that it was no longer as deep as it had been earlier in his Michigan career. University Hospital on Catherine Street, suboptimally planned from its start, was poorly suited to the growing ambulatory and inpatient functions demanded of it 20 years later and furthermore it was poorly maintained, indicative of inattention by leadership. Flexner, in 1909–1910, had mainly evaluated educational programs, library size, and teaching roles of medical schools and affiliated hospitals rather than hospital operations, scientific capacities, and leadership attention. The historical stress of a lack of a state-of-the-art clinical facility to match the educational needs of the medical school had returned again to Ann Arbor.

Reflecting this dysfunction, the hospital was placed under the direct supervision in 1911 of Regent Walter H. Sawyer (1861–1931), a Michigan Homeopathic College graduate of 1884 and Hillsdale physician, who had been elected regent in 1905 and followed the tradition of former regent Dr. Herman Kiefer as the "guardian" of the medical school.[ii,iii,2] Sawyer would serve for 24 years through 1930.

Reuben Peterson, head of obstetrics and gynecology, already experienced with his own private hospital operations, became medical director of University Hospital from 1911 to 1918, reporting to a Hospital Committee of the Board of Regents. Inevitably, tensions between hospital and expectations of faculty grew as the facilities became increasingly out of date, in spite of Peterson's position as its director. Medical faculty demanded a better hospital and in 1915 the heads of the clinical departments asked an architect to initiate plans for a new building. The faculty persuaded the regents in 1916 to seek a state appropriation of $1,000,000. Although the need was acknowledged and funding was

---

ii Herman Kiefer (1825–1911) was born and educated as a physician in an area that is now the southwestern part of Germany. After military service as a volunteer in the March Revolution, he moved to Detroit in 1849 as a political fugitive, where he practiced medicine and embraced his new country, becoming a member of the Detroit Board of Education in 1866 and a University of Michigan regent in 1889 through 1901.

iii Sawyer practiced in Hillsdale and served as trustee of Hillsdale College from 1896 until his death in 1931. He was politically active as a member of the Republican State Central Committee from 1904 to 1908. Elected regent in 1905, he was reelected three times. His five linear feet of papers in the Bentley Library reveal a fair man in passionate support of the university. He corresponded closely with presidents James Angell, Harry Hutchins, Marian Burton, Clarence Little, and Alexander Ruthven as well as other regents, revealing much of the backstory of the University of Michigan, its medical school, and the personalities thereof. One folder, in Box 5, is devoted to Hugh Cabot although, curiously, little detail related to Cabot's abrupt termination in 1930, is revealed.

approved at the rate of four yearly increments, the project was delayed for four years by World War I.

de Nancrede was well past his prime by the time of Flexner's visit, although still operating and teaching. No successor was ready to take his place and a search committee was in place by Darling's interim appointment in 1914. The old professor's legacy was largely based on his success as a teacher, his book on antisepsis, his surgical range, his gunshot authority, and his international reputation, although he failed to develop leaders for the next generation and most unfortunately, a successor at Michigan. Of the 46 surgeons who studied as medical students under de Nancrede, all went into private practice in Michigan or neighboring states, except for Max Peet. With the recent departure of Albion Walter Hewlett to lead internal medicine at Stanford, Michigan was left without leadership in its two main medical school departments, medicine and surgery.

At his interim appointment in 1914, Darling had been doubly insulted to be told not only that he was a placeholder for the next chair but also expected to lead the committee to find his replacement and successor to de Nancrede. In spite of Dean Vaughan's extensive national connections with the leaders of surgery throughout North America, advice from notables such as Halsted, and consideration of some young surgeons who later became great in their careers, the search was unfruitful. One name that might have been considered at that time, although no records to support this have yet been found, was Hugh Cabot, who had gone on from his AUA presidency to become president of the AAGUS in 1914, following the path of Arthur Tracy Cabot in 1892. The Cabot family was prominent far beyond Boston, weighing in heavily in national politics. Cabot's career in Boston was nearing its peak and as conflict in Europe was heating up around this time, he was likely thinking about the urology textbook that would be in print in four years.

World War I broke out in Europe in July 1914, and the debate over America's entry into the conflict was echoed in Ann Arbor. By September of 1914, with the first trenches dug on the Western Front, fundraisers for the Red Cross and beleaguered nations were held at the University of Michigan Hill Auditorium. On December 2, students and Ann Arbor citizens secured 1,000 suits of clothes to send to Belgium.[3] [Figure on next page.] President Wilson favored staying out of the war, while Cabot's relative, Henry Cabot Lodge (1850–1924), was one of the most prominent national advocates for engagement.[iv]

---

iv Henry Cabot Lodge was an important political factor in national politics as a senator from Massachusetts from 1893 to 1924. He favored the 1898 intervention in Cuba and entry into the fight in Europe with the Allied Powers, in opposition to Woodrow Wilson's

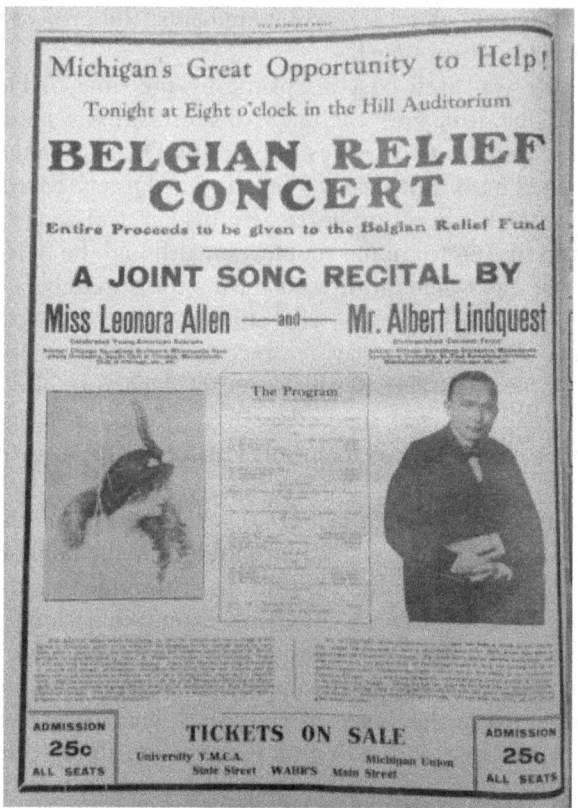

Hill Auditorium Benefit Concert, 1914, *The Michigan Daily*, Bentley Historical Library, University of Michigan.

Americans living in Paris organized a neutral military hospital, the American Ambulance Hospital, that opened September 1914 at the Lycee Pasteur in Neuilly with 170 beds at first and later 1,000 at full capacity. American subscriptions helped support the effort and its three services, the third of which became a University Service, staffed by rotating American teams for three-month stints. George Crile organized the first university service unit, staffed from Lakeside Hospital and Western Reserve University in Cleveland. Before sailing for France in January 1915, he secured the support of Harvard Medical School whereupon a Boston businessman offered to defray all expenses of travel and outfitting.

---

efforts to keep America neutral. After the Armistice, Lodge battled fiercely with Wilson over the 1919 Treaty of Versailles. The following year the League of Nations formed without U.S. participation, largely because Lodge favored signage insisting on the prerogative of reservations in governance of the league while Wilson favored none. In the long run, Lodge's reservations were carried out in the United Nations veto system.

Harvey Cushing and Elliott Carr Cutler were among the Harvard University Service volunteers that followed, serving in April, May, and June of 1915 until replacement by a staff from the University of Pennsylvania. The diaries of Cushing and Cutler are available online.[4]

The U-boat sinking of RMS Lusitania in May 1915, with 128 Americans on board, nearly brought the United States into the war, but President Wilson continued to keep the country on the sidelines, as his reelection campaign slogan promised again in 1916. The use of poison gas by Germany in 1915 elicited collaborations between the University of Michigan, Dow Chemical, and the War Department. Encouraged by the University Service experience with the American Ambulance Hospital, Sir William Osler and U.S. ambassador to France, Robert Bacon, suggested a similar program to bolster the depleted medical resources of the British Expeditionary Forces (BEF). The first contingent, a Harvard surgical unit, began work in mid-July 1915. Plans for rotation with units from Columbia and Johns Hopkins didn't materialize and Boston personnel carried the load for the rest of the war, as will be later discussed in more detail with Hugh Cabot's story. Notably, the University of Michigan was absent from these premier academic surgical teams. Hugh Cabot was among the Third Harvard Unit, sailing to Europe in May 1916 as the *Boston Daily Globe* reported, "Third Harvard Unit Going: Dr. Hugh Cabot in charge of surgeons and nurses to sail for war zone on May 20." Later that year the newspaper reported, "Denounced call to remain neutral insult to country, says Dr. Hugh Cabot."[5] Cabot knew how to capture attention from the press. He remained in Europe with the BEF for the next 2.5 years.

Germany resumed unrestricted submarine attacks and in April 1917, Wilson and then Congress finally declared war. Patriotic sentiments dominated at the University of Michigan and when its ROTC unit was activated 1,800 men signed up, the largest then for any American university.[6] Reacting to student enthusiasm to join the fight, Hutchins wrote General Leonard Wood (with whom de Nancrede had served in the Spanish American War) for advice and received this response on April 23, 1917:[v]

> I should advise the student body not to enlist until the plans of the government are definitely known. Enlistment now means enlistment in the militia or the regular army. College men should make every effort to serve as officers. . . . The best thing to do at present is to go

---

v de Nancrede intersected with Wood during their service in Cuba in the Spanish American War. Wood was a career officer who organized the volunteer cavalry Rough Riders Regiment with Theodore Roosevelt and was promoted to brigadier general during the war. He served as military Governor of Cuba after the war. In 1910 President Taft named him Army Chief of Staff and was a candidate for Commander of the American Expeditionary Forces in World War I but President Wilson selected John J. Pershing.

on with the college work, especially where the university has a military instructor as yours has.[7]

The Selective Service Act of 1917 became effective on May 18, requiring men 21–30 to register for potential military service, and a year later the age range was expanded to 18–45. On July 5, 1917, the American Expeditionary Forces (AEF) was established by the U.S. Army under the command of General John J. Pershing to join French, British, Canadian, and Australian Army units against the German Empire, and a small contingent fought alongside Italian Army units against the Austro-Hungarian Army. Chief surgeon General Alfred E. Bradley appointed Major Hugh Young as director of urology. Young soon became colonel and was assisted by Edward L. Keyes ("Jr.") and a half dozen other notables in the field.[8] Well over 100 base hospitals of the AEF were created on the Western Front, encompassing hospitals of the British Expeditionary Forces. Boston carried much of the load with a Brigham unit under Harvey Cushing leaving for Europe on May 11, 1917, soon becoming Base Hospital No. 5 at Camiers and then Boulogne. An MGH unit became Base Hospital No. 6 at Talence and a Boston City unit became Base Hospital No. 7 at Joué-les-Tours.

The first contingent of Ann Arbor draftees assembled at Hill Auditorium for a farewell meeting on September 4, 1917, to hear President Hutchins and other dignitaries. de Nancrede, proud veteran of the Spanish American War, was ready at 70 years of age to serve again at the start of the war, but Dean Vaughan, then a colonel on the Executive Committee of the General Medical Board in Washington, blocked de Nancrede from active duty. The old surgeon "bitterly resented" his exclusion.[9] More than 12,600 Michigan students and alumni served in the army and navy in World War I, and of that number 38 percent were officers.[10] The Students' Army and Navy Training Corps (SATC and SNTC), conceived early in 1918, allowed college students to study and train at the same time, with pay as privates. The army program at Michigan became largest in the country, but the mixed study and drill never meshed well with the university and was cancelled two weeks after the armistice.

In the midst of the war, the largest man-made explosion the world had seen occurred on December 6, 1917 in Halifax, Nova Scotia, just after 9:04 AM when Norwegian SS *Imo* collided with SS *Mont-Blanc*, a cargo ship entering the harbor from New York, packed to the brim with explosives destined for battlefields in Europe. John U. Bacon's book, *The Halifax Disaster*, tells the story in riveting detail, including its connections to the University of Michigan Medical School, and explains how the disaster brought the United States and Canada, previously somewhat estranged mutually in spite of their common origins and border, closer together.[11] The war affected all parts of the

Western world, some more than others, but the shocking catastrophe in Halifax was experienced personally and viscerally by the adjacent American communities in New England. Medical professionals, a large number from Boston, quickly mobilized to Halifax as volunteers, including Ernest Codman, who closed his hospital and rushed people and supplies to the levelled Halifax. Codman, who became a key figure in the concept of measuring surgical outcomes and created his hospital purposefully to that "end-result idea," never reopened the facility and soon after ended his career.

Urologic concerns during the war centered around venereal disease and spinal cord injuries. Gonorrhea dominated among the sexually transmitted diseases that were prevalent in 11 to 25 percent of Allied forces, causing 416,891 hospital admissions among British and Dominion troops. National beliefs shaped venereal disease policies: while the American troops were ordered to be chaste, the British issued condoms and allowed troops to visit brothels.[12] In World War I, only 20 percent of American soldiers with spinal cord injuries survived long enough to return home for treatment, but ratio totally reversed in the next war with up to 88 percent of spinal cord-injured soldiers returning home for treatment.[13] Work at Michigan between World War I and the Vietnam War would make a world of difference to tens of thousands of spinal patients through the latter efforts of Reed Nesbit, Frederick McLellan, Jack Lapides, and Edward McGuire.

With all that happened in 1917, it was an inconvenient time to start a new medical specialty journal, but that's exactly what Hugh Young chose to do on behalf of a specialty with its new name only 15 years old at the time. Young explained his goal in the forward: "The title of this publication *'The Journal of Urology, experimental, medical, and surgical'* expresses briefly the aims, hopes and ambitions of the editors." An Executive Editorial Committee of three with an editorial board of 18 began the monthly publication on February 1917 that continues to this day under ownership of the AUA. Michigan then and later would have substantial representation on the journal: Hugh Cabot was one of four members of the editorial board who represented Harvard University; Albion Walter Hewlett, one of the two board members from Leland Stanford Junior University, had just left the University of Michigan to lead internal medicine at Stanford; John J. Abel at Johns Hopkins was also on the board and he had led the world's first department of pharmacology in his earlier Michigan years; and Nellis B. Foster was the sole representative from Michigan at the time in 1917.[vi]

---

vi Foster, professor of medicine, and chemistry professor William Hale tendered their resignations to the University of Michigan in late 1918 for immediate military service. Hale's military attention was largely related to the study and amelioration of poison gas warfare, while Foster may have found the military service at the time more fulfilling than his work in the medical school. Foster in 1919 wrote an article for *JAMA* on

While the board of 18 had other great names outside of urology, it included principal leaders of the new field, E. L. Keyes ("Jr.") of Cornell, John H. Cunningham, Jr., of Harvard, and J. Bentley Squier of the New York Postgraduate College and later Columbia.[vii]

The year 1917 is also recalled for an important book relevant to physiology and urology called *Secretion of the Urine*. This provided a new take on uroscopy, namely consideration of its physiologic origin. Hippocratic uroscopy was a matter of attention to the sensory evaluation of urine; medieval uromancy was the speculative linkage of urine findings to diagnosis and prediction of outcome; microscopic uroscopy opened new levels of visual detail; chemical and microbial analysis of urine offered therapeutic opportunity; and Cushny's book, *Secretion of the Urine*, explained how urine was formed in health and disease. Arthur Cushny (1866–1926) had come to the medical school in Ann Arbor in 1893 to replace John Jacob Abel, a UM graduate from 1883 who had studied under Vaughan and then pursued further graduate work in chemistry as applied to medicine at Johns Hopkins and then in Germany, Austria, and Switzerland. In 1890, Abel wrote Vaughan to ask for a position as a professor of pharmacology and Vaughan made him an offer. Abel accepted but first returned to Leipzig for further work on the study of calcium carbonate crystals in the urine of animals. He returned to Ann Arbor in 1891 to teach and perform research in the medical school, where he created the first Department of Pharmacology. Abel transformed the formal and ancient lectures on materia medica and toxicology into pharmacology instruction with demonstrations applicable to clinical practice of his time. His stay was short-lived because Johns Hopkins lured him away in 1893, but that opened the door for Cushny. Vaughan found Cushny in Berne where he was investigating the issue of death from chloroform anesthesia and developing methods of titrating the delivery. Cushny was an effective teacher and a very productive researcher in Ann Arbor but returned to Europe for an attractive job as professor at University College London in 1905 where much of his work culminated in his most important book and biggest contribution of physiologic and urologic significance. He retired to his native Scotland in 1918.[14]

---

medical education and war; N. B. Foster, "Medical Education as Revealed by the War," *JAMA* 72 (1919): 1540–1542.

vii Edward Loughborough Keyes, son of Edward Lawrence Keyes, was not actually a "junior," although he used the term; E. D. Smith, E. D. Vaughan, E. S. Belt, and D. A. Bloom, "Edward Lawrence Keyes: A Pivotal Early Specialist in Modern Genitourinary Surgery," *Urology* 62 (2003): 968–972; P. J. Stahl, E. D. Vaughan, E. S. Best, and D. A. Bloom. "Edward Loughborough Keyes: An Early Twentieth Century Leader in Urology," *Journal of Urology* 176 (2006): 1946–1951.

The influenza epidemic hit with little warning in the spring of 1918 and may have first emerged in the United States, even though it became known as the Spanish flu, an inaccuracy due to a strategic detour around the American *First Amendment*, when claims of national security suppressed newspaper reporting of the initial outbreaks.[viii,15] A recent accounting of the *Great Influenza* by John M. Barry includes eight references to the University of Michigan, which felt the impact of the virus substantially among students, faculty, and local citizens.[16]

In April 1918, noncollege draftees began to come to University of Michigan in batches for two-month tours as gunsmiths, machinists, motor mechanics, blacksmiths, telephone repairmen, and carpenters, supervised by the College of Engineering. By November of that year, over 2,200 had received this technical training. While this was good from the perspective of the national needs and the workforce, the experiment strained the university. On December 1, 1918, the government cancelled the program and defaulted on payments to instructors, although the university completed the payouts.[17] During the war, Vaughan was a colonel on the staff of the surgeon general, dermatology chief Udo Wile was a major at the first American hospital in England, Moses Gomberg of the chemical laboratory served as a major investigating poison gases, and many other medical and general university faculty also served.

Cabot's textbook, *Modern Urology*, was a tour de force, although it is hard to understand how Cabot completed it and took it to publication in 1918, while he was occupied near the Western Front in France. Harvard Medical School purchased a copy on June 18, 1918, so Cabot must have been assembling it during his time in Europe when not engaged in military work. Volume 1 included 18 contributors, 722 pages, plus an index. Volume 2 with 11 other authors consisted of 671 pages plus an index. Cabot's three personal chapters were on bladder stone, bladder foreign bodies, and stones of the kidney and ureter.[18]

Modern Urology was the third authoritative urology text in the twentieth century, and Young's in 1926 would be the fourth, to embrace the new term. The *Journal of the American Medical Association* reviewed Cabot's book:

> These two volumes will be found useful and valuable as a standard reference work. One only needs to look over the list of contributors to know that each subject is covered by an authority. The numerous engravings and plates are very instructive. One can safely state that

---

viii The causative strain, an H1N1 virus, continues to circulate as a seasonal influenza but without the morbidity and mortality of the 1918 subtype. Subsequent pandemics recurred in 1957, 1968, and 2009; J. A. Belser and T. M. Tumpey, "The 1918 Flu, 100 Years Later," *Science*, 359 (2018): 255.

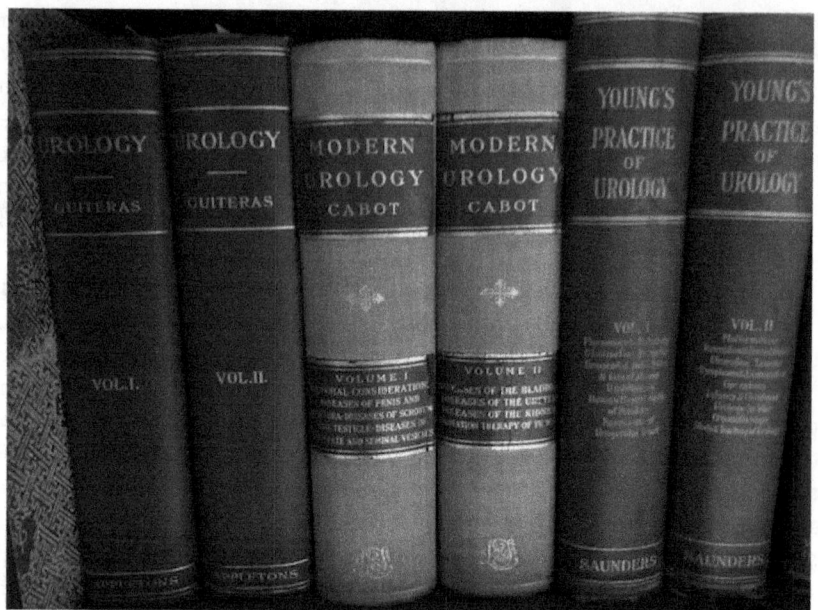

Three early twentieth-century American urology textbooks.

the work accomplished its intention, namely that "it gives articular expression to American urology."

The *JAMA* review indicates that not only was urology well-established as a specialty of surgery but it was also demarcating into very specific subsidiary areas of expertise. The book was reviewed favorably by other journals and an advertisement the following year in *Surgery, Gynecology and Obstetrics* listed 10 other favorable reviews.[19] Coincidentally, on the page next to that advertisement in *SG&O* was another advertisement for catgut sutures, an observation that Cabot must have noted with irony inasmuch as that particular suture material had been the topic of his first academic paper back in 1901 in the *Boston Medical and Surgical Journal*.

The Armistice of November 11, 1918, ended fighting between the Allies and Germany, after other armistices had been signed with Bulgaria, Ottoman Empires, and the Austro-Hungarian Empires—geopolitical entities that have largely faded away and are little known to students of medicine and specialty trainees today. *The Treaty of Versailles* formally ended the state of war on June 28, 1919, in a ceremonial room still standing that coincidentally hosted a peaceful international pediatric urology meeting almost precisely 91 years later.[ix]

---

ix The Society of Pediatric Urological Surgeons, hosted by Henri Lottmann, met in Versailles in 2010, for its 48th meeting.

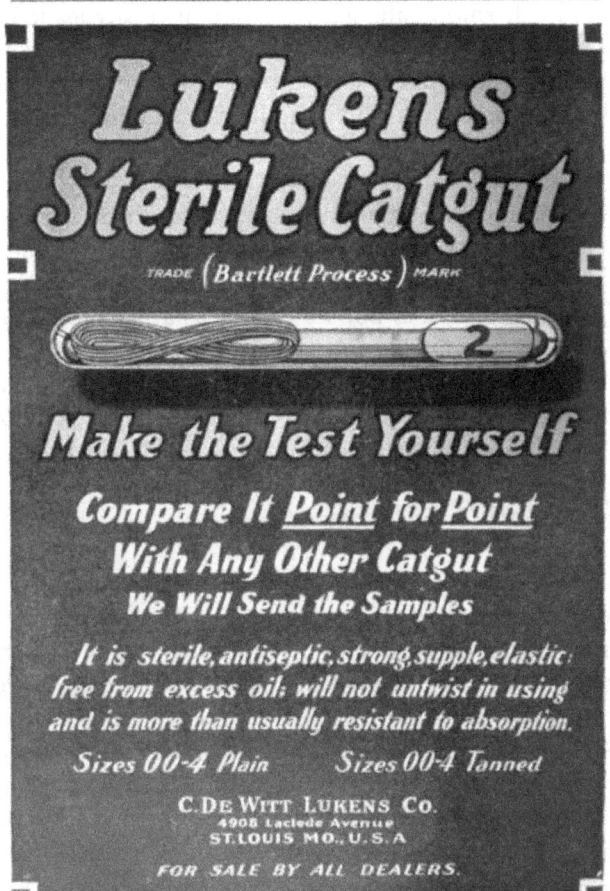

Advertisement in *Surgery, Gynecology and Obstetrics*, 1918.

Postwar years brought a new world order, higher cost of living, and a new hunger for education that added new pressures to universities. As true for all wars, the lessons learned in casualty management translated to civilian medical practice and education, and World War I accelerated the evolution of surgical specialties. Michigan's Catherine Street Complex, not even 30 years old at the end of the war, was insufficient for the postwar demands of emerging healthcare specialties and technologies. Few among the university leadership and medical school faculty recognized those impending changes. President Hutchins was well beyond his prime and anxious to see his replacement in office. Dean Vaughan was not just past his best years but so distracted with national duties that the medical school was falling behind the peer institutions of Flexner's report a decade earlier.

Interim surgery chair Darling, marginalized by Vaughan's lack of respect, was furthermore falling away from university leadership around this time. A letter to President Hutchins on November 30, 1919, regarding the unfilled internal medicine professorship after the departure of Hewlett for Stanford, reveals both familiarity and estrangement:

> My Dear Friend,
> Several attempts have been made to select a professor of internal medicine and another serious mistake will be made unless you use your guiding influence in this matter. The Faculty has been manipulated as usual and does not see clearly what should be done. I wish you would call in Dr. Newburgh and have him explain the situation which is becoming very serious. Dr. Newburgh is too valuable a man in his research for the university to lose. Having as you do the future of the Medical School at heart I have taken the liberty of addressing you in confidence concerning this important question.
> Very Sincerely, CG Darling.

"Harry" Newburgh, as he was known (L. H. Newburgh), was a Harvard-trained internist who had studied further in Vienna, ending up on the Michigan faculty as an early hire in 1916 of Nellis B. Foster, Hewlett's successor as a "metabolically oriented physician." Foster, however, had a very short stay in Ann Arbor, joining the Medical Reserve Corps at the end of the 1916–1917 academic year and then resigning in November 1917 to extend his military service, although differences in expectations from Vaughan may have been the main factor.[20] Newburgh served as acting head of medicine and was a powerful investigator but not much of a teacher. He was, however, a valued colleague as Darling's note attests. It was not until 1922 that the next dean, Hugh Cabot, found a permanent head of internal medicine, Louis M. Warfield, at which time Newburgh became professor of clinical medicine. Ira Dean Loree was the busier genitourinary surgeon at Michigan compared to Darling but was dissatisfied with the lack of resources he felt were due for the scale of his practice. His traditional nineteenth-century title (professor of genitourinary surgery) and his small stature on the rapidly enlarging national stage of urology were more clues that Michigan was falling behind in the world of clinical specialties.

The search for the next head of surgery was an essential step in bringing the medical school into the twentieth century. The full-time compensation model had been the critical attraction for de Nancrede and it turned out to be so for his successor, although it was not attractive to many candidates. Dallas Phemister, one prospect for the surgery chair, complained that the full-time model had two faults: it deprived a surgeon of contact with the world outside the university and even as generous as a university might offer, it likely would fall short of the opportunity of private practice. Michigan, accordingly, answered the second challenge by offering two salaries—a university salary and a clinical salary.

In 1919, Hugh Cabot accepted the job with a professorial salary of $5,000 and a clinical salary of $10,000. He claimed his yearly income in Boston had been around $30,000 but the Michigan model of direct disconnection from practice, anticipated new hospital building, and opportunity for an academic life would better suit him at this new stage in his life. Cabot was an international celebrity in surgery and urology, and how he came to Ann Arbor is an interesting story. He had finished training under his cousin Arthur Cabot and by 1909 was practicing the full gamut of urology, a term he had embraced. He published frequently, writing case reports, opinions, and clinical series and became a national leader. Returning to Boston after distinguished and long service on the Western Front in World War I he was disillusioned by the mercenary nature of the practice environment. The full-time employment model that had attracted de Nancrede 30 years earlier appealed to Cabot and he accepted the Michigan position as chair of the Surgery Department. In Ann Arbor, he opened up the modern era of academic clinical urology at Michigan.

When Cabot arrived in Ann Arbor, the University of Michigan was already more than 100 years old and differed from any other institution the Bostonian had experienced. The university was further unusual in that it was a public institution (birthdate 1817) that preexisted its own state (birthdate 1837). Medical education in Boston had been based on medical school relationships with separate private and public hospitals. With its own teaching hospital, since 1869, Michigan invented a new and different model of medical education, becoming a wholly owned and operated integrated health system containing a full range of medical practice and a research enterprise to provide a rich milieu for professional healthcare education.

While Vaughan brought the University of Michigan Medical School to the world stage as an educational and research institution in the early twentieth century, Ann Arbor's clinical impact remained local, for the most part, and held back the other two missions. Michigan indeed had some note worthy clinicians toward the end of the *Fin de siècle* particularly Cowie, Dock, Hewlett, and Peterson.

George Dock, an MD from the University of Pennsylvania in 1884, had stayed at Penn to study under new faculty appointee William Osler, and after a period of European study was called back by Osler to run the new clinical laboratory and serve as a clinician. Dock came to Michigan in 1891 to replace Alonzo Palmer, becoming Michigan's first major league internist. Unsatisfied with instructional and clinical resources, and distrustful of Vaughan, who had initially tried to relocate the clinical practices of the faculty to Detroit, Dock left in 1908 for Tulane and moved to Washington University in St. Louis in 1910 where Flexner and Rockefeller funds were infusing the medical school. Dock's loss was yet another indication of the inability of UMMS to embrace a shared vision of mission balance, with the understanding that world-class education and research in a medical school required a world-class clinical engine. Nevertheless, Dock's 18 years at Michigan greatly benefitted the university.

In 1896, Dock asked David Murray Cowie (UMMS 1896) to assist him in clinical duties. Cowie, as a medical student, had cared for the animals in the pharmacology laboratory, worked in Dock's clinical lab, and functioned as a subintern. Developing a private practice in Ann Arbor after graduation, Cowie maintained strong ties to the medical school, studying gastroenterology and infection, caring for internal medicine patients, and publishing papers. He had publication savvy. One example was a debilitated woman with an abdominal mass, but only after waiting for a photographer to record the physiognomy did Cowie catheterize her and remove over two quarts of urine thereby eliminating the mass.[21] In time, Cowie specialized in the pediatric sector which was still then housed in the Department of Internal Medicine, supervised inpatients on the Palmer Ward at the Catherine Street Hospitals, and built up the pediatric curriculum. Cowie headed the Pediatric Section in 1905. In 1912, he opened a private 12-bed "Cowie Hospital" on South Division. A "Contagious Hospital" in 1914 was a joint venture between the city of Ann Arbor and the university. Cowie and Reuben Peterson were its main proponents and overseers. A separate Pediatric Department in 1921 expanded Cowie's legitimacy as a pediatrician and when the new University Hospital opened under Dean Cabot in 1925, Cowie would have 110 beds for children (including those in the Contagious Hospital) with an additional 90 for pediatric surgical patients.

Reuben Peterson was another faculty member with major national visibility. Boston trained, he began practice in Grand Rapids, becoming superintendent at St. Mark's Hospital as it was about to be renamed Butterworth, where he established a nurses' training school, built a city-wide medical library, and specialized in obstetrics and gynecology. He published vigorously and innovated surgically, moving in 1898 to Chicago for private practice with teaching appointments at Rush Medical College and the Chicago Post-Graduate Medical School. Peterson came to Ann Arbor in 1901 where he pursued private practice in addition to holding the Elizabeth Bates endowment (see p. 54). From the start, Peterson was opposed to the full-time faculty model that de Nancrede exemplified and Cabot would later endorse. Peterson created his own seven-bed hospital with an operating room in a rented house on South University in 1901 and the next year leased another house on Forest Avenue with nine beds and another operating room (below).

Within a few more years he had 40 beds, a nurses' training school, a diet kitchen, and a clinical laboratory. In addition to his antagonism to the full-time model, Peterson had strong opinions against resurgent pressures to move some clinical teaching to Detroit, surprisingly with the backing of Dean Vaughan in 1906 as evidenced in a letter to Regent Sawyer.[22] Peterson and Dock became allies in frustrating Vaughan's efforts to bring clinical teaching of the medical school to Detroit. Ten years later, Vaughan tried again, writing his son who was a surgeon in Detroit and on the Detroit College of Medicine faculty. The city of Detroit offered its Receiving Hospital to the University of Michigan, but the faculty, led by Peterson, vetoed the idea.[23] Peterson became a major player in his years at Michigan, serving from 1911 to 1918 as hospital director. He became president of the American Gynecological Society and was a founding member of the American College of Surgeons. Peterson later changed his mind about the full-time model and asked Cabot for such an appointment in 1925, but Cabot had no use for him.

Dock's replacement in 1908 by Albion Walter Hewlett, however, was a gain equivalent to the loss. Hewlett had grown up in San Francisco,

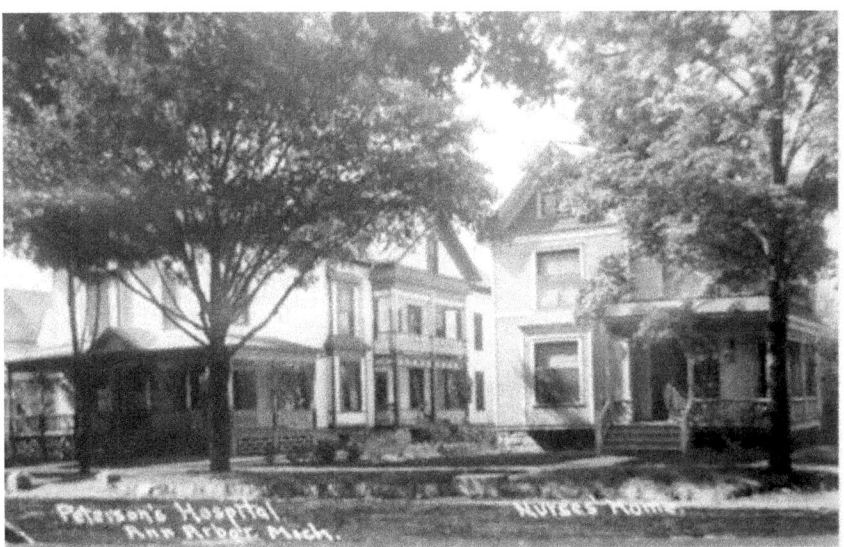

Peterson's Hospital, 620 S. Forest.

started medical school at Cooper Medical College (before its linkage to Stanford), and transferred to Johns Hopkins at the cost of an added instructional year during which he completed a number of canine metabolic studies. After two years of internship at New York Hospital and two more years of study and research in Germany, Hewlett returned to Cooper, rising to associate professor before recruitment to Michigan. After eight mutually valuable years at Michigan, Hewlett left Ann Arbor in 1916 to succeed Stanford's professor of medicine, Ray Lyman Wilbur, who had just been named president of the university.

Max Peet was an important asset that Cabot found in Ann Arbor in 1919. Max Peet (UMMS 1910) had trained and developed a research career on the east coast before returning to Michigan in 1916 to develop a clinical career. After 1918, he limited his practice to neurosurgery and blossomed in the Cabot years, especially so after Edgar Kahn (UMMS 1925) joined him on the faculty.

Frederick George Novy would intersect powerfully with Cabot and will be discussed later in more detail. One of Novy's students bears particular mention. Paul de Kruif (1890–1971) from Zeeland, Michigan, had remained in Ann Arbor following a bachelor's degree in 1912 to obtain a PhD in 1916 and then joined the U.S. Mexican Expedition (once known as the Pancho Villa Expedition) against Mexican revolutionary paramilitary forces in 1916 and 1917. He saw service in France with the Sanitary Corps investigating gas gangrene that was prevalent in the trenches of World War I. de Kruif returned to Michigan as assistant professor in 1919 working in Novy's laboratory, publishing a paper on streptococci and complement activation. Novy's influence helped him secure a prestigious position at the Rockefeller Institute in 1920, where he studied the mechanism of respiratory infection. While there, he anonymously wrote a chapter on modern medicine for a book in 1922 called *Civilization in the United States: An Inquiry by Thirty Americans*, edited by Harold Sterns. The chapters were written by prominent authors, including H. L. Mencken, Ring Larder, and Lewis Mumford and how de Kruif, a young bacteriologist (and nonphysician), came to be included in this compilation is a mystery. He was the only anonymous author, and in the description of contributors he was incorrectly described as a physician. His 14-page chapter caused the biggest stir in the book, skewering contemporary medical practice and doctors for "a mélange of religious ritual, more or less accurate folk-lore, and commercial cunning." He called unscientific medical practice "medical Ga-Ga-ism." After he was discovered to have been the author, the Rockefeller Institute fired de Kruif in September 1922, and he became a full-time science writer and without much dispute is recognized the first in that new genre of journalism. de Kruif came in contact and collaboration with author Sinclair Lewis, for the 1925 novel *Arrowsmith* that included a central character named Max Gottlieb, significantly fashioned around Novy. The book was offered the Pulitzer Prize in 1926, although Lewis refused the award. Lewis gave de Kruif 25 percent of the royalties for his help, which seemed generous to the young bacteriologist at the time, but the unexpected popularity of the work lead to later resentment over the lack of visible authorship as much as the smaller share of revenue.[24]

While UMMS had some luminaries on the national stage of academic medicine by 1919, it was largely Cabot who gave the medical school and hospital its leap into the center spotlight of medical practice, education, and research in the twentieth century. Hugh Cabot changed the medical school at Michigan as much as anyone then or since. As a world-class *urologist*, he brought modern urology to Ann Arbor and very quickly became dean of the medical school, building a great multispecialty group practice and presiding over construction of a 1,000-bed hospital that opened in 1926. His first urology trainees, Charles Huggins from Boston and Reed Nesbit from California, did well in their careers, influencing urology, worldwide medicine, and international events. Considering the various options, it seems reasonable and convenient to declare 1919–1920, Cabot's first academic year in Ann Arbor, as the starting point for the *Centenary of Urology at the University of Michigan*.

Notes

1. L. Davis, *Fellowship of Surgeons: A History of the American College of Surgeons* (American College of Surgeons, Library of Congress Catalog Number: 59-15598).
2. H. H. Peckham, *The Making of the University of Michigan 1817–1992*. Edited and updated by M. L. Steneck and N. H. Steneck (Ann Arbor: University of Michigan Press, 1967, 1994), 123.
3. The University of Michigan and the Great War website.
4. Center for the History of Medicine at Countway Library.
5. Boston Daily Globe, "Denounced Call to Remain Neutral Insult to Country, Says Dr. Hugh Cabot," November 15, 1916.
6. H. H. Peckham, *The Making of the University of Michigan 1817–1992*. Edited and updated by M. L. Steneck and N. H. Steneck (Ann Arbor: University of Michigan Press, 1967, 1994), 143–144.
7. H. H. Peckham, *The Making of the University of Michigan 1817–1992*. Edited and updated by M. L. Steneck and N. H. Steneck (Ann Arbor: University of Michigan Press, 1967, 1994), 144.
8. J. W. Schwartz, "Historical Note." In *Medical Department, United States Army. Surgery in World War II. Urology*. Edited by J. F. Patton (Washington, DC: Office of the Surgeon General and Center of Military History, United States Army, 1987), 4.
9. H. W. Davenport, *University of Michigan Surgeons 1850-1970 Who They Were and What They Did* (Ann Arbor, MI: Historical Center for the Health Sciences, University of Michigan, 1993), 48.
10. H. H. Peckham, *The Making of the University of Michigan 1817–1992*. Edited and updated by M. L. Steneck and N. H. Steneck (Ann Arbor: University of Michigan Press, 1967, 1994), 149.

11 J. U. Bacon, *The Great Halifax Explosion*, (New York, NY: HarperCollins Publishers, 2017).
12 K. Dmytruk, Z. Klaassen, S. N. Wilson, R. Kabaria, M. W. Kemper, M. K. Terris, R. W. Lewis, D. E. Neal, Jr., and A. M. Smith, "Dr. Hugh Hampton Young's Impact on Venereal Disease during World War I: The Chaste of American Soldiers," *Urology* 99 (2017): 10–13.
13 E. Bors, "Urological Aspects of Rehabilitation in Spinal Cord Injuries," *JAMA* 146 (1946): 225–229.
14 A. R. Cushny, *The Secretion of the Urine* (London: Longmans, Green, 1917).
15 J. A. Belser and T. M. Tumpey, "The 1918 Flu, 100 Years Later," *Science* 359 (2018): 255.
16 J. M. Barry, *The Great Influenza* (New York: Viking Penguin Books, 2005).
17 H. H. Peckham, *The Making of the University of Michigan 1817–1992*. Edited and updated by M. L. Steneck and N. H. Steneck (Ann Arbor: University of Michigan Press, 1967, 1994), 147.
18 The urology texts of Guiteras (1912), Cabot (1918), and Young (1926); H. Cabot, *Modern Urology in Original Contributions by American* Authors, vol. 1 (Philadelphia, PA; New York: Lea & Febiger, 1918).
19 *Surgery, Gynecology and Obstetrics* 28 (Chicago: The Surgical Publishing Company of Chicago, chief editor W. J. Mayo, 1919) 23.
20 H. W. Davenport, *Not Just Any Medical School* (Ann Arbor: University of Michigan Press, 1999), 14.
21 D. Cowie, "Two Interesting Cases," *Physician Surgery* 26 (1904): 493.
22 Bentley Historical Library, University of Michigan, March 8, 1906, Box 1 Sawyer papers.
23 H. W. Davenport, *Not Just Any Medical School* (Ann Arbor: University of Michigan Press, 1999), 166.
24 R. M. Henig, "The Life and Legacy of Paul de Kruif," Alicia Patterson Foundation 2001.

PART III

The Roaring Twenties, Ann Arbor, and Hugh Cabot

Hugh Cabot: Family and Early Career

Hugh Cabot came from one of the most prominent families of Boston (the "Boston Brahmin") and of the first two American centuries.[i] A connection of family roots to Giovanni Caboto 1455–1498, a Venetian citizen and merchant seaman has been speculated by Labardini and De Regge. Seeking a direct route to the Orient, Caboto was refused funding by King Ferdinand of Spain who had earlier backed the efforts of Christopher Columbus. Caboto went to Bristol, England, and changed his name to John Cabot, enlisting support from King Henry VII. An expedition from Bristol in 1496 had to turn back but in May of 1497 sailing with about 20 men on the *Matthew,* Cabot reached what is now Newfoundland, Labrador, and Nova Scotia thinking it was the east coast of Asia. On return to Bristol, Cabot obtained backing for a new voyage in 1498 involving five ships and 200 men with an intended goal of Japan, but their fate remains uncertain.[1] Beyond this speculation, however, no evidence has been found to link Giovanni Cabot to the American Cabots.

The American Cabots included U.S. senators, surgeons, businessmen, philanthropists, merchants, and artists. Founding patriarch John Cabot, born in 1680 on Jersey in the Channel Islands, and his son Joseph, born in 1720 in Salem, Massachusetts, have been alternatively described as *successful merchants* or as *privateers* with cargoes of opium, rum, and enslaved people. Their descendants became Boston's most successful businessmen, educators, civic leaders, and physicians. Cabot's paternal grandfather, Samuel Cabot, Jr., and great grandfather, Thomas Handasyd

---

[i] "Boston Brahmin" was a term attributed to the most prominent families of the city and among them was Oliver Wendell Holmes, referred to earlier in this text and possible inventor of the term. Cabot's family was of the highest order of this group and Hugh Cabot grew up amidst the political and intellectual furnace his family and their friends created in New England.

Perkins (father of Mrs. Samuel Cabot, Jr.), were two of the wealthiest men in nineteenth-century Boston.

Cabot's father, James Elliot Cabot (1821–1903), known as "Elliot," graduated from Harvard College in 1845, started a law firm in Boston, taught philosophy at the college, and beginning in 1848 edited the *Massachusetts Quarterly Review*. Elliot's older brother, Samuel Cabot, III (1815–1885), earned an MD at Harvard in 1839, studied in Paris for two years, joined a Yucatan exploration as physician in 1842, and began practice in Boston in 1844 when he married Hanna Lowell. Samuel III was an abolitionist and served as a volunteer surgeon in the Civil War at 47 years of age. He became a noted ornithologist, beginning a lifelong collection of birds and eggs during his Yucatan exploration and the Chinese pheasant, *Cabot's tragopan*, is named for him. Samuel Cabot III and Oliver Wendell Holmes, colleagues in medical practice, were members of the influential *Boston Society for Medical Improvement*. Samuel III and Hannah had eight children that included one of America's first impressionist artists, a chemist, a businessman-philanthropist, and Arthur Tracy Cabot (1852–1912). Arthur studied surgery at the Massachusetts General Hospital (MGH) as a protégé of the legendary genitourinary surgeon, Henry J. Bigelow, and developed a successful private practice in Boston with strong ties to Harvard Medical School. Arthur Cabot was an original member of the first urologic subspecialty society, the American Association of Genitourinary Surgeons (AAGUS), when it formed in 1886, along with E. L. Keyes and Moses Gunn who had by then moved from Ann Arbor to Chicago. Bigelow had been sent a letter soliciting his inclusion in the AAGUS membership but never joined. Gunn was invited by a motion at the first annual meeting of the group, to be an "original member" of the group although he never participated in meetings. Arthur Tracy Cabot, however, was quite active in this organization from its earliest days as a founding member in 1886, secretary in 1888, and president in 1891, reliably presenting a paper or more at the meetings he usually attended (see table on p. 71–72). Arthur and his wife Susan Shattuck lived in an elegant Colonial Revival mansion, called Cherry Hill, they built in 1902. The childless couple had the home largely to themselves.

Elliot Cabot, Hugh's father, was a transcendentalist and Unitarian in a powerful intellectual cohort that included Henry David Thoreau and Ralph Waldo Emerson, about whom he wrote a biography and served as literary executer. Elliot married Elizabeth Dwight, from a prominent family that included cousin Charles W. Elliot (1834–1926) who later became Harvard president (in office from 1869 through 1909). Elliot and Elizabeth Cabot were blessed with boys: Hugh and his identical twin Philip born August 11, 1872, plus three older brothers, Charles Mills

(1856), Edward Twiselton (1861), and Richard Clarke (1868). Elliot's genome faithfully transcribed his facial physiognomy to at least two of his sons, Hugh and Richard, according to photographs evident today. The household was intellectually stimulating and espoused Unitarian religious beliefs. Emerson, a great American intellect of the time, was a frequent visitor to the family home, although his death in 1882 probably precluded major impact on the youngest boys, Hugh and Philip.

Twin brother Philip became a banker and utilities manager. Married for nine years with two daughters, he divorced in 1911 taking custody of the girls and remarried much later in 1937. Philip became a professor of economics at Harvard Business School. He was a critic of New Deal and a vestryman at his church. After he died on December 25, 1941, his nephew Hugh Cabot, Jr., served as an usher, representing his father.[2]

Hugh grew up with a forthright and idealistic temperament. Spence later noted Hugh Cabot's "strong inclination to speak honestly, pungently, and bluntly no matter what the consequences might be."[3] Like his father, Hugh was an out-of-doors enthusiast and naturalist. He explored local fields and woods on his own and at the age of 13 traveled the Adirondacks with a guide. Within a few years, Hugh was venturing deep into Maine woods, New Brunswick, Quebec, Labrador, British Columbia, and Alaska. He became a capable and enthusiastic sailor.

Hugh graduated from Harvard College in 1894 and entered Harvard Medical School. As a student, he worked under Arthur Tracy Cabot at the Massachusetts General Hospital (MGH) and more indirectly under his maternal relative Harvard University president Charles Elliot. Hugh had a strong intellect and was a powerful figure, so no nepotism considerations needed apply, but these connections were strongly enabling and set lofty expectations that Cabot largely fulfilled. Graduating second in his medical school class in 1898, Hugh undertook a one-year internship at the MGH and then entered private practice as an assistant to his cousin.

Hugh Cabot quickly became independent in practice and ascended the academic ranks at the medical school from instructor to assistant professor and then professor. In the clinical hierarchy, he similarly went from outpatient surgeon to assistant surgeon and then surgeon at the MGH. The Cabot practice on 1 and then 6 Marlborough Street served as Hugh's residence until his marriage on September 22, 1902, to Mary Anderson Boit (1877–1936) when they moved to their own home on 87 Marlborough where they would raise four children between 1905 and 1916: Hugh Cabot II (1905–1967), daughter Mary Anderson Cabot (1907–1924), John Boit Cabot (1909–1972), and Arthur Tracy Cabot (1916–1989) named for the celebrated cousin.

Hugh's older brother, Richard Clarke Cabot (1868–1939), was the only other physician among the siblings. Hugh and Richard were polar opposites in many ways, their mother described Richard as a "contender to sainthood," a phrase that suggested Hugh's converse and contrary nature. Richard became a highly respected internist, who advanced the field of clinical hematology. He founded the *Archives of Internal Medicine*, created the first medical social work department in the United States, and originated the *Clinical Practices Conferences* (CPC) in the *New England Journal of Medicine*.[4]

Hugh Cabot was a center-stage personality, clinician, and surgeon. He maintained academic productivity throughout his career, beginning with his first paper, "A contribution to the study of catgut as a suture and ligature material" (see p. 110) published in 1901 in the *Boston Medical and Surgical Journal*.[5] Publication so early in a career was unusual for the time, only three years after graduation from medical school, and was an early indication of both his investigative nature and appetite for recognition. After this, he never missed a year of publication except for 1919, the year he came to Michigan, until the final years of his life.

Cabot began his career when surgery was at the cusp of change. Operative procedures in the nineteenth century usually were performed in the homes of affluent "private patients" but in hospitals for indigent patients. With the twentieth century, hospitals transitioned from mere dormitories for the poor and very sick to medical factories with increasingly sophisticated services such as anesthesiology, radiology, pathology, and consultations from other specialists at bedsides of patients. Boston around the turn of the century was a rich training ground, with a population of 560,000 that was easily five times larger than Ann Arbor. In addition to the MGH, the other respected metropolitan hospitals included Boston City, Brigham, Children's, Boston Lying-In, the Free Hospital for Women, Floating Hospital, and others that provided the community with a deep bench of medical expertise for practice, education, and innovation.

Embracing *urology*, the new terminology that Ramon Guiteras introduced in 1902, Hugh joined the emerging leaders and, although he never limited his practice solely to urology, Cabot became an expert in it. His range of publications demonstrated experience, insight, and expertise that seems relevant today well more than a century later. As Cabot's practice grew so did his reputation. He was outspoken and became known as a harsh critic of medical errors. Cabot rose to leadership of the second professional association of urologists, the American Urological Association (AUA), joining at its second meeting, held at the New York Athletic Club in 1903. He became secretary in 1906 at the annual convention in Boston when membership had reached 265.

Hugh Cabot's growing reputation and mentorship under cousin Arthur made inclusion in the AAGUS inevitable and membership came in May 1907 at the 21st meeting. At the time, it was customary that candidates for membership present a thesis, and Hugh offered "The value of palliative operation for cancer of the bladder." The paper was printed in the *Transactions of the American Association of Genito-Urinary Surgeons, Volume 2*, along with the theses of fellow candidates, H. A. Fowler on ureteral calculi, Faxton E. Gardner on prostatic carcinoma, and George Whiteside's "Concerning the practicability of renal transplantation."[6] It doesn't seem that the candidates for membership were in attendance at the 1907 meeting, since the theses were not discussed in the printed transactions, although all other papers printed in the discussion engendered robust printed commentary. Cabot expanded his AAGUS thesis in a paper on bladder cancer that year in the *New York Medical Journal*.[7]

As a new member of the AAGUS in 1908, at the Homestead in Hot Springs, Virginia, Hugh Cabot presented "Varicose veins of a papilla of the kidney as a cause of persistent hematuria," later published in the *American Journal of Medical Sciences*.[8] Cabot gave two papers in 1909 at the meeting in Mount Pocono, Pennsylvania: "Treatment of stricture of the bulbar portion of the urethra by resection partial or complete," and he returned to bladder cancer in the second presentation, "Some observations upon total extirpation of the bladder for cancer."[9]

Arthur and Hugh were urologic aristocrats, and as Cabots in Boston, they were geographic *de facto* royalty, as evidenced in the famous toast by John Collins Bossidy at a dinner in 1910:

> For this is good old Boston
> The home of the bean and the cod
> Where Lowells talk only to Cabots
> And the Cabots talk only to God.[10]

This conjunction of celebrity status socially and professionally afforded Hugh uncommon opportunity and power that he exercised liberally and with ease. In June 1910, he convinced the MGH trustees to create an outpatient genitourinary clinic and it opened the next month with Cabot as surgeon in charge.[11]

Hugh attended the AAGUS annual meeting in Washington, DC, in 1910, once again offering two talks: one on distal ureteral stone and the limitations of radiologic diagnosis and the second called "Value of vaccines in the treatment of infections of the urinary tract." Hugh Cabot was an early adapter of the phenolsulphonephthalein test introduced by Leonard Rowntree and John Geraghty in 1910, discussing it in New York City at the AAGUS in 1911 and publishing a paper on it in the *Boston Medical and Surgical Journal*.[12] Cabot was 10th president of the AUA when the convention met in Chicago in 1911 and his presidential address was provocatively titled "Is urology entitled to be regarded as a specialty?"[13] Cabot expanded his MGH outpatient urology service to an inpatient service in 1911 and was given five beds on the East Surgical Service and another five on the West Surgical Service. The first admission on East was a Cabot patient with urethral stricture. That year he was named first chief of the MGH Genito-Urinary Surgical Service.

Arthur Tracy Cabot's death in 1912 was a heavy blow, leaving Hugh alone to continue to distinguish the Cabot name in the highest circles of urology. Hugh's publications that year expanded from clinical observations to reflections on medical education with "The training of the urologist" where he introduced a useful metaphor for the education of trainees: inspiring them to achieve a *tripodal capacity*:

> a mind fitted to struggle with problems, a sound foundation in general surgery with its accompanying surgical judgment, and highly developed skill in the delicate manipulations in which the cystoscope plays so large a part.[14]

A paper on spinal anesthesia that year was evidence of his efforts to bring new technology and science to urologic practice.[15] The year 1912 was also busy clinically for Cabot, as his range of urologic practice expanded deeply into the risky business of prostatectomy, reporting 22 suprapubic prostatectomies with a 20 percent mortality and six perineal prostatectomies with 33 percent.[11]

The MGH urology service grew in personnel under Cabot as chief, with J. Dellinger Barney, George Gilbert Smith, Richard O'Neill, Edward Young, and E. Granville Crabtree, Cabot's first trainee then called "house surgeon." The year was also busy with academic work reflecting Cabot's growing clinical expertise and urologic range, not just with prostatectomy but also surgical treatment of hydronephrosis.[16] At the 1913 AAGUS meeting in Washington, DC, Cabot presented his observations on bladder diverticulum and he repeated the topic two years later in the *Boston Medical and Surgical Journal*.[17] Cabot's thoughts found favorable coverage in the *Boston Globe* that reported a speech he gave to the public regarding safe sex and how the public is responsible for preventing venereal disease, "Sex Knowledge Essential," the paper headlined on March 4, 1913, and the article began with an indication of the crafted celebrity of Cabot:

> Dr. Hugh Cabot, the famous surgeon, lectured yesterday afternoon at 6 Marlborough to an audience of fashionable women which entirely filled the two large rooms of the ground floor of the building

on "The responsibility of the community for the prevalence of venereal disease."

The article concluded with direct quotes from Cabot himself, giving a sense of his respected public advocacy.

> This teaching should be done by parents, but at present few are properly equipped with the facts. When it cannot be done by parents, especially competent teachers can be found if we insist on having them.[18]

The *Globe* continued to follow Hugh Cabot and his family diligently, throughout their move to Ann Arbor, time in Minnesota, and return to Boston.

An MGH bulletin in 1914 announced that female patients could henceforth be admitted to the Genito-Urinary Service. Barney was assigned all patients with acute gonorrhea and gangrenous periurethritis, thus freeing his boss from the tiresome duties of treating patients with venereal disease. Cabot was president of the AAGUS that year, meeting nearby in May at the Red Lion Inn in Stockbridge, where he spoke on movable kidney.[19] Europe tumbled into war the next month in June 1914.

Cabot was becoming disenchanted with aspects of private medical practice and he was not the only discontent in Boston. His colleague Ernest Amory Codman (1869–1940) had opened a hospital in 1911 dedicated to tracking treatment outcomes he described as "end results," and in 1914 Codman scandalized his colleagues at a medical society meeting that January showing a cartoon of a bird (representing surgeons) with its head in the sand, blinded to surgical outcomes while laying eggs of gold. Years later, Avedis Donabedian in Ann Arbor would champion Codman's significant and long-unsung contribution to today's *health services research*.[20]

Cabot attended the 1915 meeting of the AAGUS when it met at the Greenbrier in White Sulfur Springs, West Virginia, where a joint session with the American Gynecological Society featured a symposium on urinary tract infections. Cabot had firm thoughts in that area, although there is no record of any comments from him at the time, yet not many years later he discussed "the doctrine of the prepared soil" as a factor that was equally important as the bacterial factor in causing infection.[21] Cabot did speak at AAGUS sessions on "Recurrence of stone in the kidney after operation." On October 20, 1915, Cabot addressed the Mississippi Valley Medical Association in Lexington, Kentucky, with a talk called "Medicine—profession or a trade." He was safely distant from his critical peers in Boston for the talk but nevertheless chose to rebroadcast his controversial remarks on medicine's intrinsic ethical dilemma by publication in the *Boston Medical and Surgical Journal*.[22]

The global conflict that would become World War I was well underway in Europe in 1915 and while the United States was still recusing itself, the American Red Cross was preparing for a conflict that seemed inevitable to many Americans. While President Wilson and much of the nation struggled to remain neutral, other individuals and organizations were actively trying to help. The Red Cross and Colonel Jefferson R. Keane, head of the Red Cross Military Relief Division and president of the Association of Military Surgeons began organizing American medical support for Britain and France through the University Service of American Ambulance Hospital. Sir William Osler and former secretary of state Robert Bacon in January 1915 proposed similarly that American medical schools staff and equip British medical hospitals on the front. Osler outlined the idea to Harvard president A. Lawrence Lowell that spring with the intent of rotating teams from Harvard, Columbia, and Johns Hopkins medical schools to support the Brits.

Harvard initiated the program with its first unit of 32 surgeons, 3 dentists, and 75 nurses that sailed for Europe on June 26, 1915, and arrived on the Western Front on July 16 for a six-month interval with the British Expeditionary Forces (BEF) in France. Elliott Carr Cutler (1888–1947) completed a stint with the BEF and remarked in his journal:

> Coller and Wilson have applied for enlistment in the Osler unit of American surgeons to begin work in July. From Boston comes a portion of the unit headed by Drs. Nichols, Porter, Balch and many other of our best and most promising surgeons. These men enlist for three months in the British Army and receive rank and pay the same as British Army Medical staff. They may be sent anywhere. It is sure interesting and will bring the boys into new places and experiences.[23]

Cutler would become a brigadier general in the U.S. Army Medical Corps in 1923 and later performed the world's first mitral valve repair. As Harvard professor and surgeon-in-chief of the Peter Bent Brigham Hospital, he was awarded the Henry Jacob Bigelow Award for accomplishments in surgery by the Boston Surgical Society in 1947.[ii]

[ii] The American support was well-received as indicated in a later report from a lieutenant-colonel. "The first troops to go overseas . . . were the base hospital units organized originally under the American Red Cross by Gen. Jefferson R. Keane. It was a pleasant surprise to the British to find, when their Medical Department through General Goodwin, now the Director General of the Medical Department of the United Kingdom, asked for six American base hospital units to serve in British general hospitals in France, that

The Coller that Cutler mentioned was Frederick Amasa Coller (1887–1964), whose father had graduated from Michigan's Medical Department in 1878 and went on to practice in South Dakota, where Frederick was born. Frederick studied chemistry in South Dakota, graduated from Harvard Medical School in 1912, and then began surgical training at the MGH where he intersected with Cabot, although his main mentor was Charles Locke Scudder. Scudder's seminal textbook, *The Treatment of Fractures*, went through 11 editions, of which the seventh was dedicated to Arthur Tracy Cabot, reflecting the small world of the evolving surgical subspecialties. The Coller name returned later to the Michigan story (see p. 148).[24]

The initial "three-month" period of service to the BEF "Osler Unit" turned into six months and the medical team staffing fell to Boston alone without the Columbia and Hopkins rotations. Surgeons from the MGH and Boston City Hospital kept up the effort. Osler, inspecting the unit in the fall of 1915, commented favorably on the quality of the tents, the quarters, the "A.1" staff, the X-ray work, and the extraordinary "Dental men" repairing mutilated faces. Osler further wrote,

> It was a peculiar pleasure to dine with the mess & to meet so many men of the younger generation, all of whom seem treading the same footsteps of that great group—the Warrens, Jacksons, Bigelows, & Bowditches who made Harvard famous in the past. I do hope arrangements have been made to continue the work.[25]

A second Harvard team came to support the BEF in December 1915. The displacement of talented physicians and nurses from Boston must have put some stress on the clinical programs left behind, but meanwhile, Cabot's productivity, clinical curiosity, and reputation expanded with his influential presentations and publications.[26] When it was time for the next and third contingent to go abroad for the BEF, Cabot didn't flinch.

The *Boston Globe* reported on May 6, 1916, "Third Harvard Unit Going: Dr. Hugh Cabot in Charge of Surgeons and Nurses to Sail for War Zone on May 20," and according to schedule Cabot sailed to Europe on the *Andania* with a medical unit of 22 surgeons and dentists and 33 nurses. They would serve near Camiers at the No. 22 General Hospital and boosted its beds to 1,800 and eventually to 2,380. Again, Cabot's name figured in the headlines.

---

the first unit was ready to sail in ten days and all the others only a few days later"; R. B. Osgood, "Bone and Joint Casualties and the Transport Splints," *Pennsylvania Medical Journal* vol. 22 (January 1919): 205.

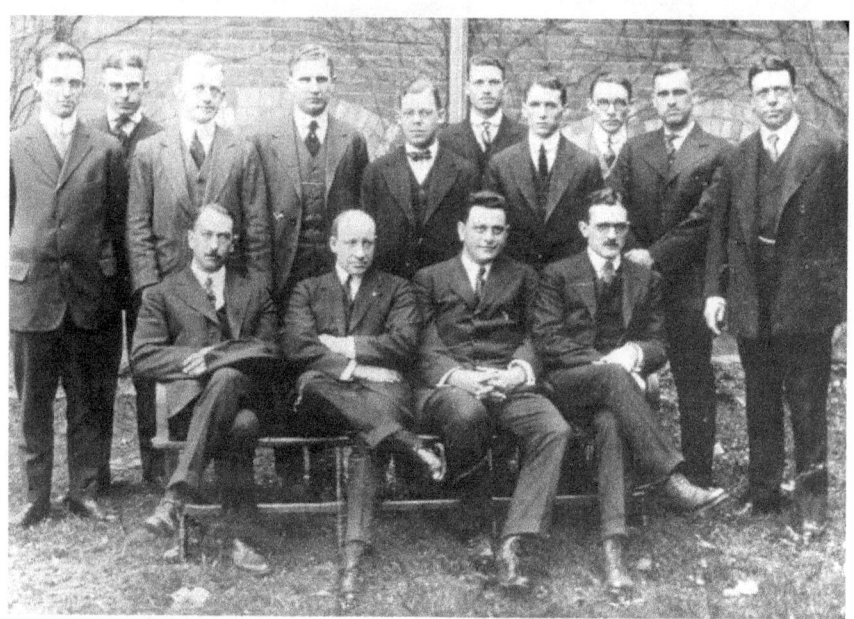

Serious young men. Medical personnel of the Third Harvard Surgical Unit. May 1916. Courtesy, Center for the History of Medicine at Countway Library. Photograph gift of Mrs. Frederick J. Caldwell to the Archives of Harvard Medical School. Seated: (l-r) Lyman Sawin Hapgood, Hugh Cabot, George Sheahan, Carl Robinson.

May 1916 was a time of negotiations between Britain and Germany to reemploy prisoners of war as well as transfer of wounded and sick to Switzerland. The world was being simultaneously reshaped that year as the Irish Rebellion collapsed, Britain and France concluded agreements to partition Asia Minor, and Mamakhatan (Armenia) having been taken by Russian forces earlier in the month was retaken by Turkey. American patriotic fever was edging a reluctant government closer to the war in which Cabot and his Third Harvard Surgical Unit were already immersed. Later Cabot wrote,

> During our three-months term of service, about 8,000 men passed through our hands, and of this number only 19 died under our care. Practically all the sick and wounded during this period came from the region of the Somme. . . . As a rule the men reached the semibase hospitals three to five days after injury. . . . All shell wounds, and to a lesser degree bullet wounds are infected, and the proportion of compound comminuted fractures of the arms and legs was very great. The universal use of steel helmets has very much reduced the importance of wounds of the head. . . . A most important part of this Unit has concerned itself with the management of dreadful wounds of the face, involving the mouth and jaws.[27]

This experience expanded Cabot's casualty expertise, administrative skill, and the confidence he already possessed in amplitude. The *Boston Daily Globe* on November 15, 1916, reported and headlined comments from Cabot in Europe with the BEF: "Denounced call to remain neutral insult to country, says Dr. Hugh Cabot."

Cabot's unit remained in place after its first three months. In November, the Harvard Corporation decided to maintain the Harvard Surgical Unit for the duration of the war under the supervision of Cabot as chief surgeon. Cabot, rarely one to simply say "yes," agreed contingent upon his extraordinary demand that Harvard drop its neutral position on the war. Harvard Corporation agreed, but doing so changed the status of the surgical unit under the Geneva Convention requiring that the unit and its staff officially join the Royal Medical Corps, with the waiver that American personnel with the BEF didn't have to take the oath of allegiance to Great Britain. After America entered the war in April 1917, members of the surgical unit had the option of transferring to the U.S. Army, but most opted to remain with the BEF until January 8, 1919. By then, the so-called "Harvard Hospital" had treated over 150,000 wounded. It is possible that Cabot returned to Boston on some occasions, although no evidence has been found for the better part of the 2.5 years he remained with the BEF. Somehow, in spite of his duties in Europe, Cabot continued academic work, from his 1916 paper on renal infections with former trainee Crabtree, to the 1918 two-volume textbook, *Modern Urology*, that cemented his academic and clinical authority.[28]

On January 1, 1919, the Great War was essentially over. Cabot was awarded Companion of the Most Honourable Order of St. Michael and St. George (Military Division) by King George himself. The unit was still abroad, and the king personally presented awards to lieutenant colonels Hugh Cabot and William Faulkner, in addition to majors Varaztad Kazanjian, E. Granville Crabtree, and Major George Shattuck, an article recalled, although seven months later.[29,iii]

Returning home from Europe, Cabot found his once-rewarding Boston surgical practice had "evaporated." Just as likely, he may have found his work even less fulfilling personally than before the wartime experience. A literate Anglophile, Cabot likely had passing familiarity with the 1906 play of George Bernard Shaw, *The Doctor's Dilemma*, an exploration of the problematic interface between professional duty and private practice. He repeated his own expostulations of that dilemma throughout his

---

iii Kazanjan's later relative, University of Michigan professor Powel Kazanjian, wrote the definitive biography on Frederick Novy; P. H. Kazanjian. *Frederick Novy and the Development of Bacteriology in Medicine (Critical Issues in Health and Medicine)* (New Brunswick, NJ: Rutgers University Press, 2017).

career voicing conflict in duties to teach, care for the indigent, and family responsibilities. Conflict in terms of cash flow and absence from his family must have also been acute during his time with the BEF, although no relevant comments have been discovered.[30] Surgical practice in Boston may have been unfulfilling, but Cabot continued to enjoy the academic connection to Harvard and on April 14, 1919, was appointed clinical professor of genitourinary surgery. The university even then was retaining the older term rather than *urology*. Cabot's appointment was backdated to September 1, 1918 possibly to cover the full academic year.[31]

The AAGUS had not met in 1917 or 1918 because of the war, so its thirty-first meeting, in June 1919 at Atlantic City, had to have been a happy reunion. The *Transactions* resumed with Volume XII in 1919 and included discussions of war activities, noting that 21 members had served as commissioned officers with many others named as consultants on medical advisory boards.

> Hugh Cabot was a lieutenant colonel in the Royal Army Medical Corps and served with the British Expeditionary Force as Chief Surgeon of a general hospital; E. L. Keyes, Jr. was a colonel in the Medical Corps with the American Expeditionary Force and director of a base hospital; Herman Kretschmer was a captain in the Medical Corps; William Wishard, Sr. served on the Council of National Defense and Hugh Hampton Young was a colonel in the Medical Corps in the A.E.F. where he was in charge of all urological work. He was awarded the Distinguished Service Medal. It was further noted that Major Harold W. Beal of Worcester, while serving with the First Division of the A.E.F. was wounded in action near Soissons, France, in July 1918 and died 2 days later.[32]

Several papers of military concern presented at the 1919 meeting included nocturnal enuresis in enlisted men, hematuria in solders, "observations of a consulting urologist," and infections of the GU tract following influenza. A positive review of Cabot's book appeared in *Surgery, Gynecology, and Obstetrics* this year.

Cabot didn't wait long after his return to the United States before returning to the podium. In June, he delivered the annual meeting oration at the Bunker Hill Monument Association at the Vendome and the *Boston Daily Globe* reported that "it consisted mainly of a review of some of the activities of the British Naval Intelligence Department in ferreting out German propaganda during the war related to the United States." Cabot then made a strong plea for the League of Nations, stressing "the absolute interdependence of the people of Europe upon each other."[33] The Monument Association was a politically potent group, electing at this meeting ex-president Taft and Elihu Root as honorary members, along with two of the Warren surgeons at the MGH as principal officers. For reasons unknown, it wasn't until August that the *Globe* reported the delayed news: "Harvard unit decorated by Britain. Col. Cabot, with several of his surgeons and nursing staff, win personal thanks of King George." That actual event had occurred on January 1, 1919, when the Harvard unit was still abroad.

With the war, influenza epidemic, and initial exhilaration of returning home behind him, Cabot found reentry into the profession and business of medicine unfulfilling, as he later recalled in his books of the 1930s. News of the potential full-time academic position in Ann Arbor must have reached him by the summer of 1919, if not before, and by September he had already lined up the job. Possibly Cabot had enough independent financial resources to turn his back on a yearly surgical income he later claimed was $30,000 a year, although subsequent complaints about housing costs in Ann Arbor seem to negate that idea, as did his references to "practice evaporation" after the war.[34] For whatever reasons, Cabot found the offer of a full-time academic job as director of the Surgery Department in Ann Arbor, at $10,000 a year, attractive and timely. When he moved to Ann Arbor with his wife Mary, their children were around 3, 10, 12, and 14 years of age. The family side of the Hugh Cabot story, including the Boston years, the war years, the Michigan era, and beyond would be an entirely different and compelling narrative of far greater complexity than this one.

Notes

1 M. M. Labardini and G. De Regge, Giovanni Caboto (c1455-c1498) and Hugh Cabot (1872-1945), MD of the University of Michigan, Nesbit Alumni Society presentation, September, 2017.
2 *Daily Boston Globe*, December 28, 1941.
3 H. Spence, "Hugh Cabot: Founder of the Urological Service at the Massachusetts General Hospital," AAGUS, 1994.
4 P. S. Ward, "The Medical Brothers Cabot," *Harvard Medical Alumni Bulletin* 56 (1982): 30–39.
5 H. Cabot. "A contribution to the study of catgut as a suture and ligature material." *Boston Medical and Surgical Journal* Vol. CXLVI, No. 13 (1901) 327–330.
6 *Transactions of the American Association of Genito-Urinary Surgeons, Volume 2* (New York: Grafton Press, 1907), Cabot 301, Fowler 323, Gardner 333, Whiteside 371.
7 H. Cabot, "Diagnosis of Tumors of the Bladder," *New York Medical Journal* 25 (1907): 1019–1022.
8 H. Cabot, "Varix of Papilla of the Kidney as a Cause of Persistent Hematuria," *American Journal of Medical Sciences* 137 (1909): 98–102.
9 H. Cabot, "Some Observations upon Total Extirpation of the Bladder for Cancer," *Transactions of the American Association of Genito-Urinary Surgeons* 4 (1909): 125–133; H. Cabot, "Treatment of Stricture of the Bulbar Portion of the Urethra by Resection Partial or Complete," *Boston Medical Surgical Journal* 161 (1909): 848–850.

10 J. Foreman, "Big Old Houses," *New York Social Diary*, December 9, 2014.
11 W. S. McDougal, *A History of Urology at the Massachusetts General Hospital 1821–2011*, pamphlet (Boston, 1996), p. 14.
12 H. Cabot and E. L. Young, "Phenolsulphonephthalein as a Test of Renal Function," *Boston Medical and Surgical Journal* 165 (1911): 459–461.
13 L. W. Jones, *The American Urological Association Centennial History* (Baltimore: American Urological Association, 2002).
14 H. Cabot, "The Training of the Urologist," *New York Medical Journal* 95 (1912): 1075–1077.
15 H. Cabot, "Subarachnoid (Spinal) Anesthesia," In *Surgery, Its Principles and Practice*, ed. W. W. Keen, vol. 8 (Philadelphia, PA: W. B. Saunders, 1912), 8560–8867.
16 H. Cabot, "Suprapubic Prostatectomy," *Surgery, Gynecology & Obstetrics* 17 (1913): 689–692; H. Cabot, "The Diagnosis and Indications for Operation in Early Hydronephrosis," *Journal of American Medical Association* 60 (1913): 16–20.
17 H. Cabot, "Some Observations upon Diverticulum of the Bladder," *Transactions of the American Association of Genito-Urinary Surgeons* 7 (1913): 62–72; H. Cabot, "Some Observations upon Diverticulum of the Bladder," *Boston Medical Surgical Journal* 172 (1915): 300–302.
18 "Sex Knowledge Essential," *Boston Daily Globe*, March 4, 1913.
19 H. Cabot and L. T. Brown, "Treatment of Movable Kidney with or without Infection, by Posture," *Boston Medical and Surgical Journal* 171 (1914): 369–373.
20 A. Donabedian, "The End Results of Health Care: Ernest Codman's Contribution to Quality Assessment and Beyond," *Milbank Quarterly* 67, no. 2 (1989): 233–256.
21 H. Cabot, "The Doctrine of the Prepared Soil: A Neglected Factor in Surgical Infections," *Canadian Medical Association Journal* 11 (1921): 610–614.
22 H. Cabot "Medicine—Profession or a Trade," *Boston Medical and Surgical Journal* 173 (1915): 685–688.
23 Countway Library. Center for the History of Medicine. OnView: Digital Collections and Exhibits. "Harvard Surgical Unit."
24 H. W. Davenport, *University of Michigan Surgeons*, (Ann Arbor: Historical Center for the Health Sciences, University of Michigan, 1993), 90.
25 Countway Library. Center for the History of Medicine. OnView: Digital Collections and Exhibits, "Osler reports on the unit."
26 R. H. Miller and H. Cabot, "The Effect of Anesthesia and Operation on the Kidney Function, as Shown by the Phenolsulphonephthalein Test," *Archive of Internal Medicine* 15 (1915): 369–391.
27 Countway Library. Center for the History of Medicine. OnView: Digital Collections and Exhibits, "Hugh Cabot and the Harvard Unit."
28 H. Cabot and E. G. Crabtree, "The Etiology and Pathology of Non-Tuberculous Renal Infections," *Surgery, Gynecology, and Obstetrics* 23 (1916): 495–537; H. Cabot, *Modern Urology* (Philadelphia, PA; New York: Lea and Febiger, 1918).
29 "Harvard Unit Members Decorated by Britain," *The Boston Globe*, August 4, 1919.
30 A. L. Lowell, "Introduction," in *The Doctor's Bill*, ed. H. Cabot (New York: Columbia University Press, 1935), xv–xvi.
31 Twenty-Fifth Anniversary Report, 1894–1919, Harvard University, Class of 1894.
32 H. M. Spence, *A History of the American Associations of Genito-Urinary Surgeons, 1886–1982* (Dallas, 1982), 21–22.
33 "Vote Bunker Hill Monument to State," *Boston Daily Globe*, June 18, 1919.
34 A. L. Lowell, "Introduction," in *The Doctor's Bill*, ed. H. Cabot (New York: Columbia University Press, 1935), xv–xvi.

Hugh Cabot Comes to Ann Arbor, 1919

On September 26, 1919, Dean Victor Vaughan, backed by a unanimous vote of the medical faculty, asked the regents to appoint Hugh Cabot "full-time Professor of Surgery." Vaughan had quietly preferred internal faculty members Frederick Novy and G. Carl Huber but when Cabot surprisingly jumped at the opportunity, the dean joined the supporting queue.[1] Cabot, then 47 years old, had recently visited Ann Arbor for three days to study the conditions and left impressed with the idea that the teaching faculty could be independent of "commercial medicine." Vaughan provided the regents details of Cabot's career and qualifications, along with a note from Cabot requesting a salary higher than initially offered. Vaughan concluded with this statement:

> I believe that this is an opportunity which has seldom come to the University of Michigan, at least to its Medical School, to secure one of the most eminent men in the world for the Chair of Surgery, and in behalf of the Medical School I beg you to grant this very reasonable request on the part of Dr. Cabot. With him at the head of our surgical department it will not be necessary to explain who is professor of surgery in the University of Michigan, it matters not in whatever part of the world one may be. I regard this as a rare opportunity, and one which cannot be neglected without great detriment to the Medical School in particular/and to the University as a whole. A few medical men who have been in the Service and have had charge of large military hospitals have seen the possibilities of the medicine of the future. Dr. Cabot is such a man. He is not only a distinguished surgeon but a man, as I have stated, of wide culture and broad vision. I hope that the request of the Faculty will be granted by you, and that Dr. Cabot will receive the appointment and be authorized to begin his work as soon as he possibly can.[2]

After negotiations with Vaughan, Cabot accepted the job at a salary of a third of what he claimed to have made in Boston in his private practice ($30,000 to $10,000). Given that Cabot had spent most of the three previous years with the British Expeditionary Force engaged in Europe during World War I and that in the eight months back in Boston he found his practice had "evaporated," that claimed figure must have been historic or hyperbolic. The *Boston Daily Globe* dutifully reported the surprising emigration of one if its Brahmins, noting the simultaneous resignation of Dr. Darling with the generous comment that likely came from Cabot himself.

DR CABOT ELECTED MICHIGAN PROFESSOR

Special Dispatch to the Globe

ANN ARBOR, Mich. Sept 26—Dr Hugh Cabot of Boston was today appointed professor of surgery at the University of Michigan. The resignation of Dr Cyrus G. Darling, head of the surgery department, was accepted with regret. It was largely through his efforts that Dr Cabot was secured. He is expected to assume his new post early next week.

Boston Daily Globe, Cabot takes Ann Arbor job.

Cabot's immersion was immediate as Vaughan's response to his acceptance indicated on September 30, 1919:

> I have just received your telegram and am enclosing herewith some leaves torn from the announcement covering the schedule for surgery. Substituting your name for Dr. Darling's, you will see the work which is laid out for you by this schedule. . . . Dr. Darling has resigned and you take his place.[3]

Clearly, Darling was out the door of the Surgery Department in no time and turned over his scheduled surgical cases to Cabot immediately. The *Michigan Daily* reported the arrival of Dr. and Mrs. Cabot on October 11,

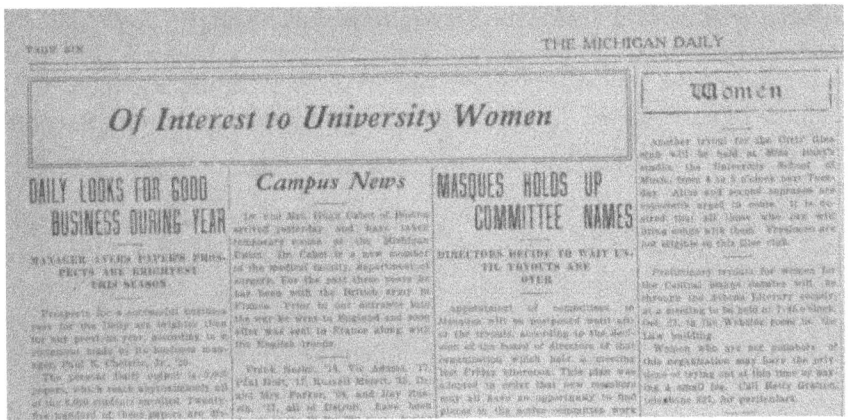

Cabot arrival announced in *Michigan Daily*, October 12, 1919.

residing in the newly constructed Michigan Union and apparently leaving their children ages 3–14, behind for a time in Boston.

Cabot thus began a remarkable 11 years in Ann Arbor that would transform the University of Michigan Medical School and bring it to the top level of medical education, clinical practice, and research. Cabot restructured the school, built a cadre of superb faculty and clinicians, educated thousands of medical students who impacted the world, but all that came with the cost of political warfare and personal animosities. Cabot created new clinical departments, dissolved the homeopathic school, and initiated the first steps to multispecialty group practice. He presided over the construction of a new iteration of the University Hospital that became Michigan's first state-of-the-art clinical facility. His campaign for "geographic fulltime" clinical faculty to operate and lead the clinical practice exacerbated faculty discord and the corporate sense of mission balance. The ultimate Cabot debacle made it clear that not even the most forceful leader can impose a formula for precise mission balance on a faculty body. It has become clearer, over the succeeding century, that mission balance is a very personal arbitrage in a free society, best played out under a set of generally accepted values, principles, rules, and shared sense of corporate purpose. Under Cabot, Ann Arbor finally gained a world-class hospital and all of this would happen under five university presidents, including Hutchins, over 11 intense years. The details that follow comprise an epic saga.

After the regents approved his appointment as chair of surgery, Cabot got to work quickly and was soon in the operating room covering Darling's scheduled cases and new cases as they arose. A letter among the papers of President H. B. Hutchins in 1919 explained the successful care of a patient, perhaps a student, known to and likely referred by Hutchins, as Cabot reminded the president that the procedure was performed "with your advice." Cabot found and removed an acutely inflamed appendix "in the Surgical Clinic October 13" and helpfully pointed out to the president (as seen below):

> Since the operation patient has progressed very satisfactorily and we see no reason why he should not make an uneventful recovery. Twenty-four hours later this case would have been a complicated one and the prognosis would not have been as hopeful.
> [Bentley Library, Hutchins papers]

The letter was typed on stationary that read: "University of Michigan, Department of Surgery, University Hospital" (nearly identical to what this senior author found on arrival to the medical school and hospital 65 years later). The departmental faculty listed were C. G. DARLING, M.D. GENERAL SURGERY; I. D. LOREE, M.D. GENITO-URINARY SURGERY; C. L. WASHBURNE, M.D. ORTHOPEDIC SURGERY; AND

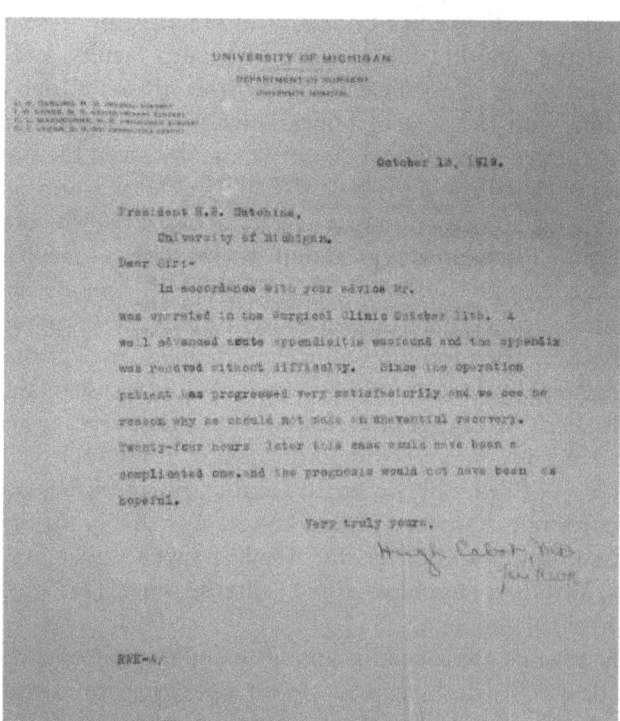

Cabot's letter to Hutchins, repeated from Preface.

C. J. LYONS. D.D.Sc. CONSULTING DENTIST. This short list seems to describe the surgery department faculty such as it was at the time.

Matters of clinical credentials and hospital privileges were not the speedbumps to practice that they would become and this appendectomy took place barely two weeks after Cabot's appointment by the regents. If organizational stationary is to reflect mindsets of its people, neither Darling nor Loree embraced the new terminology of urology, although the neologism of Ramon Guiteras had been in play since the formation of the American Urological Association in 1902 and was so clearly favored by Cabot. Ira Dean Loree was the professor of genitourinary surgery when Cabot arrived in 1919, Loree's "clinical" prefix having been dropped in 1914 when Darling took over from de Nancrede. With Cabot as his new superior, Loree continued to press for a separate genitourinary surgery department, but this made little sense to Cabot, the far more accomplished urologist, although simultaneously still a general surgeon. Loree resigned on March 9, 1920, and moved his practice to the nearby St. Joseph Mercy Hospital where he practiced until his death.

Davenport observed that Cabot was the first University of Michigan surgeon with European experience, although that shortchanges Maclean, earlier, who had been trained in Scotland. Cabot's European connections, however, were more substantial politically, initially coming from his clinical experience in Boston, a hub of international medical innovation and center of medical orthodoxy where European leaders frequently visited, and later from his time in World War I on the Western Front when he worked with leaders in British surgery, notably Major General Sir Anthony Bowlby who had been head of surgery in London's St. Bartholomew's Hospital and then chief surgical consultant to the British Expeditionary Force. In the Cabot years and even later at Michigan, Bowlby would send young surgeons to Ann Arbor for advanced neurosurgical, orthopaedic, and urologic experience, while Cabot and his successors sent some of their young trainees to Europe. Many of these individuals became leaders in their later careers on both sides of the Atlantic.

Cabot was troublesome for the university from the start. While embracing the full-time salary principle, he complained about the discrepancy from his previous income, although that discrepancy must have been from his peak private practice years before World War I. Somehow, he persuaded Dean Vaughan to ask President Hutchins and the regents for use of the university presidential residence. Both the dean and the president were at the end of their terms in office and must have found Cabot's persistence tiresome, but the presidential home was empty at the time. The house had been one of the original four professorial homes that inaugurated the Ann Arbor campus, designed by Harpin Lum and completed in the summer of 1840 at a cost of $26,900 according to Anne

Duderstadt's study of the residence.[4] From 1841 to 1852, the university had been governed by a faculty committee, but by the end of that span it became clear that an executive president would be necessary to run the school and Henry Tappan, the first university president, moved into the vacant southwest professorial house in 1852, installing gas lighting in 1858. The regents fired Tappan in 1863 and his successor, Erastus Otis Haven, added a one-story kitchen and then a third story. Haven left for Northwestern in 1869, but his successor *pro tempore*, Henry Simmons Frieze, didn't occupy the residence. James Burrill Angell, the next president, accepted the job only on the third offer and then contingent on living in the house. The next university president, faculty member Harry Burns Hutchins, preferred to stay in his own home on Monroe at Packard, so the presidential home remained empty until World War I when the Red Cross used it as a local headquarters. The house was empty again when Cabot first came to Ann Arbor, staying for a time in the new Michigan Union.

The regents meeting of October 17, 1919, recorded that "Dean Vaughan, Dr. Cabot, and Dr. Parnall appeared and conferred with the Regents." The next item of business was a motion of Regent Murfin to authorize the employment of Miss Catherine M. Fraser as nurse assistant to the professor of surgery at a salary of $1,000 per year on a 12-month basis, with board and lodging at the University Hospital. Communications to President Hutchins from Dean Vaughan and Cabot regarding the presidential residence were ultimately answered by University Secretary Shirley W. Smith (a man) in a letter dated October 18, 1919, directed to Dr. Hugh Cabot, Department of Surgery, University Hospital.

> My dear Dr. Cabot:
>
> At their meeting October 17, the Board considered the questions of the use of the President's House on the campus as suggested by you. As you doubtless know there has always been a sentimental objection on the part of the Regents to use the President's House for any other purpose than as a president's house. It has stood vacant for a number of years with the exception of its occupancy by the Red Cross though there have been insistent demands for its use by several departments for class room purposes. Some doubts were expressed whether an exception should be made even in the present case, much as every member of this Board desired to accommodate you. There were also some fears expressed that you might yourself be embarrassed in using the house, by the same sentimental objections referred to above, among your colleagues in the several faculties. However, the Board desired to meet your views and authorized the use of the house by you until June 30 [1920], without charge, with

the provision that you would take care with your own expenses in making repairs or alterations which you might require and on condition that the Board would have the right to re-possession at any time on thirty days' notice.
Yours very truly,
SW Smith
Secretary.

The letter was copied to Superintendent Pardon of the Buildings and Grounds Department. Cabot was not embarrassed by his outrageous request or the regents' gracious acquiescence, and he further challenged Hutchins regarding the specifics of the personal expenses and responsibilities that the house might incur. The discussion of the regents was more controversial than revealed to Cabot, as some outright objections had been made; however, after further negotiations, Cabot and his wife moved into the property late in 1919 and no problems occurred during their occupancy.

The house was not Cabot's only disruption in his first months in Ann Arbor. In December, he proposed to President Hutchins that private patient fees generated by faculty be directed to the hospital and pooled to support "full-time" compensation. This concept, meant to support mission balance, threatened the delicate economic environment of faculty livelihoods. If Hutchins and Vaughan were having any second thoughts, a letter of support from William Mayo to his old teacher on December 2 might have dispelled any buyer's remorse:

Dear Dr. Vaughan,
I am interested to learn that Hugh Cabot has accepted the Professorship of Surgery at the University of Michigan. He is a man of scientific imagination, great force, and has splendid training. It is certainly good augery for the future that a man of his type should be willing to leave a great center containing Harvard and the Massachusetts General Hospital to take up a western teaching position. I wish to congratulate you upon the event.
Yours very sincerely.
W. J. Mayo.[5]

Throughout the drama of Cabot's recruitment and his first months in Ann Arbor, the university had been actively recruiting a new president and Hutchins was ready to move on with his life after 11 years at the helm. Marion Leroy Burton, president of the University of Minnesota for only two years, had been in negotiation for the Michigan job and already had a daughter, Theodosia, studying on the Ann Arbor campus.

The regents offered Burton the job in December 1919, with a salary of $18,500 and the offer was accepted, with Burton explaining somewhat lamely to the University of Minnesota that he couldn't resist the better salary. The Burton family anticipated living in the President's House after renovations and knew of the Cabot occupancy.

As 1919 came to a close, Cabot and the University of Michigan were just beginning a decade that would change each other greatly, just as the world at large was changing. President Wilson began the year hopeful of building a new world order but ended the year debilitated after a major stroke. In Michigan, Edsel Ford succeeded his father as head of the family company. Congress passed two amendments to *The Bill of Rights*: a foolish *18th Amendment* of prohibition that would subsequently be reversed and a long-overdue *19th Amendment* for women's suffrage that was not fully ratified until the following year. On December 26 of the year, the Boston Red Sox sold Babe Ruth to the New York Yankees for $125,000, a figure around 10 times the salary of Burton or Cabot.

Notes

1 Bentley Historical Library, University of Michigan, TN8122 BN-726-N UM Medical School records 1850-2010 (N-Z) Box 35 folder T,U,V,W,X,Y,Z. Victor Vaughan Letter to son Warren Vaughan, November 18, 1920.
2 Bentley Historical Library, University of Michigan, Vaughan's statement to Regents, September, 1919.
3 Bentley Historical Library, University of Michigan, Vaughan VC1919 Box 33 Folder C-Car.
4 A. Duderstadt, *President's House* (Ann Arbor: The Millennium Project, University of Michigan, 2000).
5 Bentley Historical Library, University of Michigan, Medical School series, Box 33.

Hugh Cabot, President Burton, and 1920

With the war and flu epidemic behind, 1920 was a time of national optimism, heightened belief in higher education, and a new era of medical specialization and technology. The University of Michigan was encountering its own paradigm changes. A letter dated February 2, 1920, from incoming President Burton to Regent Clements addressed issues regarding the president's residence noting, with unabashed irony, that Burton "should dislike during these times of high building cost to expend funds for a president's house" and "I do not want to do anything which will inconvenience Dr. Cabot." Nonetheless, Burton explained that he wanted to have all the renovations completed, so he and his wife could move in by June before the commencement. The initial renovations he wanted included a third-floor bathroom, new windows created on the second and third floors, changing partitions, adding sleeping porches, fitting the house for steam or hot water heat, vacuum piping on all floors, a water softener in the basement, moving the laundry room, adding a recreation room for "our pool table," and building a garage. Furthermore, the letter requested, if it could be arranged with the Cabots, that the Burtons "get a good look at every part of the house" to see what else might be needed.

Even in the grand residence, the Cabots seemed to be cranky according to some rumors. A letter from Regent Clements to Hutchins on February 4, 1920, concluded with this paragraph, dropping Angell's second "l." (The residence was sometimes called "The Angell House" in honor of its third presidential occupant, James Angell.)

> My sister has written me about the housing conditions at Ann Arbor, and possibly it is only gossip, but there must be some truth in the fact that the Cabots, who are now in the Angel house, are talking about moving back to Boston, as they cannot get a house to live in at

Ann Arbor. It occurred to me that the old Sinclair-Sheehan house on Huron Street, which is for sale, could be made a very practical house, and I have had some disposition to have eyes on it myself. Do you happen to know what this house could be purchased for?

One can only imagine how it struck the weary president in the last months of his overextended second term to be asked to function as a realtor for the regent and the Cabots. Nonetheless, Hutchins on February 5, 1920, returned a letter to Clements the following day, discussing the Clements Library concept and also including further mention of the new chief of surgery:

> You speak of the housing situation as affecting the Cabots. I have heard nothing of the rumor to which you refer, that of their talking about moving back to Boston I do not think there is anything in it. I know they are looking at various places. Among other places they have examined the Sheehan house. Mrs. Cabot is quite in favor of their taking it, but the Doctor is opposed. He would like to live in the eastern part of the city. In 1918 Mrs. Sheehan offered to sell the property for $15,000. I have no recent advices in regard to the price.

Salary details remained in contention after the initial job offer the previous September and a letter from Dean Victor Vaughan to Regent Walter Sawyer on February 4, 1920, requested a $5,000 salary as professor of surgery and $10,000 "to be charged to the hospital" based on Cabot's consultation fees. Vaughan relayed to the regent that Cabot cannot "make ends meet with the present salary." However, the dean noted, "I am opposed to the salary of any professor being placed on a percentage basis, to be determined by the amount of money taken in by the hospital." Dean Vaughan wrote Regent Sawyer on February 6 with concern over the condition of the medical school, confidence in the full-time plan, but hedging his bets on Cabot:

> Dear Doctor:
> I want to make a report to you. The Medical School is, in my opinion, now in a critical condition. If we can carry on with the full time plan, I feel confident that everything will come out alright, but I must admit that we must take some chances. Dr. Cabot promises to be a powerful factor in our future, for good or for ill. Dr. Parnall tells me that the fees taken in through Dr. Cabot's consultations already amount to about $1,000 a month. If this can be done with one department in the hospital as it now stands, it does not require a wild visionary to see what may be done in a new hospital with all the

departments on a full time basis. Doctors and patients from various parts of the State are now seeking Dr. Cabot's advice. He is a strong personality and if given the opportunity will be another Will Mayo in building up a great clinic. However, we must comply with reasonable demands that he makes. His salary for next year must be materially increased.

New university president Burton was eagerly anticipated and outgoing president Hutchins was anxious to get on with his life but probably took special pleasure in issuing this *Special Executive Order* to the campus:

Having been advised by the health authorities of the University that the danger from the influenza epidemic is practically over, by special order I remove the ban on student dances, this order is to take effect Monday noon, February 23, 1920.[1]

A few days later, Cabot explained to the *Michigan Daily* that influenza dates back to the Middle Ages and no vaccine was effective.[2] As seen earlier with the *Boston Daily Globe* interviews, Cabot was adept at leveraging the media for his own promotion. The personal residential issues, however, remained unresolved and reverberated even beyond Cabot and incoming president Burton. Regent Clements, in a letter to Hutchins on March 5, 1920, discussed the President House renovations, estimated at over $40,000 and suggested other properties could be found for Burton, hoping perhaps that the old Angell residence site could be turned over for a new building to house the envisioned Clements Library.[i]

Hutchins replied on March 6 explaining that Pardon thought the renovations would cost $50,000 and, in spite of the disclaimer that "I have no right to express an opinion," the sitting president said that the site was ideal for Clements Library and "it would be unwise to put even $40,000 into the old residence."

Further letters between Hutchins, Burton, as well as the university secretary and the hospital director in the spring of 1920 indicated the delicate balance of the renovations, impending arrival of the new president, ideas for renovation, and the elephant in the house, namely the Cabots.

---

i A paragraph in the letter stated, "Further, I am not looking at my own interest at all, but of course I would be greatly gratified if the present site of the President's house was selected for my library. In that event, the building would face University Avenue, and would well occupy it. My library building will be approximately 70' by 100', and I trust will be an architectural addition to the campus. This plan should not influence our decision as to remodeling the President's house." It is unclear whether Clements meant for his library to stand on land adjacent to the President's House or to replace it.

A five-page letter from Burton to Hutchins on March 29, 1920, tells of Burton's lunch in New York City with regents Clements and Murfin who voiced approval of a $30,000 renovation expense, followed by a meeting in Detroit with Superintendent Pardon who was overseeing the renovation. The lengthy letter included details of a proposed east sun parlor, sleeping porch, boiler in place of tunnel connection, bathrooms, north porch, flooring, fireplaces, wall papers, light fixtures, and basement. Burton concluded, "I assume that the work on the house will go forward rapidly now. Believe me, sincerely yours." It seemed that one prima donna was replacing another in the old professorial residence. One letter from President Hutchins to incoming president Burton on April 1, 1920, expressed awareness of the time crunch.

> My dear President Burton:
> I have yours of March 29th with enclosures. I am sending a copy of your letter to Mr. Pardon and have an interview with him tomorrow. I shall advise him to correspond with you directly in regard to the changes you suggested. I trust that the wishes of yourself and Mrs. Burton can be fully carried out. I know that the Regents will attempt to do so.
> Work upon the house will be pushed as rapidly as possible. As you can well understand, Mr. Pardon will be embarrassed somewhat by the difficulty in securing labor and material."

Another letter from Hutchins April 22, 1920, addressed some academic matters and concluded,

> Work on the house seems to be progressing. Mr. Pardon, I am sure, is pushing it to the extent of his ability.
> With kind regards and best wishes, I remain,
> Sincerely yours,

Cabot wrote to Burton directly twice that April but didn't bring up the topic of the residence. Pardon, the building and grounds superintendent, sent a number of letters to Burton regarding the residence: one on April 26 noting the Burtons' intent to arrive by May 29 and another letter on May 4 observing that "Dr. Cabot will move on May 6."[3] Some drama likely lay behind that innocuous sentence. A letter on May 1, 1920, from University Secretary Smith to Burton, still in Minneapolis, discussed an upcoming meeting in Chicago with Dean Effinger of the College of Literature, Sciences, and the Arts, and concluded with the phrase:

> Repairs are progressing on the house as rapidly as circumstances, including Dr. Cabot's necessities, will permit, and I think the house

will surely be habitable, with doubtless some hardships to the occupants, by the first of July.

Burton, the sixth University of Michigan president and second to preside over Cabot, took office and residency occupancy in the summer of 1920. The president's home was redecorated and remodeled according to his plan with a sleeping porch and *porte cochere* (carriage porch).[4] Burton was 46 years old and like his predecessors Angell and Hutchins, he was the classic university presidential phenotype for the time. Evidently though, Burton was the most personally needy of Michigan's university presidents to that time. The men were Congregationalists and ministers by education. Burton was notably affable and persuasive and a contrast to the older and more frugal Hutchins and Secretary Smith. Burton believed the university should "spend boldly rather than conserve expediently" in order to expand and grow to fulfill the postwar public mandate for higher education.

The Cabots found local accommodations and personal correspondence shows a 2031 Hill Street address, a house built in 1915 with eight bedrooms and five baths (ultimately becoming a fraternity house in the 1950s). The worldviews of Burton and Cabot synergized well, but whereas Cabot was irascible, bullied people, and made enemies, Burton expanded his visions and beliefs to faculty, the state legislature, and donors.

Burton became university president on July 1st and his inauguration was planned for the autumn. A request to Will Mayo to attend the ceremony was respectfully declined and Mayo's letter of regret illustrated the conjoined history of genitourinary surgery, general surgery, and medical academia:

> The annual session of the Congress of the American College of Surgeons is to be held in Montreal October 11 to 15 and as President of the organization I must be there. Immediately following I am to attend a special meeting of the Boston Surgical Society in Boston, when I am to be awarded the Jacob Bigelow gold medal, an honor which I value, for this medal is given in recognition of contributions to the advancement of surgery, and I shall be the first to receive it.[5]

Burton found more than ceremonial matters on his plate that summer. No sooner than starting his presidency, Burton and his family headed back to Minnesota for vacation at Cass Lake, where he soon learned of a problem in the Homeopathic College. A Committee of Five representing the State Homeopathic Medical Society produced a critical report that instigated the resignation of Dean Hinsdale, who had held the post since 1895. A comment in Burton's correspondence from then mentions "a confidential record of telephone conversation with Dr. Hugh Cabot,

July 23, 1920." This fragment is too circumspect to understand whether the issue of concern is the homeopathic situation, the full-time plan, or some other matter that came up at the regents' meeting. It is clear, however, that alignment with Cabot mattered to Burton and they stayed in touch.

Cabot intended to build a modern surgery department and knew he also had to supply the total urological clinical expertise and teaching because Darling and Loree were both gone from the medical school by March in 1920. At this stage in his career, Cabot was heavily focused on urology and needed a full-bore general surgeon to manage the overall teaching and surgical load. This early faculty recruit, Frederick Coller, turned out to be one of his finest. As an MGH surgical resident, Coller joined Harvey Cushing's Harvard Unit that went to replace a Cleveland unit of volunteers in April 1915, at the American Hospital in France. Cushing's group included five senior surgeons (one also serving as anesthesiologist), seven house officers (including Coller), and four nurses. When the group was replaced by a Philadelphia unit at the end of June, Coller remained in Europe to join the British General Hospital No. 22, where he met Osler on his visit and perhaps because of that association, Coller later moved to the American Women's Hospital in Devon, serving from October 1915 to June 1916 when Coller returned to the United States to join his father's private surgical practice in Los Angeles. That relationship didn't last long and Coller moved to Los Angeles County Hospital to help develop its neurosurgical service. With the formal entry of the United States into World War I, Coller was commissioned in the Medical Reserve Corp and returned to France in July 1918 for field hospital work near the Western Front until April 1919. He went back to Los Angeles for another brief try at surgical private practice, until Cabot rescued him and made him assistant professor of surgery in 1920. Coller was exactly what Cabot needed throughout the rest of the decade and he would remain at Michigan long after Cabot, continuing much of the best parts of the Cabot legacy, while repairing much of the damage Cabot had incurred.

Wars perversely advance the civilian medical practice in their wakes and World War I, accordingly, advanced the devolvement of general surgery into the surgical specialties. In Ann Arbor, Cabot had urology and general surgery well covered between himself and Coller, but orthopaedics and thoracic surgery needed individual champions. LeRoy Abbott shared surgical experience on the Western Front in World War I with Cabot, Alexander, and Coller, but Abbott remained in Europe after the war, going to Edinburgh for further orthopaedic training. He became an early adapter of new surgical techniques and Cabot brought him to Ann Arbor in 1920 as assistant professor of surgery. Dissatisfaction with the full-time plan led him to leave for St. Louis Shriners Hospital in 1923 and then San Francisco, although returning often to Michigan as a visiting professor.

John Alexander also came in 1920 as assistant professor in surgery. Born in Philadelphia and educated in medicine at the University of Pennsylvania, he served in France with volunteer Americans at a French unit and transferred to the U.S. Army Medical Corps, after neutrality ended, serving until the war's end and then remaining in France to learn thoracoplasty in Lyon. Returning home briefly to the surgical staff at the University of Pennsylvania, he was quickly snapped up by Cabot.

Even amidst his busy first full year at Michigan, Cabot was expostulating strong ideas on national health care in the highly charged American political atmosphere that was fearful of socialist inclinations.[6] He relentlessly pushed his full-time salary model, was dismantling the Homeopathic College, assembling a multispecialty academic group practice, and demanding a standard of clinical excellence in everyone around him that smacked of ivory tower elitism. As Cabot was blazing new trails, a posse of enemies began forming.

Toward the end of the year, Cabot spent three days in Rochester, Minnesota, most likely as a visiting professor and as a guest of the Southern Minnesota meeting in Mankato, speaking to hundreds of physicians. While Cabot and Mayo had known each other for many years, this visit expanded their friendship and prompted Mayo to write to President Burton, complimenting Cabot's teaching, knowledge, and ideals. Mayo was specifically taken with Cabot's ideas for bettering rural medical care.

> Few doctors at the present time can be induced to engage in rural practice. The lack of modern appliances and inability to do work which satisfies the scientific conscience undoubtedly constitute the cause. There are enough doctors but badly distributed. Two quack remedies are being employed to meet the situation: First registration and licensing of low-grade peoples of various cults, osteopaths, chiropractors, etc., and second, State medicine, with its lack of scientific perspective, deterioration of medical ideals and political control. Dr. Cabot has a perfectly workable plan whereby the University, which will always be the seat of learning and culture, takes upon itself the function of seeing that rural communities are supplied with efficient medical attention, community hospitals, etc., that the lives of the most important citizens of this country, for the results of the work of the farm enable life to go on, may be protected efficiently and attractively.
>
> It is just the sort of work that you would be delighted with, and I know no one who could equal you in furthering the matter. When you have time I wish you would discuss the question with Dr. Cabot.

I should like very much to develop something of the same system in this state.

With kindest personal regards, I am

Very sincerely yours,

W. J. Mayo[7]

This letter applies just as poignantly today, 100 years later. The ideas of Cabot and Mayo regarding this larger responsibility of the university align perfectly with belief in its obligation to serve the public (public goods) that the Stenecks called the *third thread*.

The University of Michigan was on a progressive and expanding path as 1920 closed out, while the world beyond was experiencing disruptions and instabilities that would continue to grow. The description of this decade as the "roaring twenties" encapsulates the social, cultural, and economic turbulence of these times. Warren G. Harding was elected U.S. president, the first with legitimate votes from women. The Olympic symbol of interlocking rings was implemented this year. In spite of Woodrow Wilson's efforts, the U.S. Congress refused to verify the *Treaty of Versailles*, thus limiting the future of the League of Nations. A Red Scare in early 1920 resulted in the arrest of 4,025 communists and anarchists across the United States, and a Bolshevist uprising in Russia redefined that country for much of the century. Ann Arbor and the University of Michigan were not immune to these larger currents of the time.

Notes

1 *Michigan Daily*, "Special Executive Order", Ann Arbor. Friday, February 20, 1920, vol. 30, no. 97.
2 *Michigan Daily*, February 27, 1920.
3 Bentley Historical Library, University of Michigan, Burton Box 3, Cabot letters to Burton, April 26 and May 6, 1920.
4 H. H. Peckham, *The Making of the University of Michigan 1817–1992*. Edited and updated by M. L. Steneck and N. H. Steneck (Ann Arbor: University of Michigan Press, 1967, 1994), 152.
5 Bentley Historical Library, University of Michigan. Burton papers, Letter from Mayo, 1920.
6 H. Cabot, "Compulsory Health Insurance, State Medicine or What?," *Boston Medical Surgical Journal* 182 (1920): 595–601.
7 Bentley Historical Library, University of Michigan, Burton papers, Mayo letter to President Burton, December 2, 1920.

Dean Cabot, 1921

The year 1921 started off with bad news on a number of fronts: the Tulsa race riots, the Sacco and Vanzetti trial, and the rise of Adolph Hitler as Germany's Führer. Michigan's athletic peer group, the Big Ten, took a hit when the University of California, Berkeley, soundly defeated Ohio State 28–0 at the Rose Bowl. The Irish Free State was established but hardly resolved intrinsic tensions of the Emerald Island. On the positive side of the ledger, that year Einstein received the Nobel Prize in physics, insulin was discovered by Banting and Best in Toronto, and BCG vaccination began for tuberculosis. Long-standing genitourinary surgeons at the University of Michigan, Darling and Loree, had moved their private practices to St. Joseph's Mercy Hospital rendering Cabot as the sole medical school urologist. The state legislature and Burton were dismantling the Homeopathic College just as they were planning a new University Hospital and extending the full-time medical faculty model.

Cabot, meanwhile, started his second year at Michigan in good form. He traveled down to Cleveland in late January for the inaugural Clinical Society of Genito-Urinary Surgeons meeting with a dozen of the country's most prominent genitourinary surgeons including Edwin Beer, John Caulk, Arthur Chute, John Cunningham, Francis Hagner, Frank Hinman (the Hinman father), Edward L. Keyes (the Keyes son), Herman Kretschmer, William Lower (the host and chief of urology at the new Cleveland Clinic), and William Quinby. Absent according to the minutes were William Braasch, J. Bentley Squier, and Hugh Young. The main purpose of the group was to participate in surgical demonstrations to share ideas and skills of their rapidly advancing young specialty. These "operative clinics," echoed the general surgical clinics that evolved into the American College of Surgeons and were held on Friday, January 28, at Mt. Sinai Hospital in the morning and Western Reserve University Medical School in the afternoon. George Crile, not a genitourinary surgeon but a reigning authority in American surgery and one of the world's great thyroid surgeons, hosted a dinner at his home. The next morning, a Saturday, Crile was included ("by invitation," according to the program) at an operative clinic at Lakeside Hospital with demonstrations by Lower and his associates. After lunch at Lower's home, the group inspected the new clinic building.

Back in Ann Arbor, Vaughan retired as dean in 1921 after 30 years of remarkable leadership in medical education, science, and politics. When Vaughan's predecessor, Corydon Ford, resigned as dean in June 1891, the regents superseded the faculty tradition of electing their dean and directly appointed Vaughan as dean. The regents repeated their prerogative again in 1921, appointing Cabot medical school dean but not before exploring other options. Huber, Novy, Peterson, and Warthin were long-time and well-regarded members of the faculty, any of whom would have been a secure and excellent choice. During the explorations of the regents, Cabot positioned himself well for the job, working largely behind the scene without overt campaigning at least according to the visible historic record. With a new university president at the helm, plans and funding for a new hospital in place, international peace, no global plagues, and postwar confidence in play, the medical school and its new urological arena would see major changes.

Correspondence to Burton in February included a note from Cabot about public fears of "state medicine" (from "howlers of Detroit"), reminding the president that "it is teaching and not money we are after."[1] These fears may have reflected growing national anxiety about the growing spread of socialism that in 1921 was manifested in the rise of communist parties in China, Czechoslovakia, Portugal, Spain, and other nations. The multispecialty group practice Cabot was assembling at the University of Michigan may have been viewed by some ("the howlers") as a step on the path to state (socialized) medicine. In March, Burton sent letters to leaders of other universities asking for help or suggestions regarding selection of a new medical school dean. He carried the question to the April regents meeting asking whether the dean should be a clinical man, a preclinical man, a general executive, or a local-versus-outside man. *Man* was the only gender mentioned. The hospital on Catherine Street, that had opened in 1891, was functionally problematic and had been moved from control of the medical school to direct supervision by the regents under Sawyer since 1911.

The relationship of hospital to the medical school was a major concern. A straw vote by 17 medical school faculty at the time found eight opposed to continued separation from the medical school, one in favor, and no comments from seven others, including Cabot. Hospital superintendent, Dr. Parnall, was the only one in favor of separation.[i] The poll also considered both the full-time plan, with seven in favor and no comment from nine, and queried opinions regarding desired characteristics for the next dean. Four faculty (including Cabot and Parnall) favored a "clinical man," eight (including Vaughan) wanted a preclinical person, and five preferred a "general executive." Eleven faculty stated a preference for a local candidate, four wanted an outside person, and two had no preference. Cabot was present at the April regents meeting where these issues were discussed but he was quiet on the separation issue, presumably saving his impact to support the following discussion on his full-time plan, where the faculty straw vote showed seven in favor and no comment from nine. It appears that no one dared to speak against Cabot's cherished full-time plan so early in his tenure or else the leaders were ambivalent, although the latter seems unlikely.[2]

The selection of a new dean was a high priority for the medical school in 1921 and Regent Sawyer and President Burton took charge of the issue. Burton wrote leading medical schools and received names for consideration including Will Mayo, two faculty from Johns Hopkins, and Cabot. Mayo sent two letters to Burton in April but did not offer himself for the job. Novy and Huber from the Michigan faculty also had considerable support. A letter from Burton to President Goodnow at Johns Hopkins on March 29 revealed,

> We are committed to the full time plan and pushing the new hospital. . . . In regard to salary, I think we are in a position to offer a reasonable remuneration. While Dean Vaughan's salary has only been only $7,500 we confidently assume that we shall have to pay more for his successor. The present Superintendent of the hospital is receiving $12,500 and Dr. Cabot on full-time is receiving $15,000.[3]

A letter from Burton to President Hadley at Yale on April 11 brought up the idea of combining the dean and hospital superintendent positions, recognizing that this would require a rare skill set:

> just one man in the country that I think might be interested in that type of work and who would also commend himself to a medical faculty.

---

i Christopher Gregg Parnall (some records spell his name "Parnell") graduated from UM in 1902 and the medical school in 1904. He served the school in the Department of Obstetrics and Gynecology and became medical superintendent of the hospital in 1918, resigning in 1924.

Subsequent correspondence suggests that Burton was not thinking of Cabot in that regard. Sawyer wrote to Burton a few days later asking him to "secure a dean distinguished in medicine and with executive ability" and that "full-time for the heads of all clinical chairs should be our object." Burton asked Johns Hopkins associate professor Thomas Boggs by letter on May 2 to discuss "the medical situation here at the University

Burton's letter to Thomas Boggs concerning a prospective visit.

of Michigan" with himself and Sawyer on their anticipated visit to Baltimore May 11.[4] [On previous page: Burton's letter to Boggs.]

Charles de Nancrede died in April 1921 and the University of Michigan's *Encyclopedic Survey* recorded, "He died in Detroit in 1921, leaving, as do most physicians, little tangible evidence of the great service he had rendered to humanity." Warthin, Peterson, and Lloyd wrote de Nancrede's memorial and it was read to the faculty senate.[5]

In May, the dean and regent visited Johns Hopkins, Yale, and interviewed a candidate in New York at the Commodore Hotel. A letter from a highly placed Hopkins leader to Burton supported two Hopkins faculty but said of the one who was a pathologist, the "only thing that can be said against him is his race," although noting that the man mixed well with gentiles.[6] Dr. Welch, however, separately voiced strong support for the impugned pathologist. A private letter from Vaughan to Burton supported Novy for dean. Interestingly, few prominent external authorities recommended Cabot. Huber as well as Novy had much support among faculty in addition to Vaughan's private preference for either of the two as expressed in a letter to his son Warren Vaughan on November 18, 1920.[7] A number of other faculty offered several names, including Cabot's. Cowie recommended Cabot and Wile from Michigan and Harvey Cushing from the Peter Bent Brigham Hospital in Boston. Cowie noted, regarding his recommendations, "but it would be unfortunate to disturb either in their practice and very consuming work."[8]

J. G. Van Zwaluwenburg also recommended Cabot to Burton with the qualification, "but I fear his unfortunate temperament."[9] Van Zwaluwenburg (UMMS 1908) had joined the faculty under Dock and would develop cardiac roentgenology with Dock's successor, Albion Hewlett. Cabot reciprocated the respect of Van Zwaluwenburg, describing him as, "Lean, lank, and uncouth in appearance, there was nothing either lean or uncouth about his personality." Hospitalized for pneumonia at University Hospital the following January, Van Zwaluwenburg died a few days later at 48 years of age.[10] Professor L. H. Newburgh, with Harvard Medical School and MGH roots, also recommended Cabot, endorsing his full-time plan and an end to the separation of the hospital and medical school.[11] Wile also backed Cabot, which is surprising given their differing thoughts on private practice. Burton moved expeditiously and brought Cabot's name to the regents, and they appointed him dean effective July 1, 1921.

Medical politics had demanded much attention from the new president, given that Dean Vaughan had been well past his prime in attention and energy. Burton had more on his plate than the medical school in 1921 and must have hoped that Cabot as a strong new dean would shield him from the quotidian medical school issues. One notable innovation of Burton's at the time was the launch of a fellowship in creative art with its own "full-time salary." Robert Frost was the first appointee and a gift from Chase Osborne (1860–1949), former regent (1908–1911) and Michigan governor (1911–1913), financed the program at the start. Nevertheless, Burton could never keep far from the medical school.

Cabot first addressed the faculty as dean when the medical school term opened and after sincere deference to Victor Vaughan identified a vision of the three main teaching audiences of medical schools: undergraduates (meaning medical students), "graduate physicians and the advancement of the boundaries of medical knowledge," and the "teaching of the public in matters of public health and health policy and assisting in working out the relation of physicians and hospitals to the people of the state." The address was printed in the state medical society journal.[12]

The full-time (salary model) that had enticed de Nancrede to Ann Arbor 30 years earlier was contested by many faculty, but Burton, the regents, and Cabot held firm to it. The plan was effective at the start when Cabot recruited Frederick Coller, Leroy Abbott, and John Alexander to the Surgery Department. These men became major forces in defining their emerging subspecialties, but Cabot had no compulsion to bring in another urologist. At the time, his text, *Modern Urology* of 1918, was the latest and most authoritative book in the field and it was logical that he didn't immediately need a competitive authority in the field but rather a proper disciple before long.

In spite of the machinations over the deanship and its new responsibilities, Cabot found time to advocate his strong clinical beliefs. A speech in early June to the Michigan Hospital Association, meeting in Ann Arbor, "urged avoidance of psychological damage in the case of patients admitted to hospitals." University Hospital director C. G. Parnall was also serving as president of the Michigan Hospital Association. Cabot's public remarks sometimes included prejudicial stereotypes that offended some stakeholders and his speech to the hospital association was emblematic:

> "In the war, one constantly saw well men the victims of suggested diseases and injuries, suffered by their companions in arms," said Dr. Cabot, who was himself in charge for a time of the medical corps of the British expeditionary forces. "Especially was that true of the French soldier, no less brave than the British soldier, but less stolid, more impressionable. The most frequent suggested disease, was paralysis."[13]

Cabot carried his academic duties beyond Ann Arbor and the *urology brand of the University of Michigan*, for the first time in its history, entered into robust national and international conversations. In Halifax that year, he spoke on "the doctrine of the prepared soil: a neglected factor in surgical infection," a phrase that would echo through his successors at Michigan for the next century.[14] The *Detroit Free Press* reported, on June 8, 1921, "Dr. Hugh Cabot sees need of psychological safeguards for patients," reflecting his worry about the mental health of his hospitalized patients, especially those affected by the war. In October, he was an honored guest at the first annual meeting of South Central section in Kansas City and spoke on "the management of some renal and ureteral calculi."[15] Every appearance broadened the reputation and influence of the University of Michigan, the medical school, and their national impact in general surgery and urology. The *Michigan Daily* reported his advocacy of bringing private patients ("pay clinics") to the University Hospital and its facilities on November 5, 1921:

> So long as the state charity patients receive the same careful attention that they have heretofore received, I see no reason on earth why we should not conduct this pay clinic in connection with our hospital.[16]

This was a contentious issue at the time. Many people in the state, particularly physicians in private practice, viewed the University Hospital as a public good, supported by taxpayers, but now with Cabot in charge it was unfairly competing economically with them.

Duties as dean added to Cabot's work and expectations. A Department of Pediatrics was established this year in the medical school, extracting that discipline from the Department of Medicine, where pediatrics had been taught and practiced since at least 1890. A gift from the widow of Alonzo Palmer in 1901 had provided Michigan's first building for children's care, opening in 1903, although the structure also encompassed other endeavors for much of its long history. David Murray Cowie, a disciple of William Osler, was Michigan's first instructor in pediatrics (1905) and became the longtime pediatric teacher, clinician, and researcher at the university. Cowie had established his own private hospital in 1912 and, with Reuben Peterson, developed the university's Contagious Hospital, opened in 1914. In spite of Cabot's affinity for children's surgery, he would frequently clash as dean with Cowie over budget matters for the Pediatrics Department.

A letter from Regent Clements to Cabot in October (on the next page) is typical of the requests for special consideration in terms of admittance to educational programs or faculty hiring that come with leadership in academia. This request was a mild prelude to feverish contortions of parents to secure educational opportunities at elite universities for their children a century later.

Dean Cabot, 1921

Letter of recommendation to Dean Cabot. Bentley Library.

The state legislature passed a resolution in 1921 carefully "advising" the university to consolidate its medical school and Homeopathic College, in the interest of "economy," and it discontinued the long-standing homeopathic appropriation. Homeopathic supporters protested strongly at a public hearing with Dean Hinsdale of the Homeopathic College, but the legislative advice prevailed and over the next year Burton reached out to other major universities to see how they viewed homeopathic medicine (below).

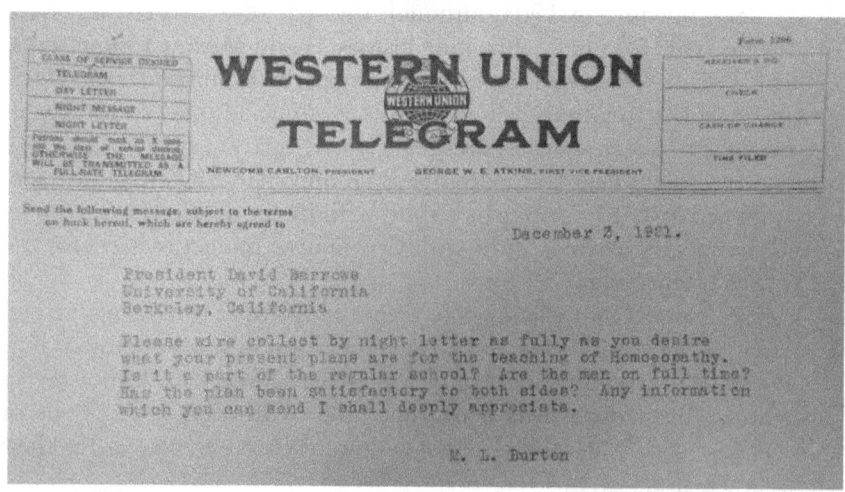

Telegram from Burton to President David Barrows of University of California, December 3, 1921. Bentley Library.

Notes

1 Bentley Historical Library, University of Michigan, Burton Box 1, Note from Cabot to Burton, February 1921.
2 Bentley Historical Library, University of Michigan, Burton Box 3, Folders 1, 2.
3 Bentley Historical Library, University of Michigan, Marion Burton Papers Box 3, Letter from Burton to President Goodnow at Johns Hopkins, March 29, 1921.
4 Bentley Historical Library, University of Michigan, Illustration: Burton to Boggs.
5 A. S. Warthin, R. Peterson, and A. H. Lloyd, "Charles Beylard Guerard de Nancrede 1847–1921," *Michigan Alumnus* 27 (1921): 567, 570, 573; D. A. Bloom, G. Uznis, and D. A. Campbell, "Charles B. G. de Nancrede: Academic Surgeon at the fin de siècle," *World Journal of Surgery* 22 (1998) 11: 1175–1181.
6 Bentley Historical Library, University of Michigan, Burton Box 3, W. G. MacCallum to Burton, May 13, 1921.
7 Bentley Historical Library, University of Michigan, TN8122 BN-726-N UM Medical School records 1850-2010 (N-Z) Box 35 folder T,U,V,W,X,Y,Z. Victor Vaughan Letter to son Warren Vaughan, November 18, 1920.
8 Bentley Historical Library, University of Michigan, Burton Box 3, Cowie, April, 25, 1921.
9 Bentley Historical Library, University of Michigan, Burton Box 3, J. G. Van Zwaluwenburg, April 21, 1921.
10 J. Tobin, "X-Ray Vision," *Medicine at Michigan* 21, no. 1 (2019): 50–51.
11 Bentley Historical Library, University of Michigan, Burton Box 3, L. H. Newburgh, April 25, 1921.
12 Bentley Historical Library, University of Michigan. Burton papers; H. Cabot, "Address of the Dean at the Opening of the Medical School—University of Michigan," *Journal of Michigan State Medical Society* 20 (1921): 431–435.
13 "Avoid Hospital Shock, His Plea," *Detroit Free Press*, June 8, 1921.
14 H. Cabot, "The Doctrine of the Prepared Soil: A Neglected Factor in Surgical Infection," *Canadian Medical Association Journal* 11 (1921): 610–614.
15 L. W. Jones, P. C. Peters, W. C. Husser, *American Urological Association Centennial History* (American Urological Assn Inc, 2002), 275.
16 "Cabot Describes Pay-Clinic's Aim," The *Michigan Daily*, November 5, 1921.

Hugh Cabot, 1922–1926

Cabot, 1922

For Cabot, now chief of the Department of Surgery and dean of the Medical School, matters of medical education and clinical care remained a priority and he never succumbed to becoming primarily an administrator. He was quick to recognize new roles for emerging technology in practice and teaching. He brought motion picture technology to the medical school, as the *Detroit Free Press* reported on March 22, 1922: "Film surgery to aid classes: U of M first in world to get projection machine for operation study." It is unlikely that the University of Michigan was truly the first in the world to film surgery, but that's beside the point that Cabot was an early adaptor. Furthermore, Cabot distained gratuitous observers in the operating room.

> The practice of having medical students present at operations is a very ancient but a very inefficient method of teaching surgery as no one but the surgeon himself and his assistants can see what he is doing.[1]

The Homeopathic College was dissolved on June 30, 1922, although the medical school continued two elective courses in homeopathy for a time. Dean Hinsdale resigned and went over to the Museum of Anthropology to pursue Indian archeology for another 22 years of service to the university.[2] As an ideology-based program, homeopathy had no legitimate standing at a public university school, but its disassembly left hard feelings throughout the state. Ironically, its initial inclusion and later dissolution were directed by the unseemly (and unconstitutional) meddling of the state legislature.

The full-time faculty continued to receive two salaries, one from the medical school and another from the hospital, based on professional fee collection and hospital revenue. A strong dean, Cabot, leveraged his efforts toward the educational and clinical sides of the triple mission more than to laboratory investigation, although it cannot be said that he was "not academic." He resurrected the medical school thesis, requiring a 5,000-word text with bibliography: "designed to make the student conversant with the methods that are useful in preparing the subject for publication."[3]

An article in the *Detroit Free Press*, November 5, reported an interview with Cabot's wife Mary, who explained her intention to open a "tiny tea shop." The subheading of the article read,

> Mrs. Hugh Cabot tires of social life and decides to enter business. Wants to do something which is worth while, she tells interviewer.

The author noted a recent trend of "women of the British aristocracy" and "American women of considerable social position" to do something more than the "entertaining and being entertained" typical of academic social life:

> But until this fall, Michigan faculty women have not ventured the step, although several have made no secret of the fact that business has its appeal, and that mere social life paled upon them. The war, of course, is blamed. It has been rather hard for many of them to go back to the old order, now that war is over, and the need for their services outside the home ended.

The interviewer asked, "Is Dr. Cabot proud of his wife's ambition, and is he pleased?" "Just about as pleased as a bear with a sore paw," the writer answered personally, revealing that Cabot himself had been sitting nearby quietly in the room: "Dr. Cabot smiles a crooked smile, and says nothing," which translated means "We'll wait and see."[4]

Mrs. Cabot opened her tea shop and called it the Cosy Corner Tea Room on November 22, 1922. It was at 330 Maynard Street across from Nickels Arcade and as reported in the *Michigan Daily* was "known to all Ann Arbor residents." The owner was described as "one of the most efficient and successful tea room managers."[5] Mrs. Cabot needed help to run the shop, which became more than a tea room, in that it served lunch and dinners seven days a week.

Cabot, 1923

Faculty recruitment, retention, and replacement occupied much of Cabot's attention, a common experience for most medical deans of the time and equally so a century later. Cabot's first big problem of the year involved Warren Plimpton Lombard, a great physiologist yet "an intolerably dull teacher," who announced intention to retire at the end of the term, later in the year. In January, Cabot created a search committee of C. W. Edmunds, F. G. Novy, and H. B. Lewis. By May, Cabot had recruited Robert Gesell from Washington University.[6]

The Homeopathic College issue persisted. Burton, worried if the university had taken the right direction and perhaps second-guessing his decision to close the college, continued to query other universities by letter to

23 of them on March 1 to see if they had such programs. Three schools responded that they had discontinued homeopathic programs (Iowa, Nebraska, and Minnesota). Northwestern noted that a homeopathic school had sought to join the university but was denied. The University of California School on Parnassus Avenue had taken over "a Hahnemann program" and told Burton that even though its homeopathic program was not presenting any immediate problems, the university would be fine if it dissolved. The remaining 19 universities including Columbia, Penn, Charlottesville, Kansas, Harvard, Missouri, Johns Hopkins, Yale, Wisconsin, and Missouri gave emphatic responses of "never" having homeopathic instruction. Princeton noted that it avoided the issue entirely by having no medical program of any sort.

Ann Arbor was the site of the Thirty-Third Annual Meeting of the Association of American Medical Colleges on March 2 and 3, with Michigan Union serving as headquarters. The locations of national organizational meetings are usually deliberate choices, and the situation of this particularly significant program at the University of Michigan Medical School reflected Vaughan's long-standing influence in the organization as

Referred to in Diary March 2, 1923   Exhibit

Program

of the

Thirty-third Annual Meeting

of the

Association of
American Medical Colleges

to be held at

Ann Arbor, Michigan

MARCH 2 and 3, 1923

HEADQUARTERS
MICHIGAN UNION

AAMC Annual Meeting 1923, Ann Arbor. Bentley Library, Sawyer Box 5. Letters March 1, 1923.

well as Cabot's celebrity as a surgeon, urologist, and newly as a medical educator. Cabot, in the opening session, presented the *Report of Committee on Education and Pedagogics*. The opening session program gives an indication of the issues of concern to medical education at the time (below).

> March 2, 9:30 A. M.
>
> PRESIDENT'S ADDRESS: *The Moral Qualifications of the Medical Student.*
> > C. P. EMERSON, Dean Indiana University School of Medicine.
>
> *Problems of the Two Year Medical School.*
> > HARLEY E. FRENCH, Dean University of North Dakota School of Medicine.
>
> *Four Years in Medicine.*
> > THOMAS ORDWAY, Dean Albany Medical College.
>
> *The Teaching Hospital.*
> > CHARLES N. MEADER, Dean University of Colorado School of Medicine.
>
> *Shall a Fifth or Intern Year Be Required for the M.D. Degree and for Admission to the Licensing Examination?*
> > AUGUSTUS S. DOWNING, Assistant Commissioner of Education of New York.
>
> *The Place of Anatomy in the Medical Curriculum.*
> > WM. S. KEILLER, Acting Dean University of Texas Department of Medicine.
>
> *Shall the Premedical Requirement Be Increased?*
> > THEODORE HOUGH, Dean University of Virginia Department of Medicine.
>
> *The Medical Curriculum.*
> > Report of the Committee on Education and Pedagogics. Presented by HUGH CABOT, Chairman.

AAMC first morning program, March 2, 1923.

Cabot argued for curricular reform,

> Your committee believes that sounder and, so to speak, rounder development of students will take place with a lesser amount of assigned teaching, giving more time for general outside reading not

necessarily of a medical character, for exercise and, perchance, for contemplation. We think that there is evidence that on the present system of what might be called "forced feeding," considerable intellectual indigestion has resulted and that students come to the later years of their medical course intellectually fagged.[7]

He submitted a curricular plan for four years encompassing 3,600 to 4,400 hours of assigned or supervised work. General surgery instruction included components of urology in addition to orthopaedic surgery, ophthalmology, otolaryngology, and roentgenology. [Below: from the Program of the 33rd AAMC meeting. Bentley Library, Sawyer Box 5. Letters March 1, 1923.]

Required schedule hours in 4 calendar years
3600 - 4400 distributed as 900 - 1100 hours per year.

1.	Anatomy including Embryology and Histology	14 - 18%
2.	Physiology	4½ - 6%
3.	Biochemistry	3½ - 4½%
4.	Pathology, Bacteriology and Immunology	10 - 13%
5.	Pharmacology	4 - 5%
6.	Hygiene and Sanitation	3 - 4%
7.	General Medicine	
	Neurology and Psychiatry	
	Pediatrics	
	Dermatology and Syphilis	20 - 26½%
8.	General Surgery	13 - 17½%
	Orthopedic Surgery	
	Urology	
	Ophthalmology	
	Otolaryngology	
	Roentgenology	
9.	Obstetrics and Gynecology	4 - 5%
		76 - 100%
	Electives	25 - 0%

Cabot's UMMS curriculum 1923.

Dissatisfaction with the salary models persisted within the faculty. Udo Wile, professor of dermatology with a salary of $4,000 per year, complained to Cabot of the need to supplement the salary by seeing patients on nights and during weekends and proposed to Burton that similar "part time men" should be allocated beds at the University Hospital for their private patients.[8] Insufficiency of the full-time salary prompted orthopaedic specialist Abbott to leave this year, after only three years in Ann Arbor. He was replaced by his former trainee, Carl Badgley (UMMS 1919), who would leave in 1929 but return in 1932. Fluidity among the emerging subspecialty lines and perhaps ultimate confidence in the skills of certain surgical generalists such as Coller, explain the referral of a Detroit patient, who had written to Dean Cabot the previous September requesting an orthopaedic specialist, to Coller.[i]

The death in 1923 of Detroit iron industrialist Thomas Henry Simpson due to pernicious anemia gave Cabot a big opportunity, after Mrs. Simpson offered the university nearly a half million dollars for a hematology research building. Another death that year had larger national impact when, on August 2, President Warren G. Harding died in San Francisco during a speaking tour. Vice president Calvin Coolidge was awakened at his family home in Vermont by reporters to learn of the death, whereupon Coolidge's father, a justice of the peace and notary public, administered the oath of office at 2:47 AM on August 23, by kerosene lamp. The new president then went back to bed, but a chain of events would soon extend to the University of Michigan.

The *Detroit Free Press* saw fit to report in September that Hugh Cabot, Jr., was taking entrance exams for Harvard College, evidence that the Cabot children were living in Ann Arbor, and that this family was newsworthy.[9] In an interview published in the *Los Angeles Times* on December 13, titled "Men teachers are preferred," Cabot observed that women might be as good as men teachers, "but they should know they'll be responsible for undesirable students." He was implying that the disciplinary side of their job might be more than they might expect, with perhaps a hint that they might not be up to the task.[10]

Cabot, 1924

On February 6, 1924, a letter to Regent Sawyer from former dean Vaughan repeated a claim from hospital superintendent Parnall that Cabot's fees of around $1,000 per month could continue to support the "full time plan." Clements noted Cabot's "strong personality" was like that of Will Mayo (UMMS 1883) and suggested Cabot's salary "must be materially increased." It is likely that Cabot was doing some effective

---

i The requestor, McCotter, was likely related to UM anatomy professor Rollo Eugene McCotter. Bentley Library, September 19, 1922. UM Medical School Records 1850–2010, Box 35, Folder AtB1922.

personal lobbying to the regents going around the president to at least one of them. The question of having the hospital continue to report directly to the regents or returning it to Medical School supervision was raised again and likely it was Cabot who raised it. On February 16, 1924, Sawyer wrote a number of other medical schools regarding the reporting relationships of their hospitals and received replies from 13 including Minnesota, Montreal, Iowa, University of Chicago, Harvard, Johns Hopkins, New York's Mt. Sinai, and San Francisco. Responses were mixed, not surprisingly given the idiosyncratic situations inherent to each school and proving once again the familiar adage, "if you see one academic medical center, you've seen just one."

Spring 1924 was a terrible time for the Cabot family. Mrs. Cabot had taken 16-year-old daughter Mary on a round-the-world cruise through the Panama Canal and across the Pacific but in April the *Boston Globe* reported,

> Miss Cabot and her mother sailed from New York last Jan 15 on a cruise around the world, going through the Panama Canal, across the Pacific Ocean and touching at various Oriental ports. While in India the girl became seriously ill and her father, now identified with the University of Michigan Medical School, was notified by cable of her condition.
>
> Mrs. Cabot succeeded in getting her daughter to Naples, where she had been for the past three weeks at the International Hospital, but various complications, including bronchial pneumonia, had set in, and it was impossible to save her life. Dr. Cabot sailed for Naples the last week in April, arriving there in time to meet his wife and daughter on their arrival from the Orient.[11]

The *Michigan Daily* announced the story on its front page (below). Mary was cremated and her remains placed in the Cabot family plot in Brookline.

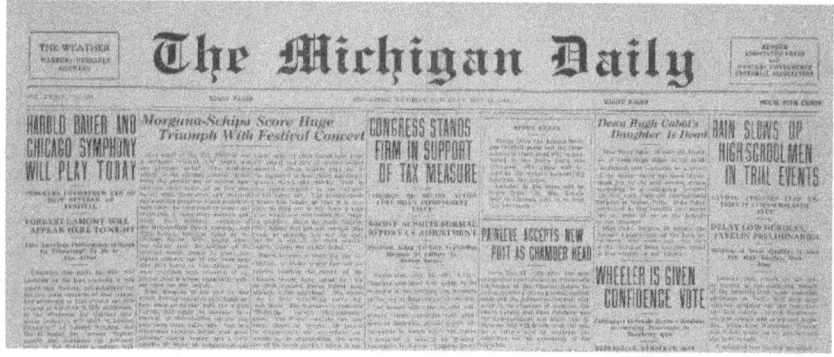

Hugh Cabot's daughter Mary dies on cruise. *Michigan Daily*, May 24, 1924.

It was a proud moment for Ann Arbor and the University in June 1924, when UM president Burton made the nominating speech for Calvin Coolidge at the Republican National Convention in Cleveland, Ohio, on June 10–12, and Coolidge was elected on the first ballot. Burton was mentioned as a potential running mate, among others, but ultimately Coolidge favored Herbert Hoover. It took the university community by surprise when Burton suffered a heart attack in October, four months after his speech, and angina confined him to bed for the rest of the year. Coolidge won the election and Burton died the following February at 51 years of age.

The surgery training program attracted promising new interns to Ann Arbor, in response to Cabot and Coller's influence, and anticipation of the new hospital. Charles Huggins was one of the first new trainees, arriving in Ann Arbor in the summer after completing Harvard Medical School. While Coller heavily influenced this stage of Huggins' education, the young man became the first Michigan trainee to develop a urology career under the stamp of Cabot. After leaving Michigan as an instructor in surgery from 1926 to 1927, Huggins went to the University of Chicago. Huggins was also the first Cabot trainee to lead a urology department and the only one to achieve one of the highest accolades of mankind, the Nobel Prize.

Ethylene anesthesia was introduced to Ann Arbor in September 1924 and had significant advantages, although it could be very explosive in certain conditions. Laura Davis Dunstone, instructor in pharmacology who had worked with de Nancrede, was the main authority and resource for anesthesiology at Michigan and when Cabot arrived, she was using mixtures of nitrous oxide, oxygen, and ether. Ethylene was a big advance and Cabot favored the new agent but with strict precautions that not everyone among his faculty followed. Cabot could not resist implementing a technical advance and then writing about it, and accordingly wrote a paper on anesthesia this year with Dunstone.[12] Clinical faculty unkindly blocked Cabot's efforts to include registered nurse Dunstone in their clinical departments, but she loyally remained at UM. Her appointment was finally transferred from the Department of Pharmacology to the Department of Surgery in 1934 and she retired in July 1938.

Cabot produced a second edition of *Modern Urology* this year, solidifying his claim to clinical authority and academic prominence. Without access to his calendar or other means of knowing how he apportioned his daily work, it's difficult to understand how he managed to put this book together, corralling the multiple authors, reading their chapters, writing his own parts, and assembling the two volumes, given his multiple other responsibilities. Yet, this had to have been easier than the first edition, produced during Cabot's overseas service during World War I. The new edition, also in two volumes, of *Modern Urology in Original Contributions by American Authors* was described on its title page as "Second Edition, Thoroughly Revised." Like its predecessor, it was dedicated to his late cousin: "Dedicated to the memory of Arthur Tracy Cabot to whose skill and integrity as a surgeon and to whose wisdom, gentleness and force of character I desire to express my debt of gratitude." The preface explained the timing and the authors that Cabot selected:

> The five years which have elapsed since the appearance of the first edition have brought no peace to those who would keep abreast of this department of surgery. Revision has become inevitable. It is to be regretted that changes have had to be made in the list of contributors, but death is no respecter of persons. Walter J. Dodd has joined the long and still lengthening list of martyrs to the development of the science of roentgenology, and the sudden death of Paul Pilcher has deprived us of a sound and respected colleague.
>
> In order to avoid great increase in the size of the volumes it has been found necessary to omit the "Historical Sketch of Genitourinary Surgery in America," by F. S. Watson. This has perhaps served its purpose in forming a background to the first edition, but nevertheless we, in company with many readers, shall miss this brilliant essay by its distinguished author.
>
> I wish to express my appreciation of the complete cooperation of my many colleagues in revising their Chapters.
>
> Hugh Cabot.
> Ann Arbor, Mich., 1924.[13]

One wishes a time machine to discover how and when he put this work together, cajoled his contributors, and penned or dictated his own three chapters in Volume II: "Stone in the Bladder," "Foreign Bodies in the Bladder," and "Stone in the Kidney and Ureter." The only other author with as many as three chapters was Hugh Hampton Young who produced "Cancer of the Prostate," "Sarcoma of the Prostate," and "Calculus Disease of the Prostate." Young was undoubtedly working simultaneously on his own textbook that would appear two years later. *Modern Urology* was well received in its field and attracted favorable attention outside urology, as with a favorable review in the *American Journal of Obstetrics and Gynecology*. The reviewer complimented Cabot: "The smooth and continuous text, from twenty-seven well-known contributors, gives evidence of careful editorial supervision," faulting only the absence of coverage of vesicovaginal fistula.[14]

William Mayo (UMMS class, 1883) and Cabot were more than passing acquaintances. Both were leaders of American surgery and they shared the commonality of the Midwest and the University of Michigan. For some reason, 1924 was the year Mayo picked to give a gift to Cabot's Surgery Department to establish an annual lecture in a "subject closely related to surgery." Mayo offered to give the first few lectures himself to allow the fund to accumulate.

Other notable events that year in Ann Arbor included the planning of the Thomas Henry Simpson Research Building. This year the university joined TIAA.[ii] This program had been set up by the Carnegie Foundation in 1918 to attract and retain faculty in the professoriate. At this time salaries were $2,200–$2,600 for assistant professors, $2,700–$3,000 for associates, and $3,200–$6,500 for professors, the higher ranges going to law professors. The range for deans was $6,250–$7,500. Tensions persisted in the medical school regarding full- and part-time salaries and the differential between income in the private practice sector.

Cabot, 1925

The Cabot home on Hill Street must have seemed empty after young Mary's death.[15] Cabot was immersed in his work as dean, chief of surgery, and national visibility.

On January 23, 1925, Cabot addressed the University of Colorado School of Medicine and Colorado General Hospital at the dedication of a new building. The talk offered a wide view of academic medicine and was printed in *Colorado Medicine* with the title "Organized Clinical Teaching." Cabot first praised the state and university, recognizing the importance of their provision of context and resources for medical education.

> This school has at its back the atmosphere and power of the university as is yet so constructed as to place at the disposal of the student all of the necessary component parts in a well balanced medical curriculum.

He contrasted German and British systems:

> The great strength of the German contribution in medicine was, in the earlier day, in the medical sciences and from these the clinical teaching was an outgrowth added gradually and piecemeal as time

---

ii TIAA – Teachers Insurance and Annuity Association of America – College Retirement Equities Fund was founded in 1918. Its conservative investing strategy helped it survive the 1929 stock market crash and the Great Depression and matched a 5 percent for retirement contribution of faculty with another 5 percent from the university.

went on. . . . In Great Britain during a somewhat similar period, the outstanding development was on the clinical side and the epoch making figures in British medicine were essentially clinicians. . . . It is not more than fifty years since all of the teachers in the medical schools of this country [the U.S.A.] either were or had been clinicians. I can, myself, remember the days at Harvard when anatomy and physiology were taught by Oliver Wendell Holmes, long a practitioner of medicine and co-discoverer with Semmelweis of the origin of puerperal fever.

Michigan's dean didn't quite get it right with Holmes and Semmelweis, who were years apart in their observations. Cabot argued for a hybrid "American System" of clinical teaching that combined the German reliance on science and discovery with the British focus on the patient "not so much as an experimental animal, but rather as a human individual." He offered thoughts on the "full time" plan as well as the potential of American democracy to build better models of medical schools and health care.[16] Cabot's lofty thoughts notwithstanding, he didn't leave clinical urology behind at this time in his career, discussing catheter cystitis in an article for Michigan's medical journal around the same time.[17]

Cabot understood the British system through his service in the BEF alongside English physicians during the war and his close friendship with Sir Holburt Waring (1866–1953) who became dean at St. Bartholomew's in London. Cabot visited St. Bart's on several occasions later. Further opportunity came with a two-week visiting professorship in 1925 at the legendary hospital and medical school. From this tour came a relationship that brought exceptional British surgeons-in-training to Ann Arbor. These men, Basil Hume, Rupert Corbett, Arthur Visick, Herbert J. Seddon, Norman Capener, and Henry Philbrick Nelson, became leading general surgeons, orthopaedists, and thoracic surgeons after returning home.

Corbett and Coller became close friends and the training exchange continued well after Cabot's era in Ann Arbor. When John O'Connell of St. Bart's became a Rockefeller scholar in the United States in 1936, he came to Ann Arbor to visit Max Peet before returning as neurosurgeon at Bart's, where he carried out the first separation of conjoined twins joined cranially. Coller's memoir mentions one British rotator "was a man called Nelson, an inspiring thoracic surgeon, who died at an early age from septicemia following a cut during an autopsy." Ironically, nearly a century after Oliver Wendell Holmes gave evidence in Boston regarding the germ theory and prevention of septicemia by handwashing, as Cabot mentioned in his Colorado talk, and a half century after Lister in Great

Britain proved that carbolic acid irrigation could further minimize transmission of disease, the old ways persisted.[iii,18]

A modern hospital was long overdue in Ann Arbor. The education and research missions of the Medical School needed an appropriate milieu to fulfill Michigan's aspirations to be world class in medical education and medical care. Planning and funding had been in place for a decade, before Cabot and Burton brought the new hospital to completion. The massive facility provided over 1,000 beds that allowed Cabot to build a world-class clinical faculty to provide, teach, and innovate in the growing range of specialty care. Cabot's surgical services had 10 large operating rooms, four of which had galleries for observers, although Cabot discouraged the traditional and gratuitous medical student observation of surgical procedures unless students were part of a specific team. Additionally, the operating suite included two smaller operating rooms and space for the growing ancillary services. The surgical services had eight wards, each with 50 beds, and the hospital also allowed 75 beds for private patients shared among surgeons and all other faculty.

Burton's death came on February 9. In his short tenure, he doubled the university's income and expanded the physical plant with new buildings, in addition to the substantial changes to the president's house. President Emeritus Hutchins was called back to sign the February diplomas and Dean Alfred Lloyd of the Graduate School was named acting president.[19] A committee of three regents (Clements, Beal, Sawyer) and three professors selected by Senate Council (Huber, Reeve, Sadler) began to search for a presidential successor. A list of more than 45 names came to the committee and less than 10 made it to the second round of consideration.[20] The university selected Clarence Little, a biologist and president of the University of Maine, although in that role only for the three previous years. At Michigan he was given $15,000 a year, with $2,000 for living and entertainment and $5,000 to continue his laboratory. At 36 years of age Little was now Cabot's third university president, but the first with commonality with Cabot, both having been New England and Harvard men.

---

iii Henry Nelson, a New Zealander, was one of the most remarkable of these young trainees and "in America he was regarded as by far the most brilliant." Nelson was educated in England at Marrow and Caius College, Cambridge, then St. Bartholomew's Hospital and Medical School where he became interested in thoracic surgery. He became an instructor under John Alexander at the University of Michigan for a year, after Cabot had left, before returning to St. Bart's and the Brompton Chest Hospital. During the course of work back in England in 1936, he cut his left index finger and developed a virulent streptococcal infection, requiring an amputation above the elbow. Nonetheless, the infection became generalized and he died of streptococcal sepsis on June 24 at age 34, leaving a wife, children, and immensely saddened colleagues as evidenced by comments in the *British Medical Journal*; J. E. H. Reynolds, "Obituary," *British Medical Journal*, July 4, 1936.

During Burton's five years, Hugh Cabot introduced the University of Michigan to new paradigms that disrupted and transformed the medical school, its hospital, and the University of Michigan. Many of Cabot's changes were out of step with his contemporaries and times, and his personality and leadership style added to the growing backdraft that would limit his time at Michigan to little more than a decade.

Cabot found his way into newspaper coverage better than most chairs of surgery and deans. The *Michigan Daily* front page on April 21, 1925, headlined, "Faculty-Student Debate Held on Athletic System," where Cabot defended the role of athletics in college life, while other faculty members and students resolved that "intercollegiate athletics in their present form are objectionable and should be materially modified." The subheadline said, "Cabot lauds fellowship of athletics, cites examples of later success."[21]

James Bruce, whom Cabot had brought from Saginaw as director of internal medicine and the hospital medical service, would become a formidable adversary. Cabot gave Bruce no professorial title, reserving that for Preston Hickey, until then professor of radiology. Cabot seemed to disdain internists, even though brother Richard was one, and mainly brought Bruce on board to manage internal medicine administratively and to improve relations with state-wide Michigan physicians.[22] Bruce would soon become the inaugural head of a Department of Postgraduate Medical Education that would expand that "third strand" of public goods, carrying medical education beyond the undergraduate and graduate levels to clinical practitioners in what came to be called *continuing medical education*. This had been one of the three educational targets Cabot mentioned in his inaugural address as dean.

Reed Miller Nesbit made the journey from California by train to Ann Arbor in the summer of 1925 to train under Cabot and Coller, and he would develop a urologic career that paralleled that of his co-trainee, Huggins, in lifetime achievement. Nesbit, an MD from Stanford's medical school and a seasoned intern from Fresno County Hospital, reported for duty to a new hospital administrator Harley Haynes on August 1 and learned he would be sharing a room with Huggins. Both young men experienced the routine surgical training experience largely under Coller's aegis, but Cabot's urological practice affected Nesbit more strongly.

The dedication for the new University Hospital on November 19 featured UMMS graduate William Mayo, who had telegraphed his friend Cabot saying he would be glad to stay the day after the ceremony if tickets to the Michigan-Minnesota football game could be found. Mayo got his tickets and Michigan won.

History offers no clues about Cabot's reading habits, but his background and his writing suggest he was well-read, and as a Michigan faculty member he must have been aware of Sinclair Lewis's bestseller of 1925, *Arrowsmith*, written with the assistance of former Michigan bacteriologist Paul de Kruif, PhD, 1916 (see p. 116). A central character in the book was heavily modeled on Cabot's colleague, Frederick Novy. de Kruif's role in providing the scientific background, was acknowledged in a generous comment in the book dedication, and was rewarded with 25 percent of the royalties. Lewis was awarded the Pulitzer Prize for the work in 1926 but turned it down, rumor had it, out of anger that his previous book *Main Street* hadn't received the Pulitzer in 1921.

The year 1925 gave clues to paradigm changes that reverberated over the next century. A diphtheria epidemic in Nome, Alaska, and a dog sled run to deliver diphtheria antitoxin serum at the beginning of the year heralded powerful changes in health care and the worldwide public interest in it. In December, the opening of American's first motel, the Milestone Mo-Tel in San Luis Obispo, signaled the new mass mobility of the population that came with affordable and reliable motor vehicles. These disparate technologies, at the start and end of the year, were reshaping medical practice, education, and research. With its new hospital and Cabot's forceful leadership, the University of Michigan Medical School and clinical practice had grown beyond their former regional status.

Cabot, 1926

Hugh Cabot must have been in an optimistic frame of mind when the sun rose (if it did in Ann Arbor) on New Year's Day, 1926. As medical school dean, he was assembling a strong faculty of basic scientists and clinicians in Ann Arbor. The newly completed hospital provided an excellent clinical milieu for world-class health care, education, and research befitting a great academic medical center. As chief of surgery, he had built an extraordinary team of surgical subspecialists and as a world-class authority in urology he had initiated a training program that brought the first urology trainees to Ann Arbor. His first and only Michigan trainees to become urologists were Charles Huggins and Reed Nesbit, and if nothing else came from Cabot, they would have been a legacy hard to top. Cabot's textbook, *Modern Urology*, then in its second edition, was the iconic reference for teaching and practice, although it would get displaced by Young's book later in the year.

At Michigan for only seven years, Cabot was actually under his fourth university president. Clarence Little had been in office only for a few months on this New Year's Day, following the premature death of Marion Burton and the eight-month acting presidency of Alfred Henry Lloyd. Wasting little time, Cabot sent Little a letter voicing the same "full time" salary idea suggested previously to Hutchins in 1919. This persistent idea was a cornerstone of Cabot's belief that health care and medical education should be public goods rather than mercantile commodities and in this he had strong support among the regents. Faculty support, however, was divided and, furthermore, Cabot's adversarial personality and success in abolishing the Homeopathic College continued to enlarge the number of his detractors. No evidence exists that such darker thoughts entered his mental calculus at the dawn of 1926 or at other times.

A series of newspaper interviews in the *Boston Herald* in February featured an article, "Michigan and Harvard: a comparison" that was largely a summary of the views of Cabot and Little. The article was reprinted in the *Michigan Alumnus* with the author noting,

> it is unfortunate that considerations of academic etiquette should necessarily cripple the forceful picturesqueness of Dr. Cabot's remarks in the course of their preparation for publication. Few British colonels—even in fiction—have talked more meatily, or with greater tang than this brisk, stocky scientist, and the written record of his words, unhappily can give only a faint flavor of his personality.[23]

As with each modern new year, the world changed recognizably for better and for worse in 1926. At this point in this narrative, it is useful to take stock of the state, nation, and world as they swirled around Cabot, the university, and urology, as graduate education in urology at Michigan was beginning. Calvin Coolidge was U.S. president, Alex Grosbeck was Michigan governor, and John Smith was Detroit mayor. Ford Motor Company had 191,948 U.S. employees. Police raided prohibition violators and gambling resorts throughout the state and nation. Detroit Tigers under Ty Cobb as manager had a 79–75 season. Sports were better in Ann Arbor with the Wolverine football team in its 25th and final season under Fielding Yost, tying for the Big Ten Conference championship that year, as coincidentally did the basketball team under E. J. Mather. March saw the first liquid fuel rocket launch (Robert Goddard in Massachusetts) and that month Richard DeVos, cofounder of Amway, was born in Grand Rapids. Bessie Coleman, the first African-American and Native American woman to hold a pilot's license, died testing an aircraft in Jacksonville, Florida. In June, American painter Mary Cassatt died in France at age 82. The Kuomintang's military unification campaign began in northern

China in July, the month that John Dingell, Jr., Michigan's great U.S. representative (1955-2015), was born in Colorado Springs. In September, the Weimar Republic joined the League of Nations. A. A. Milne published *Winnie-the-Pooh* in October, the same month Harry Houdini died at age 52 after ruptured appendicitis in Room 401 at Detroit's Grace Hospital. Route 66, also known then as the Will Rogers Highway or Main Street of America, joined the United States Numbered Highway System on November 11. The Japanese Shōwa period began on December 25, when Emperor Hirohito's father died. The 1926 Nobel Prize in Medicine or Physiology was deferred for reasons explained later (see p. 180).

Amidst that reshaping world, Cabot wrote a profile in *Michigan Alumnus* detailing the UM Department of Surgery in optimistic terms.[24] This would be the first full year for Cabot's Department of Surgery to stretch its wings in the university's first great teaching hospital. This might have been a good time to transfer the chair of surgery to Frederick Coller, who was loyally performing most of its day-to-day teaching, administrative work, and surgery, but such was not Dean Cabot's style.

Eddie Kahn later offered priceless recollections of his cohort of young bucks in training under Cabot and Coller:

> July 1, 1926, four of us were appointed first-year residents in Surgery. Russell Mustard was older than the rest of us and one of the two top students in my [medical school] class. He played an important role in getting me through the first year. Reed Nesbit, from California, was from the start an outstanding technician. He later became chief of Urology and President of the American College of Surgeons. Charles Huggins, who had come from Harvard, was an individualist, had a marvelous sense of humor, and was excellent company. He and I realized we were behind Mustard and Nesbit technically and arranged with George Adie, an instructor in Surgery, to do some operating in the Dog Laboratory. When we finished our work, Charlie turned to me and said, "I'll tell you one thing, Eddie. We'll never be surgeons." He was only partly right, as he later, while at the University of Chicago, became one of the only two surgeons I ever knew of who won the Nobel Prize.[25]

Kahn would later become the head of neurosurgery at Michigan.

An Advertisement in the *Michigan Daily* on October 24, 1926 promoted the Cosy Corner Tea Room with luncheons from 11:30-1:30 at 50 cents and 65 cents and dinners daily from 5:30-7:30 at 85 cents and $1. Sunday dinners of chicken or steak were served from 12:30 to 2 o'clock for $1.50. Mrs. Cabot by this time had delegated operations to a manager. One worker for a time at the Tea Room was a young lady from Texas, Mabel Ophelia Wilkins who had come to Ann Arbor to study to be a hospital dietitian and would marry Reed Nesbit. Nesbit family lore has it that one of the manager's duties was the daily preparation of the Cosy Corner's signature chocolate sauce. (Nancy Nesbit p.c. 2019)

In November, Cabot and Harley Haynes, the new University Hospital director, asked the regents to revisit the mandatory full-time faculty model with a base academic salary for teaching and a clinical supplement from a pool created from private practice fees, that while lower than clinical incomes in the "commercial" world, would make the academic job not unattractive in comparison.[26]

While Cabot forcefully pushed the full-time model, he wasn't particularly generous with it. Personal animosities perhaps were in play for some cases, such as with Reuben Peterson, who had initiated resignation in 1922, out of dislike for Cabot, but rescinded the gesture and remained on the faculty, part-time. In 1926, however, he asked to become full time, expecting a $2,000 per year raise, but Cabot denied the request, explaining in a letter to President Little that Peterson, at 64 years of age, should be retired. Peterson did retire in 1931 and, according to Davenport, "moved to Duxbury, Massachusetts, where he amused himself with the

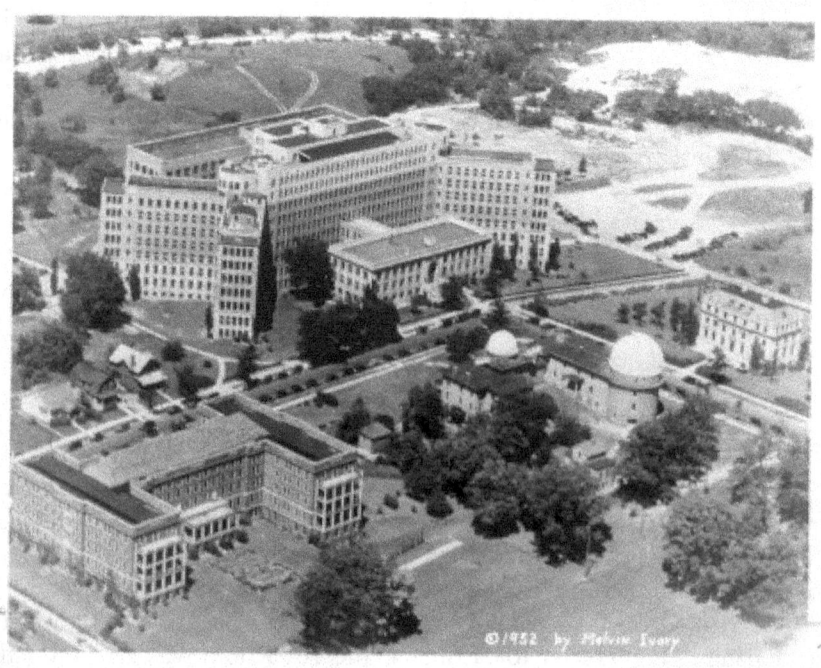

Simpson to right of white-domed Observatory, 1932 photo. Bentley Library.

occupation characteristic of a superannuated professor: writing a history of the University Hospital."[27]

The Simpson bequest from three years earlier was fulfilled partially in June 1926, with an Albert Kahn building that opened across the street from the Detroit Observatory, but Cabot had to fill it to complete the bequest. Chairing a committee, he developed a long list of candidates for director of the Simpson Memorial Institute. One particularly attractive candidate, Raphael Isaacs was identified in some external correspondences as "unsuitable" for reasons related to religious identity.[28] The Simpson search continued to occupy Cabot as 1926 drew to a close, while the medical campus was expanding.

Notes

1 "Film Surgery to Aid Classes," *Detroit Free Press*, March 2, 1922.
2 H. H. Peckham, *The Making of the University of Michigan 1817–1992*. Edited and updated by M. L. Steneck and N. H. Steneck (Ann Arbor: University of Michigan Press, 1967, 1994), 164.
3 H. W. Davenport, *University of Michigan Surgeons 1850–1970 Who They Were and What They Did* (Ann Arbor, MI: Historical Center for the Health Sciences, University of Michigan, 1993), 72
4 "U Dean's Wife Plans to Open Tiny Tea Shop," *Detroit Free Press*, November 5, 1922, page A6.
5 "Vocational talks will end today," *Michigan Daily* 35, no. 136 (April 1, 1925): 5.
6 H. W. Davenport, *Not Just Any Medical School* (Ann Arbor: University of Michigan Press, 1999), 64.
7 H. Cabot, *Report of Committee on Education and Pedagogics*, Association of American Medical Colleges, Proceedings of the Thirty-Third Annual Meeting, held at Ann Arbor, Michigan, March 2 and 3, 1923, 143.
8 Burton: Clements Library (1923).
9 *Detroit Free Press*, September 30, 1923.
10 "Men teachers are preferred," *Los Angeles Times*, December 13, 1923.
11 "'Mary A. Cabot' Dead in Naples," *Boston Daily Globe*, May 24, 1924, 20.
12 H. Cabot and L. B. Davis, "A Preliminary Report on the Value of Ethylene as a General Anesthetic Based on the Study of 500 Cases," *Journal of Michigan Medical Society* 23 (1924): 372–376.
13 H. Cabot, *Modern Urology* (Philadelphia, PA; New York: Lea and Febiger, 1924).
14 T. R. Frank, "New Books," *American Journal of Obstetrics and Gynecology* 9, no. 1 (1925): 130–140.
15 *The Ann Arbor Street Guide*, 1925 version, gives the Cabot's address as 2031 Hill Street.
16 H. Cabot, "The Development of Organized Clinical Teaching," *Colorado Medicine: The Journal of the Colorado State Medical Society*. Western Newspaper Union, Denver 22 (1925): 130.
17 H. Cabot and J. L. Loomis, "Etiology and Prevention of So-Called Catheter Cystitis," *Journal of Michigan State Medical Society* 24 (1925): 32–38.
18 F. A. Coller, The University of Michigan and the Department of Surgery.
19 H. H. Peckham, *The Making of the University of Michigan 1817–1992*. Edited and updated by M. L. Steneck and N. H. Steneck (Ann Arbor: University of Michigan Press, 1967, 1994), 155–174.

20 H. H. Peckham, *The Making of the University of Michigan 1817–1992*. Edited and updated by M. L. Steneck and N. H. Steneck (Ann Arbor: University of Michigan Press, 1967, 1994), 177.
21 "Faculty-Student Debate Held on Athletic System," *Michigan Daily*, April 21, 1925.
22 H. W. Davenport, *Not Just Any Medical School* (Ann Arbor: University of Michigan Press, 1999), 168.
23 S. Griscom, "Michigan and Harvard: A Comparison," *The Michigan Alumnus* 32, no. 22, #21 (March 13, 1926): 421–425.
24 H. Cabot, "UM Department of Surgery," *Michigan Alum* 32 (1926): 516.
25 F. A. Coller, The University of Michigan and the Department of Surgery, 53.
26 Bentley Historical Library, University of Michigan, Regents Communication Box 135. Folder: Admissions requirements and salaries 1925–1927, November 4, 1926.
27 H. W. Davenport, *Not Just Any Medical School* (Ann Arbor: University of Michigan Press, 1999), 228–229.
28 H. W. Davenport, *Not Just Any Medical School* (Ann Arbor: University of Michigan Press, 1999), 168.

Hugh Cabot, 1927–1930

Cabot, 1927

Cyrus Sturgis (1891–1966) of the Peter Bent Brigham Hospital was considered carefully as the best candidate for the Simpson Institute by Cabot and President Little, who traveled to Boston to make an offer in January 1927. Sturgis accepted the job with the private understanding that he would also become head of the Department of Internal Medicine after a year. Sturgis asked Raphael Isaacs to start the work of organizing the institute and Sturgis didn't move from Boston to Ann Arbor until the summer of 1927. A year later, the additional responsibility of heading internal medicine materialized for Sturgis, eclipsing Bruce who may have felt due the title.

The matter of quotas, in terms of representation of disfavored ethnic groups in medical school classes and faculty, was an issue of the time and factored into the popular discussions of human eugenics and fantasy ideas of "ethnic purity." Cabot was susceptible to those notions. The University of Michigan had no limits or quotas and Cabot sought advice of new university president Little, by letter in June, ostensibly on the basis of preclinical faculty complaints that the medical class sizes of over 200 included large fractions from central or southern Europe. Davenport later studied documents of the time and recognized the flavor of the considerations was that these students and faculty were "undesirable" from their ethnic origins and, even though many were very well-qualified academically, limits or quotas should be applied to certain categories or people. Davenport wrote, "Cabot was worrying about Jews." These apprehensions extended beyond the dean among some others on the faculty and applied to other groups of people including "out-of-state" students, women, and African Americans. The upshot of these ethnic anxieties and prejudices was that applicants with satisfactory credentials were asked to interview in person for medical school, beginning in 1927. Midwest students came to Ann Arbor, while others had interviews in New York, Denver, or Los Angeles where they took a standardized test that included vocabulary, reading, and "interest" examination as well as having to write a short essay on a nonmedical topic. This speedbump was effective, for in its first year of 589 qualified applicants, only 300 came for interviews with the largest attrition at the New York site. Arthur Curtis, faculty secretary, assembled data by 1934 showing that non Christian students were not only disproportionate in the classes but more ominously were preferentially favoring Christian hospitals rather than Jewish hospitals for their internships.[1]

As a surgeon, Cabot had a keen interest and firm ideas regarding anesthesiology, as evidenced by his papers on the topic. After a patient on the Obstetrics Service was killed by an ethylene explosion because an old anesthesia machine was not grounded, Cabot blamed the service chief Reuben Peterson publicly. Peterson was respected among the faculty and this blame added to the dissatisfaction with Cabot that was building up. A letter to President Little in 1927 revealed the hostility of medical faculty members, Huber, Novy, and Gessel in particular.

Cabot didn't win all of his battles. Novy's bacteriology curriculum was one example. An accreditation visit from the Association of American Medical Colleges revealed that Novy had garnered 384 hours of the curriculum for bacteriology, in contrast to 150–160 hours at peer institutions, leading Cabot to reply that Novy was beyond his control.[2] Cabot challenged the post-Flexnerian curricular structure of two preclinical years, followed by two clinical years, in a paper called "A plea for the further extension of clinical opportunity into earlier years of the medical course."[3] He didn't abandon his clinical contributions, first-authoring a new anesthetic paper with Henry Ransom, a young man he had earlier brought to the Surgery Department.[4]

Causation of gastric cancer was a hot topic of the time and central to the deferred Nobel Prize of 1926. Cabot and George Adie had published their thoughts on its etiology in 1925, quoting some views of their colleague, Aldred Warthin.[5] The 1926 Nobel Prize for medicine was disputed because some committee members favored Katsusaburō Yamagiwa of Japan for his work inducing cancer in rabbit ears by means of coal tar, while others favored Johannes Fibiger, Danish pathologist who had shown that a roundworm he called *Spiroptera carcinoma* (properly called *Gongylonema neoplasticum*) caused gastric cancer. The deferred 1926 award was announced a year late on October 27, 1927, and presented to Fibiger on December 10, although reassessment proved his conclusions were erroneous, while those of Yamagiwa have been confirmed. The year 1927 also featured the Lindbergh flight across the Atlantic in May. In August, Coolidge said, "I do not choose to run for president in 1928."

The Cabot's social events were regional news, as when they hosted a musical event in November, according to the *Detroit Free Press*, "The Matinee Musicale, to which Ann Arbor's very interesting society members belong will meet next Tuesday at the home of Mrs. Hugh Cabot of Hill Street."[6] American musical theater was about to experience a new phenomenon when on December 27 Kern and Hammerstein's *Showboat* debuted on Broadway.

1928 and Cabot's Men

A third *Race Betterment Conference* January 2–6 in Battle Creek at the Battle Creek Sanitarium featured University of Michigan president Little, as president of the conference, and medical school dean Cabot, among other academics and luminaries. John Harvey Kellogg, president of the Race Betterment Foundation, stated this purpose of the organization:

> To bring together a group of leading scientists, educators and others for the purpose of discussing ways and means of applying science to human living in the same thoroughgoing way in which it is now applied to industry—in the promotion of longer life, increased efficiency, and of well-being and of race improvement.

This was part of the eugenics movement. Kellogg in 1906 had cofounded the Race Betterment Foundation with biologist Charles Davenport and economist Irving Fisher and they held their first conference in Battle Creek in 1914. A second conference was held in San Francisco in 1921 and presided over by David Starr Jordan, chancellor of Stanford. At the 1928 meeting, Cabot approached the topic from the perspective of medical education in his talk, "Race betterment as influenced by the selection and training of medical students." He expanded on seven main points: the passing of the general practitioner, the public setting of medical standards, the changing distribution of physicians, changing standards and methods of medical education, speculations on what the future will expect of physicians, the duty of the public to protect the medical profession from "ill-trained and irresponsible interlopers," and finally the need for caution in selecting physicians. Kellogg's Race Betterment Foundation was not the only group considering this dark topic. Three International Eugenics Congresses provided bigger stages where scientists, politicians, and pundits considered social engineering to improve humanity.[i]

---

i The First International Eugenics Congress was held in London on July 24–29, 1912, and was dedicated to Francis Galton, who had coined the term eugenics. Leonard Darwin, son of Charles, presided and Winston Churchill attended. A Second Congress, deferred

In Ann Arbor, faculty discontent with Cabot was growing. In 1928, Carl Eberbach was yet another faculty member to resign because of "salary insufficiency" and he entered private practice. Cabot's men in the Surgery Department, however, remained on board in spite of the increasingly divisive environment and they were impacting their fields far beyond Ann Arbor throughout American and international medicine. These men, in 1928, were as impressive as any surgical departmental faculty in the world.

John Alexander, an extraordinary medical student at the University of Pennsylvania, had served like Cabot on the Western Front and returned to Philadelphia for only a short time, working with Charles Harrison Frazier, before Cabot brought him to Ann Arbor, where he initiated the risky business of thoracic surgery, perfecting the methodology of collapse therapy for pulmonary tuberculosis.[7] Like many physicians of his era, Alexander incurred tuberculosis requiring a period of immobilization in a body cast at the Lake Saranac Sanitarium in New York, where he wrote *The Surgery of Pulmonary Tuberculosis*, published first in four installments in the *American Journal of Medical Sciences* in 1924 and then as a book in 1925.[8] Alexander and his protégé Cameron Haight made Michigan a world center for cardiothoracic surgery.

Carl Badgley, UMMS MD, 1919, had interned at University Hospital and stayed to train in orthopaedic surgery under LeRoy Abbott from 1920 to 1922. Badgley pursued private practice in Detroit briefly but returned to UM in 1923 when Abbott left. Then, to Cabot's disgust, Badgley went back to private practice at Henry Ford Hospital, returning to Ann Arbor again in 1932 "in the depth of the Great Depression when even orthopaedic surgeons could not earn large incomes."[9] Badgley remained at the university for a distinguished career until retirement in 1963. His old colleague from the early Cabot days, Sir Herbert Seddon, gave the introductory remarks at the first Carl Badgley Lecture in Ann Arbor.[10]

Frederick Coller, whose career was recounted earlier, remained in Ann Arbor long after the Cabot days and proved to be one of Michigan's most eminent faculty members. In 1928, Cabot brought Reuben Kahn from the Michigan Department of Health Laboratory to University Hospital to update the diagnostic laboratories.[11]

---

from 1915, was held in New York at the American Museum of Natural History on September 25–27, 1921. Alexander Graham Bell was honorary president and the U.S. State Department sent invitations around the world. Major Leonard Darwin, the guest speaker, advocated "elimination of the unfit." A Third International Eugenics Conference was held again in New York at the Museum on August 22–23, 1932, and dedicated to Mary Williamson Averell who helped fund the meeting. Charles Davenport presided over the meeting (not to be confused with Michigan's Horace Davenport several decades later).

Charles Brenton Huggins (1901–1997) was born in Nova Scotia, a 1920 graduate of Acadia University where he was the youngest student in the class and a 1924 MD graduate of Harvard Medical School.[12] He came to Michigan in 1924 to study surgery under Cabot and Coller, and a year later he was sharing duties and a room with Reed Nesbit. Charles Huggins was Cabot's first trainee to become a urologist. Huggins nearly became a faculty member at Johns Hopkins in 1927 but instead joined the University of Chicago where he practiced urology and pursued research on the hormonal dependence of prostate cancer. It was said that in his early days of practice he purchased the textbook of the younger Edward Keyes and literally memorized it in a short period of time.[13] Huggins's work on the beneficial effects of androgen ablation on metastatic disease, published in 1941 with Clarence Hodges, led to the Nobel Prize in 1966.[14]

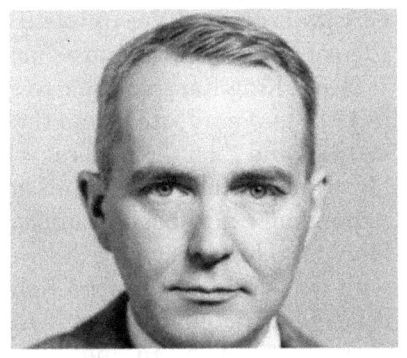

Edgar A. Kahn (1900–1985) was born in Detroit as one of four children and the only son to architect Albert Kahn, who designed a number of structures at the University of Michigan including the Simpson building, the new University Hospital, Hill Auditorium, the Burton Memorial Tower, the Graduate Library, and the Clements Library. He graduated from Phillips Andover Academy in Massachusetts in 1918 and earned concurrent undergraduate and medical degrees from Michigan in 1924, then serving as intern under Cabot and Coller in the first days of the new University Hospital. An interest in neurosurgery grew and he became the first neurosurgical resident under Max Peet and then a dedicated faculty member at the university.[15]

Reed Nesbit, the California recruit, was viewed as hardworking and quiet, while his wife Mabel, who had briefly worked at Mrs. Cabot's tea shop, was sociable and athletic. Nesbit's story will follow in our next book.

Max Peet had returned to Michigan in 1916 as a general surgeon, but had been stimulated by his mentor in Philadelphia, Charles Frazier, with whom he studied cerebrospinal fluid in canine models. Frazier had also influenced John Alexander. Peet began to develop expertise in neurosurgery at Michigan as soon as he joined the faculty, although initially managing the wider range of general surgery as well. Cabot encouraged Peet's pursuit of neurosurgical practice and Edgar Kahn who joined Peet and soon became a full partner in their academic, clinical, and research pursuits in neurosurgery. An important collaboration of Max Peet and

Charles Frazier of the University of Pennsylvania advanced the knowledge of cerebrospinal fluid as neurosurgery extended its reach.[16]

Henry King Ransom came to the University of Michigan from Jackson in 1916 and graduated from the College of Literature, Science, and Arts in 1920 and then the medical school in 1923 in the early Cabot period. He trained in surgery with an internship and assistant residency in Ann Arbor but extended his surgical repertoire with a residency at Johns Hopkins Hospital where he would have had familiarity and contact with the legendary Howard Kelly of Baltimore, who was coincidentally developing a nonmedical interest in the University of Michigan. Ransom returned to Michigan and served loyally under Coller, who succeeded Cabot as chair. Rising to full professorship in 1950. Ransom served for a year and a half as interim chair after Coller. Ransom was respected as a superb teacher, surgeon, and leader at the regional and national levels of American surgery.

Through Sir Anthony Bowlby, colleague from the British Expeditionary Forces and later chief of surgery at Saint Bartholomew's Hospital, a number of first-rate rotating British surgeons, including Norman Capener, Rupert Corbett, Basil Hume, Herbert Seddon, and Arthur Visick, came to work in Ann Arbor with Cabot and his men. Seddon was present the day that Cabot was dismissed and 15 years later would loyally author Cabot's obituary for the *Lancet*.

Cabot continued his presence on the national stage of urology. He presented "The scope of the operation of ureteral transplantation in relief of diseases" at the North Central Section of the AUA held at Columbus in November. Cabot's own family was growing up, undoubtedly still mourning the loss of the only daughter. The *Detroit Free Press* continued its "celebrity coverage" of the Cabot family, reporting in September that youngest son Arthur Cabot was returning home to Ann Arbor from summer camp in Ontario, Canada.[17] The marriage of oldest son Hugh, Jr., to nurse Louise Melanson on December 22, 1928, was covered by the *Chicago Daily Tribune*.

Cabot, 1929

This year brought big shocks to the university, starting in January with President Little's announcement to resign. The regents begged him to reconsider. Little had presided over many changes including a new iteration of education with a proposed university college, a new University Hospital, field stations in northern Michigan and Jackson Hole, expanded scholarship and loan programs, plus the construction of Michigan Stadium. Little's efforts came at great personal costs; the university college initiative had created deep dissent among the faculty and his marriage was failing. The January meeting of the regents recorded,

> The Board voted to accept the resignation of President Little as presented and further adopted the following resolution:
> Resolved, That in accepting the resignation of President Little, the Board of Regents expresses the most profound regret.
> His high ideals of educational standards, his initiative, his constructive aspirations, his frankness, courage, and sincerity have made the severing of relationships a heartfelt loss to us all. We trust that the future may have for him the richest rewards.
> [Proceedings of the Board of Regents January Meeting, 1928, 876–877]

Later, a backstory of improprieties would dampen Little's reputation.

At Little's request, the Board voted to suspend operational plans for the university college, one of his favored initiatives, pending the views of his successor. A committee for a new presidential search was formed with Sawyer, Beal, and Clements, together with the dean of administration Alexander Ruthven, a position that Little had created only a few years earlier. Ruthven effectively became an acting president as Regent Sawyer, once again, had to manage a search. Little left Ann Arbor in June, to return to Maine where he would direct the Jackson Memorial Laboratory until retirement in 1956. The laboratory had been named for UM alumnus class of 1900, Roscoe B. Jackson.

The Cabot family announced the wedding of their oldest son Hugh II, inviting 500 guests to the Michigan Union to meet the newlyweds and the event was covered by the *Detroit Free Press*.[18] Whether due to turbulence at the presidential level of the university or other matters, Cabot sent his regrets to the Clinical Society, meeting in Baltimore on January 25–26. After the first meeting of that group, there is little evidence of Cabot's participation up to 1929.

The selection of a new university president embroiled the regents and the high levels of the university, as reflected in correspondence of Regent Sawyer where a letter to him from Allen Shoenfield of the *Detroit News* on July 12 explains:

> The news of Dr. Little's marital difficulties did cause some temporary disturbance in campus circles but the more reasonable agreed that the college president is but human and is therefore entitled to avail himself of any human devices intended to settle such problems.

> Despite my newspaper connections I feel, personally, that the public has little right to inquire into or speculate about such private matters.
>
> I saw Dr. Bruce for a few moments on Tuesday as he had run down from the north for a day and was returning that night. He seemed somewhat perturbed about the general situation regarding the presidency and viewed with alarm the apparent rise of the local candidate's stock.

Ruthven was the "local candidate." A letter on July 23 to Sawyer from Bruce, then director of Post-Graduate Medicine, gives further details of the politics.

> I had a long talk with Huber yesterday and asked him frankly if he thought Ruthven the best man for the job. He replied by stating that of the men mentioned he thought Ruthven was at least as good, and his knowledge of Michigan affairs gave him an advantage, but the thought there were many men outside who are undoubtedly superior.
>
> Clements certainly put up a poor argument for Mr. Ruthven when he stated that he was not an outstanding man, and that seems to be the feeling generally. The local opinion is that someone probably outside the Board of Regents who has an ax to grind brought pressure to bear on Mr. Clements, and in that connection Doctor Curtis told Dr. Wile that if Ruthven were not elected he thought Cabot would probably resign. It is quite generally thought that Cabot is the most active of any who are pushing Mr. Ruthven's candidacy.[19]

Ruthven had come to Michigan for a PhD and joined the faculty to teach Zoology, becoming professor and director of the Museum of Zoology in 1915. A well-known herpetologist, his book on garter snakes in 1908 advanced the field and he named 16 reptile species. He rose to chair of the department and then dean of administration in 1928, in the days before Michigan's provost position. He was an effective administrative dean, but the regents favored candidates they viewed as more attractive. Resignations of Regent Ben Hanchett for "health reasons and Regent Ralph Stone, for 'nerve tension-nerve exhaustion,' according to letters to Regent Sawyer, revealed disharmony on the board that influenced the presidency search."[20]

After politicking, debate, and offers to other individuals, the regents settled on Ruthven, initially considering placing him in an acting position but ultimately going all the way in September 1929. A note to Sawyer from Udo Wile on October 11, 1929, pointed out tensions in the medical school under Cabot that were already known to the regents. Huber added another letter to the Sawyer file on November 4 as did James Bruce the same day. Bruce's note, mainly about Cabot, was typed with an additional handwritten section, noting as to a "successor to the present incumbent, I think you would be justified in suggesting a committee."[21] This may have been one of the origins of the idea for replacing the dean with an executive committee.

As regent overseeing the new hospital, Sawyer's correspondence shows the extent of genitourinary activity in the *September Revenue Classification* as providing aggregate fees for cystoscopy of $152.50 and dilatation of $19 and professional fees for Genitourinary Service A of $393.50 and Genitourinary B of $88.00 that year. It seems safe to conclude that Genitourinary A was Cabot's service and Genitourinary B at this time consisted of Nesbit and trainees.[22]

Ruthven had been in office as the appointed president barely a month before the stock market crashed, although the effect of the catastrophe was not evidenced widely in the university archives. The "Black Thursday" of October 24 that brought the Roaring Twenties to a stop bore little mention in the papers of University of Michigan leadership or in public comments of Cabot at the time who was otherwise not reticent to make public comments about major public matters. Sawyer's wide correspondence as a regent in October 1929 and the following months bear no mention of the national catastrophe, even when university finances were discussed. As the general economic depression unfolded, however, student enrollment at the University of Michigan would drop (around 10,000 in 1930–1931 and then to 8,713 in 1933–1934). The mill tax was maintained until a 15 percent reduction in 1932 when the university instituted salary cuts and hiring freezes. Peckham wrote, "The prolonged financial depression brought out the genius of President Ruthven. He proved to be a magnificent rear guard fighter, fending off legislative bills and other ill-considered proposals that would have crippled the University."[23]

Cabot had achieved much at this point in time. Ann Arbor was an epicenter for medical education, residency training, and clinical practice, especially so in urology. Cabot was recognized as a very competent urological surgeon but only an indifferent general surgeon" according to Davenport's assessment of contemporaries.[24] The surgery department included 7 professors, 15 instructors, and 15 residents, in addition to dental surgeon Lyons and a dental intern. The medical school faculty was reaching a limit to its tolerance for Cabot and his ideas in the later 1920s. Cabot was accruing more enemies than friends, and the critical algebraic formula that explains the expiration date of any dictator, when enemies outweigh friends, was nearing its resolution. Peterson's distaste for Cabot began with their conflict over the full-time model and was exacerbated by the 1927 anesthetic explosion and death that Cabot blamed on Peterson. Cabot's subsequent reprimand of Cowie and Peterson for failing to show up for medical student examinations and many other bruised feelings among the faculty further tilted the scales of disfavor. Bruce's antagonism was well known.²⁵ David Cowie and Frank Wilson complained to President Ruthven that Cabot terrorized the faculty and other letters, signed and anonymous, flowed to leadership and regents. Medical school files include an undated, unaddressed, and unsigned two-page typewritten note with five charges against Cabot. The letter, probably sent in confidence to one or more regents charged:

1. "Evidence that his coming here was to exploit his position to his own financial advantage."
2. "Has shown every evidence of absence of administrative ability . . . subterfuge and chicanery and doubtful practices . . . evidenced by his investigation and report against the work of Drs. Novy, Huber, Edmunds and others."
3. "He is untruthful, malicious and undependable as evidenced by misrepresentations and unprofessional conduct in his accusation to the President of the Taylor case, the [redacted] case, and his attack on the Health service, all of which on investigation proved that he was guilty of absolute premeditated falsehood."
4. "The maintenance of a system of espionage in which he has enlarged and tried to engage a number of young men and others, whose promotions have seemed to hinge upon the ability they showed in furthering his ends. This he has boasted about."
5. "As a surgeon he is incompetent and dangerous in that he disregards many of the most commonly recognized safeguards in surgery. This not only endangers the patient but is a most pernicious influence on the student. Dr. Coller has been much distressed over these delinquencies and has expressed discouragement in trying to get over to the student the importance of the principles of surgical cleanliness when they are violated daily by his chief . . . Dr. Cabot is entirely out of sympathy and at variance with the medical profession, both locally and nationally, and the difficulties and differences are constantly increasing. . . . For these and many other reasons he is regarded as incompetent and untrustworthy both as a surgeon and as an administrator."²⁶

Clearly, Cabot's support in the medical school had eroded. By exclusion, it might be guessed that the unnamed writer could have been Peterson, Wile, or Bruce, but others were equally motivated. The charges ring true, for the most part, although the final one regarding surgical incompetence may have been related to Cabot's unfortunate habit to sweat during surgery, when sometimes the sweat might contaminate the field. Although it was said that "Cabot's sweat is sterile," at least one postoperative infection was claimed to have resulted.²⁷ The sweating was brought up even after Cabot was fired, when his former disciple Edgar Kahn gave

Cabot a headband to wear during surgery at Mayo as a gift, fearing that nobody's sweat was sterile in Rochester, Minnesota.[28]

Adjacent to the letter of five charges in the historical files was a local newspaper clipping, also undated, with a photograph of Cabot headlined "Debates Tonight." A paragraph explains that Dean Cabot will oppose Professor Thomas Reed of the political science department in the Student Faculty debate at Hill Auditorium on the proposition "Intercollegiate athletics, in their present form, are objectionable and should be materially modified." Whoever sent the clipping and to whom it was sent are unknown, but the clipping was affixed to a sheet of paper with an amended title: "Candidate for the Presidency on the Anti-Constructive Platform." Elsewhere on the paper, the typist also wrote with equal sarcasm: "Serene alike in Peace and Danger." (below - clipping.)

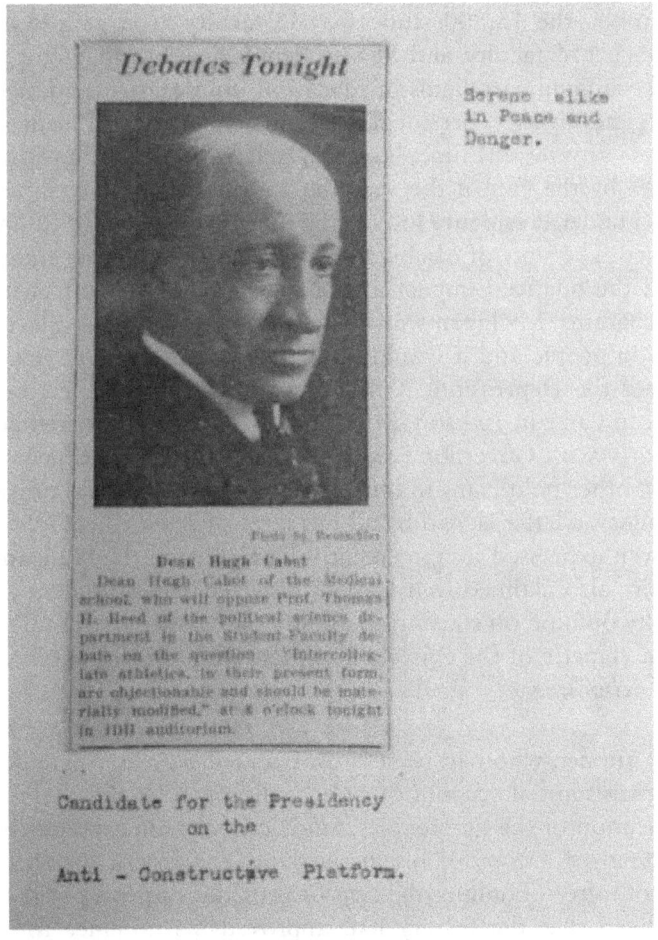

Sarcastic loose clipping in Bentley files. Author unknown.

The medical school saddened in 1929 when Victor Vaughan died on November 21 in Richmond, Virginia, from a presumed heart attack. He had published his autobiography, *A Doctor's Memories*, in 1926 and his last paper, "A chemical concept of the origin and development of life" in 1927.[29] Ruthven mentioned "the Vaughan service" in a letter to Sawyer on November 27. Other noteworthy events of the year included the start of Herbert Hoover's administration in Washington (March 4, 1929–March 4, 1933), a Dow-Jones peak of 381 before the crash (not reached again until 1954), and an unexpected earthquake of 7.2 and tsunami off the Grand Banks of Newfoundland, felt as far away as New York City.

Cabot, 1930

The stock market crash two months earlier and growing geopolitical instability must have affected New Year's celebrations in 1930 in Ann Arbor among the 15,500 students, 833 faculty at large and the medical school's 116 faculty and 585 students. The loss of Victor Vaughan signaled changing paradigms in education, clinical care, and medical science. Regents bylaws, presidential correspondence, and medical school documents around this time, however, reflect little of the national uncertainty, yet by the end of the year the national economic circumstances worsened under President Hoover and worldwide geopolitical instability heightened. The state of Michigan was hit hard by the deepening depression and the financial impact at the state level would affect its educational programs. Michigan was the seventh largest state at this time with 4.8 million people and it would grow 8.5 percent over the next decade, in spite of the Depression. Reflecting its history with the roots of the Republican Party in Jackson, Michigan, in 1854, the state remained true to the party with Governor Fred Green, Detroit mayor Charles Bowles, and most other politicians in office, including every federal office holder.

In January, a letter signed by all but three of the medical school chairs to Ruthven expressed disagreement with Cabot on the "full time" idea. The chairs also claimed that Cabot "deceived" the president regarding the faculty opinion on starting an anesthesiology department. Davenport offered a vignette of the episode in a footnote in his book *Not Just Any Medical School*:

> C. J. Tupper, who had been Dean Furstenberg's associate dean, gave a circumstantial account of Cabot's dismissal on the occasion of the dedication of the Furstenberg Study center. I am grateful to him for sending me a copy of his manuscript. The gist of the story is that Cabot, after obtaining the approval of the surgeons, told President Ruthven that the faculty had approved his nominee for the new Department of Anesthesiology. When Cabot asked the faculty for

retroactive approval of his communication to President Ruthven the faculty, led by Udo Wile, balked. A deputation of the faculty left the meeting to report to the president that the faculty had taken a vote of no confidence in the dean. It is difficult to reconcile the chronology of this story with documented events.[30]

That last sentence may refer to specifics of the Anesthesiology Department. A distinct Department of Anesthesiology didn't form until 1949. Anesthesia had been under the aegis of registered nurse Laura Davis (later Laura Davis Dunstone) appointed in the de Nancrede era and at work until 1938. Cabot was a strong supporter of her. Cabot's "methods" and "terrorization" of the faculty were also faulted in a letter found among the Sawyer papers.[31] Toward the end of January, former university president Harry Hutchins who had hired Cabot died at age 83.

Sawyer was the regent with the sharpest focus on the medical school, but oddly, his papers archived at the Bentley Library, although they revealed active correspondence throughout most university crises, personal illnesses, and the death of his wife, have a gap corresponding to the months when the faculty turned most strongly against Cabot, after December 31, 1929, until April of the following year. A few later folders offer some hints into the critical months around January and early February 1930. A critical tipping point had been reached and on Friday, February 7, the regents heard a comprehensive oral report from Ruthven and then voted to relieve Cabot of his duties "in the interests of greater harmony." This was a monumental and disruptive step, of a magnitude usually necessitated by some single major breach of law or behavior, although no evidence for such matters exists. Cabot had been accruing enemies in the medical school and university since his first moments in Ann Arbor. His restrictive full-time plan remained in place and displeased many faculty economically. The part-time plan similarly had few enthusiasts. Cabot's ideas of group practice and the perceived intrusion of his new University Hospital on private practice generated a committee of the state medical society to study what it considered the 'Cabot problem.' Retrospectively, it is difficult to find many Cabot loyalists either locally or throughout the state by this time. Clearly, he had a "tin ear" and the backlash seems to have taken him by surprise.

The first meeting of a new Medical School Executive Committee was held the next day and the minutes consisted of four paragraphs below.

MEETING OF THE EXECUTIVE COMMITTEE (No. 1)

At the meeting of the Board of Regents held Friday, February 7, 1930, (Proc. p. 169), Dr. Cabot was relieved of the duties of Dean of the Medical School and as Director of the Department of Surgery, and the President is advised to appoint an Executive Committee of *five* to direct the affairs of the School.

That night the *Washtenaw Tribune* issued a special "scoop" on the dismissal of Cabot.

Saturday, February 8, at 10:30 A.M., President Ruthven telephoned to Dr. Novy asking if he would accept appointment on the Executive Committee. Answered in the affirmative. A little later, word came by telephone that a meeting would be held at the President's House at 5:00 P.M.

Drs. Huber and Novy arrived together and found Dr. Bruce, Peet, and Wile present. These five constituted the Executive Committee with the President as Chairman. An informal discussion arose as to the division of work. Dr. Huber offered to look over the preparation of the budget and suggested Dr. Novy take over the matter of admission of students. Dr. Novy suggested that the Committee meet each Monday at 4:00 P.M. in the President's Office. After some discussion of the advisability of giving Dr. Cabot a leave of absence to July 1st, the meeting adjourned.

(Signed) F. G. Novy

The *Boston Daily Globe* broke the news on February 9 with a special dispatch: "Dean Cabot removed on faculty's revolt. As head of Medical School at University of Michigan 'Could not get along' with other instructors, says President Ruthven." The article consisted of the following headings: *Refused to Resign*; *Specific charges not made*; *Parallels Dr. Little case*; *Barred outside practice*; *'State medicine machine;'* *Specialist here, war surgeon*. Ruthven's formal statement was included:

> I very much regret that it has been necessary to make a change in the administration of the Medical School. The conditions which seem to require such action are numerous. By far the most important one is a serious incompatibility between the Dean and heads of departments.

Later, Ruthven said, "Dr. Cabot just couldn't get along with anybody on his faculty."

Cabot himself likely provided the leak to The *Globe* for its special dispatch as it included quotes from his letter to Ruthven, referring to the regents as "the gentlemen":

> I next call attention to the fact that the remedy suggested by the gentlemen is one that has in the not distant past been used to cloak the dismissal of the university faculty guilty of gross misconduct.
>
> It is not suggested any such charges are brought or are likely to be brought against me. I therefore suggest the remedy is inappropriate.

The *Globe* revealed Cabot's negative views of "State Medicine," referring more to Michigan than a national healthcare system:[ii]

> Dr. Cabot voiced objection to the entering wedge of the State medicine machine's dictating to him how to run the school, and he declared further that when Dr. Ruthven became president last September, he told the regents that he would run the school according to his own ideas or resign immediately.[32]

The *Ann Arbor Daily News* on February 10, 1930, featured an article titled "The 'Incompatibility' of Cabot." The article began,

> Much like the resignation of President Little approximately a year ago, the removal of Dr. Hugh Cabot from the deanship and surgical directorship of the University medical school appeared to be an inevitability, due to a set of circumstances that had been combined into an 'incompatible' situation.

The article praised Cabot's "progressive acts," described his estrangement from the faculty, and mentioned his refusal to resign, concluding,

> We are convinced, with the administration, that Dean Cabot's removal was in the best interests of the University, in view of the situation in its various phases that had developed, but we sincerely trust that he will be able to carry on in another capacity with credit to himself and to the school and University which he has served for a term of years that is by no means inconsequential.

A meeting of the Executive Committee on February 10, 1930, listed as "No. 2," recorded that the present staff in the dean's office "Dr. Curtis, Miss Noble, and Miss Cummings to be notified that they are to carry on their work." A discussion "regarding replacement of Dr. Cabot on the Promotion Boards" was mentioned but without further specifics. "Dr. Wile reported that Miss Noble had taken out of the safe the budgets of last year and would mail them to the heads of Departments." This implied that Cabot had maintained some level of secrecy in his management of medical school finances. Huber was assigned charge of the preclinical

---

ii We have been unable to find the letters to Ruthven or other references to Cabot's threat to the regents of it in any files as of yet at the Bentley Library or other locations. In fact, there is a dearth of Cabot-related material for the last few months of his time at Michigan.

budgets and Bruce and Wile were to look after the clinical budgets. The minutes later recorded this disruptive period:

> There was discussion of the unrest on the surgical staff and it was arranged for the President to meet the staff from Dr. Coller down to and including the senior internes, tomorrow at 3:00 or 4:00 P.M. in the Director's room at the University Hospital. (All were present except Doctors Alexander and Nesbit who were out of town.)
>
> Dr. Novy reported that the schedules for the Second Semester would be out in a day or two. Also that in the new Medical Announcement for 1930–1931, certain changes should be made. The President suggested that a blank line be used to replace the name of Dean Cabot....
>
> No action was taken regarding leave of absence for Dr. Cabot, it being deemed best to postpone this and similar action regarding Miss Hinckley who was reported to be 'packing up.'
>
> The meeting adjourned to next Monday at 4 P.M.
>
> (Signed) F. G. Novy, MD

Medical students rallied to Cabot's side, according to the *New York Times* on February 11, 1930: "Stirred by Cabot case Michigan students debate resolutions of regret," according to the lede. Cabot was a national celebrity and clearly this matter rose above the level of a Big Ten faculty fumble.[33] The third meeting of the Executive Committee (No. 3), again in President Ruthven's office, noted, "The President requested that the matter of the resignation of Dr. Cabot be left in his hands. He also stated that he would speak to Dr. Coller and offer him the Directorship of the Department of Surgery." Peet was absent for that meeting but was then appointed to the Junior Promotion Board.

At meeting No. 6 on March 17, the committee debated Cabot's leave of absence, his pay, and his request for reimbursements of $500 for instruments left behind. President Ruthven conceded that Cabot could be paid $1,400 for the month leave of absence. Dr. Peet said that Cabot's instruments would not be used, and mentioned for the minutes that Cabot tried to get Dr. Ransom to leave for a job in Virginia. Meeting #8 on March 31 noted,

> A request from the President of the Senior Class that Dr. Cabot be allowed to sign diplomas was presented. There was no objection to the request, but Dr. Cabot is to sign at the Seniority place, or at the end.[iii]

---

iii Medical school diplomas were signed individually by the dean and the faculty chairs in order of their seniority until 2017 when Marschall Runge, EVPMA and dean, decided they should be signed electronically.

The eighth meeting also recorded, "The request of the Victor C. Vaughan Society for official recognition and sanction was presented."[iv] Novy was instructed to submit details regarding officers, members, and objects to the Committee on Student Affairs.

Cabot was understandably crushed emotionally by the dismissal but maintained his composure publicly. A picture of him shortly thereafter, in Washington, DC, at the 10th annual meeting of the Clinical Society of Genito-Urinary Surgeons in late March shows a somber and strikingly less confident visage.[34] Cabot kept up his academic publications, with a paper that year "Coccus infections of the kidney" in the *Annals of Surgery*.[35] Cabot was an early adapter of the idea of adding 5 percent CO_2 to the anesthetic oxygen mixture toward the end of a procedure to minimize atelectasis and he extended that theme in another paper that year.[36]

The abrupt dismissal of Dean Cabot left the medical school struggling to manage immediate details of day-to-day operational and academic matters, and the Executive Committee minutes likely reflect only the tip of the iceberg. At meeting 11 on May 17, President Ruthven asked who would represent the Medical School at Commencement Exercises and the committee voted that it should be Novy. Another item of business at the Executive Committee reflected the quotidian disputes of academia: "The President mentioned a letter from Dr. Kampmeyer complaining about the Department of Medicine. This was referred to Dr. Bruce." By this time, it was probably clear to Ruthven that such issues are a main reason that university presidents need deans for the schools and colleges. The final two items at this meeting signaled entry of the medical school into a new era, after Cabot. The first of these discussed a new administrative structure for the Medical School Executive Committee with elected representatives from the domains of preclinical medicine, clinical medicine, postgraduate medicine, and the hospital. Some discussion was held as to whether the hospital director, Haynes, be a member of the future structure (that would become the Executive Committee) and Bruce suggested that the decision be put to Haynes to see if he wanted to serve. Last,

> Dr. Wile called attention to an order by Dr. Cabot prohibiting colored men from examining women in the medical service. It was decided to rescind the order in question, and Dr. Wile was to discuss the question with Dr. Sturgis who is to adjust the matter.[37]

---

iv The Victor Vaughan Society of medical students and faculty played an active role and was later energized by Horace Davenport and Robert Bartlett of the faculty. Under the auspices of Dr. Howard Markel and The Center for the History of Medicine, Vaughan's name was dropped in 2017 due to recognition of his support of the eugenics movement.

The new administrative structure began quickly, for meeting 12 on May 28, 1930, was the last under the old system, ending with a typed comment in the minutes, addended by handwritten notes added years later. A new Executive Committee, designated by the Board of Regents to administer the Medical School, consisted of the directors of preclinical medicine (Novy), clinical medicine (Wile), postgraduate medicine (Bruce), and the secretary of the medical school (Curtis). The hospital director (Haynes) was "advisory" to the committee, which was to elect its own chairman. Ruthven, having had enough of the mundane details of medical school administration was probably glad to step away from the daily details of the medical school. The directorship positions were described as "ex-officio" and ultimately they became elected by their cohorts.

Formalized Executive Committee per Board of Regents, June 1930. Courtesy Bentley Library.

The medical school had no dean after Cabot and functioned under its Executive Committee for the next three years. James Bruce, Harley Haynes, Frederick Novy, and Udo Wile conducted the executive business of the school from 1930 until 1933 when Novy became interim dean.[v] The full-time model yielded to a system wherein clinical departmental and section heads were allowed complete control of their clinical units and unrestricted private practices, with surgical procedures and inpatient care across the street at St. Joseph Mercy Hospital or other facilities including University Hospital. This paradigm would last up through the

---

v Arthur Curtis was secretary of the Medical School when Executive Committee (EC) started and remained on it for three years that it was running the school. He stayed for another year after Novy became interim Dean (1933). In the notes from a regent meeting in August of 1934, Curtis is then appointed to Assistant Professor in the Department of Postgraduate Medicine for the following year (July 1, 1934-June 30, 1935). Regents meeting notes from July of 1935 state "The resignation of Dr. Arthur Covel Curtis as Secretary of the Medical School, effective August 31, was accepted" but also note: "Dr. Arthur Covel Curtis was promoted from Assistant Professor of Internal Medicine to Associate Professor of Internal Medicine to date from July 1, 1935, twelve-month basis."

1980s and in spite of the obvious conflicts of interest and commitment, it allowed great clinical expertise to attract patients from afar, fuel education and innovation, and build a world-class clinical reputation in Ann Arbor with clinicians John Alexander, Frederick Coller, Eddie Kahn, Reed Nesbit, and Max Peet, among others.

With the request from the medical students for Cabot to sign their diplomas in 1930, it was logical that his picture be included with that class. Curiously, though, his picture persisted in the 1931 and again in the 1932 class picture, when his former trainee and successor as the university's urologist, Reed Nesbit, appeared as well. In 1933, however, only Nesbit was pictured.

The surgical department had been operating autonomously under Coller by this point in time and had grown large enough to divide it into two sections, red and blue services, under Henry Ransom and Eugene Potter, respectively.[38] Just as time heals most wounds, an action recorded at Executive Committee Meeting 92 on May 9, 1935, brought Cabot's face back to Ann Arbor: "Dr. Coller moved that the Executive Committee obtain a picture of Dr. Cabot so that it could be hung in the faculty Room. Seconded by Dr. Haynes and PASSED." The Executive Committee continued to meet weekly until dean Novy was in place in 1933, and it continues to meet on alternate weeks to the present day continuing to list the sequential number of its meetings. The first January meeting in 2020 was number 2884.

When the Executive Committee took the place of Dean Cabot in 1930, none of its members regretted his absence. Bruce, although initially hired by Cabot, never had an easy relationship with him and had been displaced in 1928 to head postgraduate medicine. Haynes, the hospital director, had crossed swords with Cabot over various matters. Novy, a former contender for the 1921 deanship, became further estranged from Cabot over salary matters and curriculum issues early in the Cabot era. Wile was never fully aligned to Cabot. A one-time student of Osler, Wile had been recruited to Ann Arbor in 1912 to teach dermatology and syphilology and initially asked permission to open a private office in Detroit, but after faculty debate he was allowed to open only a free clinic in Detroit. However, as soon as he moved to Ann Arbor, he opened a private office on Liberty and Maynard, continuing to operate it for the next 35 years. This was all before Cabot arrived, but their relationship never was warm. Many others at the university and throughout the state were glad to see Cabot gone.

The Mayo Clinic was a logical destination for Cabot's next step. William Mayo and Cabot were well known to each other, and the Mayo salary model was in accord with Cabot's beliefs. Furthermore, the clinical prowess of the Mayo Clinic was much that the University of Michigan (and Cabot in particular) had aspired to achieve. It was telling that Herbert Henry Dow died at Mayo Clinic on October 15, 1930, where he was being treated for liver disease, presumably because equivalent expertise was not available nearer his home in Midland or even in Ann Arbor, Detroit, or Grand Rapids. A very successful industrialist, Dow, could have gone wherever he wanted or where reputation directed him. In terms of clinical care reputation, Ann Arbor was a relative newcomer to the field with its 1925 modern hospital and the clinical expertise that had accrued largely in the Cabot era. The delicate balancing act of the academic mission against the economics of clinical practice did not fall apart after Cabot was dismissed but the full-time model was disassembled. The Surgical Department and other faculty units rebalanced their missions and found a compensation model that succeeded for many decades, wherein the clinical departments controlled their individual professional revenues.[vi]

A cursory scan of the events of the time shows great change in the world around Ann Arbor. The 1920s may have come in with a roar of optimism, novelty, and new technologies, but the decade concluded with shifting realities, economic uncertainties, geopolitical realignments, and new celebrities. Mickey Mouse made his first appearance in 1930; Pluto was confirmed as a celestial body; and the Communist Parties of Vietnam, Indo-China, and Panama were established. Gandhi initiated his civil disobedience campaign and broke British India's salt laws. Danish painter Einar Wegener began sex reassignment surgery in Germany, Britain returned leased lands to China, and Haile Selassie began a 44-year rule of Ethiopia. Volcanic island Anak Krakatau appeared in the Sunda Strait. Earthquakes and hurricanes disrupted lives and property, as did revolutions and rebellions in Brazil, Peru, and Kurdish Turkey. Anglican bishops approved limited birth control, while Papal encyclical *Casti connuni* prohibited it. Neoprene was invented by Dupont and penicillin achieved its first recorded cure, an eye infection treated by George Paine at the Sheffield Royal Infirmary. The United Kingdom Mental Treatment

---

vi Mission imbalance would plague the Ann Arbor health system just as at all other medical centers for the ensuing century and would be exacerbated by the infusion of federal money through research grants after World War II and later dominance of third party payees including the government. It has been long obvious that education, research, and clinical care comprise the mission of academic medical centers, but the recognition that the clinical piece is the essential deliverable—the moral epicenter, the financial engine, and the milieu for research and education—has not been widely understood. The essential deliverable underpins everything in the healthcare industry and at a moment's notice rightly trumps other activities, 24 hours a day, 7 days a week, and 12 months a year. Robust teams, mission-oriented faculty, excellent systems, and believable leaders balance the mission and deploy the essential deliverable: kind and excellent patient-centered care.

Act provided free treatment for psychiatric conditions and discarded the term *asylum* for *mental hospital*. On December 2, President Herbert Hoover asked Congress to fund a $150,000,000 public works program to create jobs as the Great Depression deepened. The University of Michigan Medical School closed out the year without a dean and having dismantled Cabot's full-time dream. The clinical programs had reached new levels of excellence, but with the school run by committee, aspirational potentials were constrained. Gradual national and state-wide recovery from the Great Depression would slowly fortify the university barely in time for the next international catastrophe.

Notes

1. H. W. Davenport, *Not Just Any Medical School* (Ann Arbor: University of Michigan Press, 1999), 29–30.
2. H. W. Davenport, *Not Just Any Medical School* (Ann Arbor: University of Michigan Press, 1999), 49.
3. H. Cabot, "A Plea for the Further Extension of Clinical Opportunity into Earlier Years of the Medical Course," *Bulletin of the Association of American Medical Colleges* 2 (1927): 105–108.
4. H. Cabot and H. K. Ransom, "Ethylene as an Anesthetic for General Surgery," *Annals of Surgery* 86 (1927): 255–259.
5. H. Cabot and G. C. Adie, "Etiology of Cancer of the Stomach," *Annals of Surgery* 82 (1925): 86–108.
6. *Detroit Free* Press, November 20, 1927.
7. J. Alexander, "New Instrument for Subperiosteal Costectomy," *Journal of American Medical Association* 83 (1924): 443.
8. J. Alexander, *The Surgery of Pulmonary Tuberculosis* (Philadelphia, PA: Lea and Febiger, 1925).
9. H. W. Davenport, *Not Just Any Medical School* (Ann Arbor: University of Michigan Press, 1999), 207.
10. H. W. Davenport, *University of Michigan Surgeons 1850-1970* (Ann Arbor: Historical Center for the Health Sciences, University of Michigan, 1993), 191.
11. H. W. Davenport, *University of Michigan Surgeons 1850-1970* (Ann Arbor: Historical Center for the Health Sciences, University of Michigan, 1993), 106.
12. Picture courtesy William P. Didusch Center for Urologic History.
13. R. M. Engel, Charles Brenton Huggins, MD. Retrieved from http://www.urologichistory.museum/content/collections/uropeople/huggins/p2.cfm, William P. Didusch Center for Urologic History, AUA (2003).
14. C. Huggins and C. V. Hodges, "Studies on Prostate Cancer," *Journal of Urology* 167, no. 2 (1941): 948–951.
15. R. C. Schneider, A. Edgar, and M. D. Kahn, 1900–1985. *Journal of Neurosurgery* 64, no. 2 (1986): 167–168.
16. C. H. Frazier and M. M. Peet, "Factors of Influence in the Origin and Circulation of the Cerebrospinal Fluid," *American Journal of Physiology* 35 (1914): 268–282.
17. *Detroit Free Press*, September 16, 1928.
18. *Detroit Free Press*, January 6, 1929.

19 Bentley Historical Library, University of Michigan, Walter Sawyer papers, Letter from Bruce to Sawyer, July 23, 1929.
20 Bentley Historical Library, University of Michigan, Letter to Sawyer September 24, 1929 and Letter to Sawyer August 14, 1929.
21 Bentley Historical Library, University of Michigan, Sawyer papers, 1929.
22 Bentley Historical Library, University of Michigan, Sawyer correspondence, 1929.
23 H. H. Peckham, *The Making of the University of Michigan 1817–1992*. Edited and updated by M. L. Steneck and N. H. Steneck (Ann Arbor: University of Michigan Press, 1967, 1994), 198–199.
24 H. W. Davenport, *Not Just Any Medical School* (Ann Arbor: University of Michigan Press, 1999), 185.
25 H. W. Davenport, *Not Just Any Medical School* (Ann Arbor: University of Michigan Press, 1999), 34.
26 Bentley Historical Library, University of Michigan, University of Michigan Medical School files.
27 H. W. Davenport, *Not Just Any Medical School* (Ann Arbor: University of Michigan Press, 1999), 185.
28 H. W. Davenport, *Not Just Any Medical School* (Ann Arbor: University of Michigan Press, 1999), 112.
29 V. C. Vaughan, "A Chemical Concept of the Origin and Development of Life. A Preliminary Presentation," *Chemical Reviews* 4, no. 2 (1927): 167–188.
30 H. W. Davenport, *Not Just Any Medical School* (Ann Arbor: University of Michigan Press, 1999) Chapter 16, Footnote #46, 344.
31 Bentley Historical Library, University of Michigan. Letter in later Sawyer papers.
32 *Daily Boston Globe*, February 9, 1930, page A13.
33 "Stirred by Cabot Case.; Michigan Medical Students Debate Resolutions of Regret," *New York Times*, February 11, 1930.
34 W. W. Scott and H. M. Spence, *The Clinical Society of Genito-Urinary Surgeons. A Chronicle 1921–1990* (Baltimore, MD: Williams and Wilkins, 1991), 76.
35 H. Cabot and R. M. Nesbit, "Coccus Infections of the Kidney," *Annals of Surgery* 92 (1930): 766–773.
36 H. Cabot and H. Lamb, "The Choice of Anesthesia with Particular Reference to the Protection of the Patient," *Ohio State Medical Journal* 26 (1930): 998.
37 Bentley Historical Library, University of Michigan, President's Office meeting no. 11 page 14, May 17, 1930, box 6.
38 *UM Encyclopedic Survey*, 949.

The Medical School after Cabot

Alexander Ruthven, named reluctantly by the regents as university president in 1929, presided over the painful termination of Cabot early in the next year and continued as university leader for 22 years of growth and maturation of its medical school. Many of the university's research accomplishments were substantial, but the biggest prizes in scholarship (Nobel and Lasker awards, for example) eluded Michigan for the most part. The medical faculty and hospital continued to draw challenging medical problems from the state and beyond as well as make significant contributions in technology and science, but regional patients of means, such as Herbert Dow mentioned earlier, tended to travel to other centers for clinical expertise, drawn by long-standing clinical reputations. The ideal apportioning of mission balance and the failure to fully embrace the essential deliverable of academic medical centers (namely, kind and excellent patient-centered care) precluded that ultimate reputational step for Michigan.

The Cabot years had so disrupted the medical school that President Ruthven appointed no successor as medical school dean, preferring instead to leave an Interim Executive Committee in charge of the daily business of the Medical School and even serving as the admission committee. James Bruce, Harley Haynes, Frederick Novy, and Udo Wile constituted that committee until 1933 when Frederick Novy was appointed interim dean. Novy retired in 1935 and Ruthven named Albert Carl Furstenberg permanent dean, absent any consultation with the faculty. This otolaryngologist was the antithesis of Cabot. He had a busy private practice with an office on Main Street, another office at St. Joseph Mercy Hospital where he operated and hospitalized private patients, and he had a similar situation at University Hospital. As Medical School dean he was given a fourth office and staff in the West Medical Building. Furstenberg, unsurprisingly, was known for being perpetually late. Cabot had left him a good situation, as Davenport recounted,[i]

> In the early years of Furstenberg's deanship there were two large basic science buildings and several hospital buildings with 1,330 beds. Sixteen thousand patients were seen each month in two outpatient clinics, and twenty-seven thousand were admitted to the hospital each year, where one thousand operations were performed each month. There were more than two hundred physicians on the hospital staff and one hundred men and women on the faculties of the basic science departments.[1]

During his entire 11 years at Michigan, Cabot retained the title of head of the Surgery Department, but his recruitment of Frederick Coller in the summer of 1920 provided an able lieutenant. In fact, Coller became the operational head of the department in its daily work without the title until Cabot left. Later, Edgar Kahn noted that Coller was a great surgeon, whom was widely "worshipped":

> Mustard and I worked under Dr. Cabot, the Dean of the Medical School and Chief Surgeon. As a technician he was not as good as Dr. Coller; but he had wonderful surgical judgement. I learned from him that "tincture of time" can cure a lot of things. He was a strict disciplinarian and tough mentally and physically.[2]

A more reasonable and kinder leader would have likely given Coller the dignity of the surgery department chairmanship sometime after becoming dean of the medical school, but not Cabot. Nevertheless, Coller never showed any evidence of resentment, nor was he visible among the anti-Cabot activists. With Cabot gone, Coller easily stepped into the official role of surgery chief. Although Coller had worked well with his chair and dean, Hugh Cabot, Coller had a very different style and was generally revered by those who worked under him. Nesbit later reminisced, nearly reverently, about Coller in rough notes likely prepared much later for the Mayo Lecture at Michigan in 1968, and retained by Nesbit's oldest daughter, Nancy:

> Frederick Coller—Brought here by H.C. after War I
> Harvard—MGH—His father

---

[i] Furstenberg's name is spelled variably in multiple sources. Even the text with the medical school class pictures features the correct Furstenberg in some years and the incorrect Furstenburg on other years.

Completely different Personality than H.C.
Master Surgeon—Relaxed in O.R
   Technique e.g., Rachmaninoff
Scholar—Med. History—Civil War, Artist
Capacity for creating friendships of all types & levels.
   My mother
   My ???with him at Conrad Hilton
Definition of Gentleman—"Have another drink"
Loose administration
   Described his methods—if-of
     Democracy with dictatorship
Log raft vs. Streamlined battleship
   His loyalty & support of his men when in trouble. The ?????
Great Leader in the organizations of Surgery
   Amer. Surg Soc. ACS.
His men—countless positions of importance
In all levels of Academic & Clin Surg.
Ideals he instilled & inspired
All reflected in the great number
Who occupy responsible positions in surgical societies
   e.g., ACS.
His Philosophy of Training
   His letter.

Some notations are indecipherable and other comments remain obscure.[3]

Cabot had been sole urologist at the university since 1920 until Huggins in 1924 and Nesbit came to train with him in 1925. Section of Urology was not established until after Cabot's departure, when Nesbit was named its head. Over the ensuing 38 years, Nesbit would train 76 residents and numerous others as fellows. As an innovator of TURP technique, he made Ann Arbor an epicenter for treatment, attracting patients from around the country and world. Frank Hinman, Sr., was a notable example, traveling with his son in 1954 from San Francisco for TURP by Nesbit.[4] The U.S. State department selected Nesbit to travel to Taiwan to treat Chiang Kai-shek (1887–1975) and thereby developed a deep relationship with the Chang family.

With Cabot gone, the Medical School ended the mandatory full-time faculty salary plan on July 1, 1931, allowing clinical faculty to conduct private practices in addition to their academic responsibilities, performing their private surgical procedures and hospitalizing their patients at University Hospital or in the adjacent St. Joseph's Mercy Hospital. Senior faculty augmented educational and research opportunities for their junior faculty and trainees from their personal funds.

The shift for the surgical faculty, however, was not immediate. Frederick Coller, the new chair of the Department of Surgery after Cabot retained his full-time status, with a salary of $8,000 per year until 1935. Alexander, Badgley, and Nesbit discarded their full-time status the following year.

Cyrenus Darling died in April 1933. He had severed his ties to the Medical School after Cabot's arrival in 1919 but retained his title of professor of oral surgery in the Dental College until 1926, when the Board of Regents named him professor emeritus. In August 1936, Ira Dean Loree died at age 67, having continued his career at St. Joes' Hospital with little further interaction with Hugh Cabot or the University of Michigan. If the transition of general surgery from Moses Gunn to Charles de Nancrede was considered "a bumpy ride," the shift from ancient genitourinary surgery to modern urology under Cabot must be described as an abrupt transition, but it smoothed out under the aegis of Coller with Nesbit at the helm of urology.

Although a Cabot disciple, Coller was diplomatic and gracious, developing a strong network of loyal referring physicians as well as an attractive residency training program, as evidenced by a robust alumni society that later formed in his name. Coller got along well with his division heads and other faculty colleagues, but their relative independence left him and his fellow general surgeons with the lion's share of surgical teaching and responsibility for the nonprivate surgical cases at University Hospital. Coller argued with the Executive Committee and the dean to increase his surgical faculty but with varying degrees of success. He didn't bring a physician anesthesiologist to the faculty until 1938 when Fenimore Davis (UMMS, 1935), after training in Iowa and Wisconsin followed by a short experience in Kansas City, returned to Ann Arbor and unceremoniously replaced his one-time teacher, Laura Dunstone.

Within a few years Michigan's Medical School was very different from what Cabot had envisioned as most senior faculty transitioned to the part-time plan. Davenport saw the disadvantage of the new order:

> Each department chairman or section head ruled his department or section with a firm hand, and his juniors were absolutely dependent upon him for professional and financial advancement. There were inbreeding and provincialism. By the end of the 1930s every member of the Departments of Physiology and Surgery was trained at Michigan, and some other departments were not much different. Because the dominant members of the faculty thought alike, they determined the tone and policies of the school.

Davenport praised the Vaughan years but disparaged those of Furstenberg:[ii]

> Dean Vaughan and those who cooperated with him made Michigan what a well-informed historian of U.S. medicine called "not just any school," and that school lasted until the bad days of World War I. Dean Furstenberg and his colleagues made an entirely different kind of school that lasted long after World War II.

Davenport, the physiologist, was of mixed opinion regarding Cabot, mainly faulting his weak commitment to laboratory investigation. Four faculty members, however, were particularly noteworthy from Davenport's perspective: Louis Harry Newburgh who had come to Ann Arbor in 1916 and Frank Wilson, Reed Nesbit, and Frederick Coller who had all been recruited by Cabot.

The 1930s were troubling times for the Medical School regarding the issue of academic refugees from Germany. Davenport found that only two surgeons, Carl List and Herman Pinkus, were accepted in Ann Arbor and then only with the stipulation that they received no pay from the university or hospital, so they were therefore brought on as researchers. Pinkus did tissue culture work for Coller and List, a neurosurgeon who had worked with Cushing, eventually became an instructor with a medical school salary, the only refugee that the school actually employed. The Urology Section remained apart from any refugee engagement.

Cabot gave Nesbit a great head start in urology. Davenport noted that in the 2.5 years Nesbit and Cabot worked together they performed 450 suprapubic prostatectomies with a mortality of 25 percent. While this seems terrible by today's standards, severe obstructive uropathy was a highly lethal condition on its own and even in those days of early anesthesiology, lacking antibiotics, and with little understanding of fluid and electrolyte balance, surgical intervention with those odds didn't seem an unreasonable choice.[5]

In 1935, otolaryngologist Albert Carl Furstenberg (1890–1969) became the next dean and served until 1959. The Executive Committee,

---

ii Davenport's phrase for his 1999 book, *Not Just Any Medical School*, came from Gert Brieger who wrote, "Michigan was not just any medical school. It was one of a handful of truly important centers of medical education in the years around 1900." The reference was a "Letter to Ms. Rebecca McDermott of University of Michigan Press" dated 30 July 1977 and quoted by permission.

however, remained an essential part of medical school governance and function, continuing to meet even to the present day, and numbering the meetings since the turbulent February, 1930.

Notes

1 H. W. Davenport, *Not Just Any Medical School* (Ann Arbor: University of Michigan Press, 1999), 295–296.
2 Coller and Kahn memoirs.
3 Nesbit notes for 1968 Mayo Lecture at Michigan, courtesy Nancy Nesbit, 2019.
4 D. A. Bloom, F. Hinman, Jr., and Frank Hinman, Sr., "A First Generation Urologist," *Urology* 61 (2003): 876–881.
5 H. W. Davenport, *University of Michigan Surgeons 1850-1970* (Ann Arbor: Historical Center for the Health Sciences, University of Michigan, 1993), 194.

Cabot after Michigan

Cabot's abrupt termination by the regents was optically framed as a resignation. A photograph of him six weeks afterward, in a group picture of the Clinical Society meeting in Washington, DC, shows nine members including Cabot seated on the far right with an uncharacteristic visage, with hands folded and seemingly lacking his expected confident expression. Somehow, however, the confident profile of his younger years persisted on the University of Michigan Medical School class pictures for two more years. Cabot is last seen at Michigan in the 1932 class picture when he is joined by Nesbit for the first time.

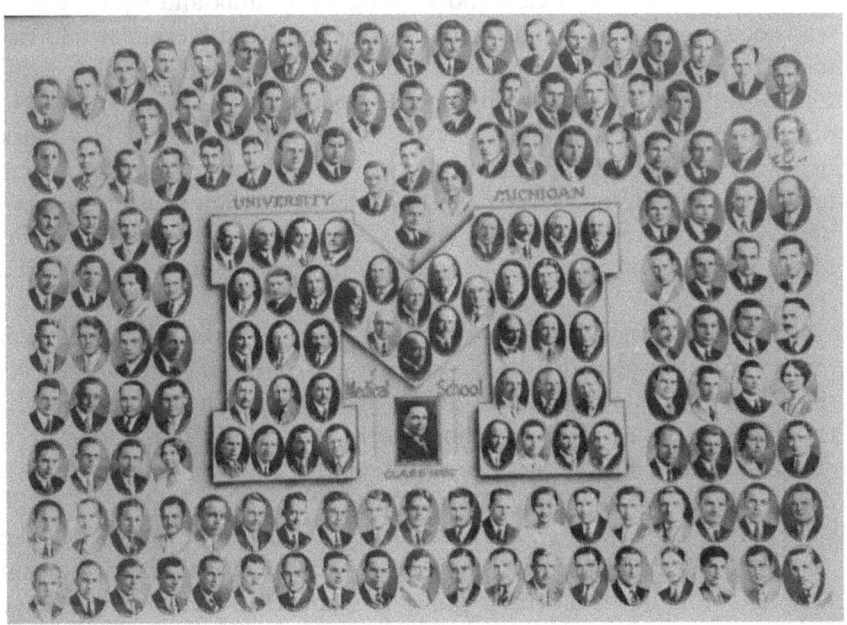

UMMS class picture of 1932 with both Cabot and Nesbit.

An article from Cabot and Nesbit in 1930 on "Coccus infections of the kidney: their frequency and their relation to the upper urinary tract" reflected continued collaboration between the two urologists as well as Cabot's belief that most renal infections were blood-borne in origin.[1]

1931–1939

Cabot appeared at the Clinical Society in 1931 where the group picture in St. Louis again showed a muted expression. When the topic of undescended testicle was discussed, it was likely that Cabot spoke up, for that was the year of his influential paper with Nesbit on single-stage orchidopexy. Cabot's work at the Mayo Clinic allowed him freedom to travel and write, including his *Surgical Nursing* book.[2] He lived at 705 Second St. SW in Rochester and seemed to have had an uncontroversial time at the clinic. The professional stationary he used displayed the simple Mayo Clinic heading at the top and on the upper left: Surgical Section of Dr. Hugh Cabot. His chronology in these years is discovered most easily through his academic travels. He missed the 1932 meeting of the Clinical Society in Philadelphia and then the 1933 one in Iowa City. Cabot was active enough among the members of the American Association of Genito-Urinary Surgeons that in 1933 in Washington, DC, at its 45th meeting he was recommended to the American College of Surgeons (ACS) as a member of the Board of Governors, along with Caulk and Squier. Cabot was not selected, but in later years his protégé, Reed Nesbit, would rise to the presidency of the ACS and later Nesbit's own protégé, Ralph Straffon, would similarly ascend. For some reason, the Clinical Society did not seem to meet in 1934, but that year Cabot appeared at the New York Academy of Medicine in April to discuss "The drainage of nephrostomy upon kidney function."[3] Later in December at the Southeastern Section in Atlanta, it was recorded: "Dr. Hugh Cabot of the Mayo Clinic, author of the textbook *Modern Urology*, spoke on 'treatment of undescended testicle.'"

Cabot missed the 1935 Clinical Society back in Cleveland. His election that year as president of the New England Section of the AUA reflects the esteem of his colleagues in his original clinical and academic territory, reversing the customary choice of having a local practitioner lead an AUA section as well as opposing the trend of being a section president before becoming AUA president. Cabot's book, *The Doctor's Bill*, came out in 1935 with an introduction by A. Lawrence Lowell, relative of Mary Cabot and until recently president of Harvard. The dedication was made to "the considerable group of students of medicine who have honored me by their confidence." This detailed and scholarly book still bears much that is familiar to health care in 2020.[i]

Cabot began the book by comparing medical practice in 1890 to that of 1930. The chapters were: "Modern medical diagnosis and its requirements, Our medical resources, The general practice of medicine, Specialists and group medicine, Group Health resources, The workmen's compensation acts, The income of physicians, The ability to pay for illness, Health insurance in continental Europe, Health insurance in the British Isles, Medical needs in the United States, Some suggested methods of improvement, Laissez faire or compulsion, and Where do we go from here?" Notes, bibliography, and a robust index followed. The University of Michigan was mentioned once and only then in passing to its Student Health Service. In the discussion on training of specialists, he wrote:

> The specialist in the fields of the senses will probably require more time [for training]. The urologist should, I think, be a fairly capable general surgeon before he undertakes the often complicated and trying surgical problems of the genito-urinary system. In the same way, the orthopedist should be a surgeon before he is a specialist, and five years will probably be less than will commonly be thought necessary for his development. In the narrower fields, as typified by the surgery of the nervous system, prolonged experience is necessary because the opportunities for broad experience will be more difficult to obtain and, and a really comprehensive view, therefore, will take more time.[4]

Cabot's wife, Mary Anderson Boit Cabot, died in 1936 at 58 years of age and was buried in Brookline, at the family plot. The Clinical Society met that year in London on September 3–4 at invitation of the British Clinical Society of Urology. Cabot sat for the group picture in the front row of the 23 participants, nine of whom were the hosts. Cabot has the same dour appearance seen in photographs since he left Ann Arbor. The London meeting cycled through St. Thomas's Hospital, St. Peter's

---

i Lowell was a serious choice for the book introduction, having stepped down as president of Harvard University two years earlier. A "Boston Brahmin," like Cabot, Lowell had a major career in academia and government, although the families had not always aligned: Lowell's debate in 1919 against Senator Henry Cabot Lodge was an iconic moment of political civility in the argument over the League of Nations. Lowell's opposition to President Wilson's choice of Louis Brandeis for the Supreme Court earlier in his career, however, was not a high point for Lowell.

Hospital for Stone, and St. Bartholomew's Hospital. That same year Cabot published a third edition of *Modern Urology* that was favorably reviewed. The *Annals of Internal Medicine* in April 1937 reported,

> Cabot's *Modern Urology* is well named for it brings up to date every phase of urology and does it very efficiently. The chapters are written by different authors who are authoritative and who well represent urology in America. The book is in two volumes, is well edited, and is profusely illustrated. The first volume is divided into six sections dealing with the lower urinary tract. It contains a chapter dealing with methods of diagnosis which is unusually informative and a chapter on transurethral resection of the prostate gland, which, while enthusiastically written, is nevertheless a well balanced description of the . . .[5]

Richard Cabot's link to that journal perhaps explains this unusual convergence of internal medicine and urology. As with the 1918 version, Cabot dedicated the book to his cousin Arthur. Cabot appeared at the AAGUS meeting in Quebec in 1937 with a paper "methods of selecting the proper operative treatment for cancer of the bladder."

Cabot's opinions regarding the social organization of medical practice continued to develop along egalitarian principles from his early days in Boston. In those days, he was an isolated iconoclast, but later in the 1930s he found like-minded colleagues, notably a group called the American Foundation Studies in Government that obtained and digested 5,000 letters from 2,100 physicians with their thoughts on the "present status and future of medical practice." The initial understanding was that conclusions would not be drawn immediately from the findings of the letters; however, the *Journal of the American Medical Association* on October 16 noted,

> Nevertheless, at the time of publication some earnest workers in the vineyard expressed the belief that certain deficiencies in the medical scheme were clearly apparent and that concrete proposals should be made which would have the approval of the medical profession and might lead to governmental action.[6]

During a conference in New York, some of the foundation participants met with Eleanor Roosevelt and later her husband. From those discussions, a resolution from the House of Delegates of the New York State Medical Society containing a set of proposals from the American Foundation Studies in Government was introduced in the House of Delegates of the AMA "and there rejected with an enthusiastic unanimity which indicated quite clearly the utter dissatisfaction of the medical profession with these proposals." Cabot and orthopaedic surgeon Robert B. Osgood,[ii] leaders in the executive committee of the foundation, wrote a letter to colleagues asking for support of the principles and proposals. Cabot's letter from August 1937 was printed in a *JAMA* editorial:

> Dear Doctor:
> A few of us who were included in the Executive Committee of the American Foundation for Studies in Government, whose Report has just appeared, are hopeful that certain basic opinions can be properly put forward based upon the weight of evidence in the report. I think it important that a considerable group of influential and well-known physicians should assent to certain fairly general propositions, the tendency of which will be to show that what is needed is a very broad attack along a wide front rather than more narrow attacks upon limited objectives. There has, we think, been a good deal of rather just criticism of the medical profession on account of its unwillingness to advise positive rather than negative action. There seems to be some evidence that legislation looking toward compulsory health insurance has attracted a good deal of favorable attention in political bodies. It seems to us that compulsory insurance attacks only a very limited portion of the problem and that legislation to put this into operation might well do serious harm not because it would not be of assistance in solving certain problems but rather it would help and might, therefore, tend to stop progress along a broader line.
> Will you read over the enclosed statement of the Principles and Proposals and after due consideration, if you feel willing to approve, sign and return to me.
>
> Sincerely yours,
Hugh Cabot.[6]

The editorial noted that some orthopaedic surgeons who signed the letter were later "indignant" at the manner of securing their signatures and on reconsideration opposed any governmental subsidy and control of medical practice. The *JAMA* editors concluded,

> Such careless participation in propaganda as has here occurred is lamentable, to say the least. Certainly the unthinking endorsers of the

---

ii Osgood's name turned up earlier in the WWI discussions and see footnote ii on page 129.

American Foundation's principles and proposals owe to the medical profession some prompt disclaimers.

No disclaimers would come from Cabot, who can hardly be characterized as "unthinking," although his style of leadership that got him into trouble at Michigan seems again in play with his statement of principles and proposals.

A *New York Times* article later that October, titled *Subsidized Medicine*, discussed the foundation report further, noting that it arose from physicians who were dissatisfied with the status quo in health care:

> ... their dissatisfaction with the medical care now available and to suggest means whereby medical science may be advanced, the standards of medical practice raised and medical education improved. The Foundation made no recommendations of its own, but let the doctors speak for themselves. On behalf of a group who contributed to the report, Dr. Hugh Cabot of the Mayo Clinic and Dr. Robert B. Osgood of Boston, two physicians of the highest standing, have circulated a letter in which they call upon their profession to "assent to certain general propositions," one of which is the propriety of supplementing inadequate private endowments by grants from public funds—local, State, and possibly Federal—to medical schools, hospitals, and research laboratories.[7]

The *New York Times* described the report, officially titled "American medicine: expert testimony out of court," as widely condemned and noted the *Journal of the American Medical Association* was "outraged at this seeming violation of organized medicine's economic interest in the treatment of disease and research." The idea of acceptance of any public funds was viewed as "a step in the direction of socialized medicine."

In response to the national hostility, *A Committee of Physicians for the Presentation of Certain Principles and Proposals in the Provision of Medical Care* representing 430 physicians and surgeons pushed back in an article in the *New England Journal of Medicine* that November (see next page). Fourteen physicians led the committee and Cabot was one of two vice chairmen. Coller was later listed among the prominent surgeons who signed the principles and proposals, although no other names came from the University of Michigan Medical School. Among the 53 prominent names in American medicine, the other person from Ann Arbor was Clyde C. Slemons, listed in the public health section.[8]

Cabot once again was dead center in the midst of controversy and at odds with most of his colleagues in the nation.

> **Principles and Proposals**
>
> Committee of Physicians for the Presentation of Certain Principles and Proposals in the Provision of Medical Care.
>
> A Summary.
>
> Principles
>
> 1. The health of the people is a direct concern of the government.
> 2. A national public health policy should be formulated.
> 3. Economic need and adequate medical care are separate problems and require different solutions.
>
> Proposals
>
> 1. First step is to minimize risk of illness by prevention.
> 2. Adequate care for medically indigent should be met from public funds.
> 3. Medical education and investigations and procedures to improve standards should be supported by public funds (i.e., "health services research").
> 4. Medical research should be supported by public funds.
> 5. Hospitals serving medically indigent people should be consistent with above principles.
> 6. Public funds should be allocated to private hospitals consistent with above principles.
> 7. Public health services at all levels of government should be expended by evolutionary process.
> 8. Investigation, planning, and execution of these proposals should be assigned to experts.
> 9. Administration and supervision of governmental health functions, implied by these proposals, should be consolidated under a separate department.

In October, 1938, Cabot returned to Massachusetts to marry Elizabeth Cole Amory in Hingham, the widow of Walter Amory who had died a year previously, having been a patient of Cabot's at the Mayo Clinic (figure on next page). Cabot soon retired from the Mayo Clinic, dropped out of clinical medicine, and returned to Boston where he and Elizabeth lived for the remainder of his life. Not surprisingly, when the Clinical Society met in Rochester and Minneapolis on December 1–3, 1938, Cabot was not present in the group picture or in the program, and no further participation of Cabot in the society is evident during the remainder of his life. Perhaps some clue to Cabot's influence, however, was the election of Reed Nesbit to AAGUS membership at its 1938 meeting (along with J. A. Campbell Colston and Archie Dean to fill the seven vacancies at the

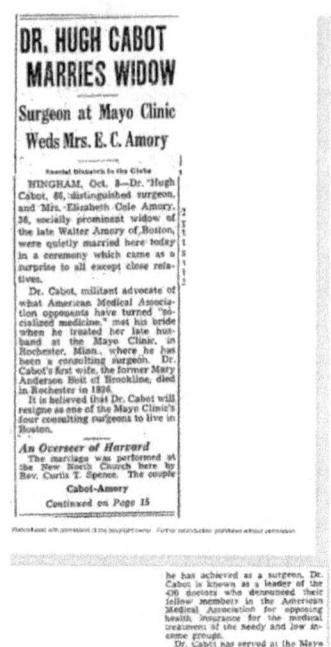

The Baltimore Sun, October 9, 1938

time). Richard Cabot died in 1939 on May 7 at age 70, and on July 28 Cabot's good friend William Mayo succumbed at age 78 to gastric carcinoma.

Cabot maintained interest in finding solutions for fair delivery and payment of medical services. In 1939, he became a founder of the White Cross in Boston, an organization developed around the concept of complete prepayment for medical services. Backlash to this from his peers was cut short by the next war.

1940–1945

In 1940, the AUA membership sharply attacked its former president Cabot at the annual meeting for his articles criticizing the cost and availability of medical care.[9] Cabot was unapologetic, doubling down that year with a book produced for the public expressing his beliefs in overarching public obligations of medical care. Unlike his other books, *The Patient's Dilemma* lacked a dedication. Perhaps, at the end of his career and toward the end of his life, sentimentality, gratitude, or deference to those who had influenced him had slipped away. The preface began with a whimsical excerpt from *Alice in Wonderland*, wherein the March Hare invited Alice to have some wine but she found only tea on the table. When Alice said that she didn't see any wine, the March Hare replied, simply, "There isn't any."

So, it was for the public, Cabot explained, who are invited to have good medical care, if they can find the health care they need and want, much less pay for it. Cabot used the figure of speech "the mythical average man" throughout the text and he described the conflict most physicians experienced, as he had in Boston, namely the "devotion of something like one-half my time to the teaching of medicine and the care of indigent patients at the Hospital," juxtaposed with "the obligations to one's family in the way of providing the wherewithal to carry on a successful struggle for existence." Resolution of that conflict "took me, just after the War, to the University of Michigan as professor of Surgery on 'full time,' and later as Dean in the Medical School." Those references to Ann Arbor are *nearly* nostalgic and seem to have been slow in coming since his rough termination a decade earlier.

The book begins with a brief discussion of the impact of scientific discoveries, then delves into the idea of "good medical care" with its costs, delivery systems, and standards. A chapter on the cost of medical care in relation to delivery allowed him to make a pitch for private group practice and the importance of bringing a new area of expertise, what is today known as the social worker, into the delivery systems, giving Cabot a chance to mention his brother.

> Here we saw the beginning of medical social service in this country, initiated by the late Richard Clarke Cabot in an attempt to humanize the contact between the busy and sometimes senior physicians and the confused, worried patients who seek their care.[10]

Cabot devoted one chapter to medical security and another to the government and medical care, ending with a chapter on medicine of the future and his personal journey, largely framed by the conflict he described in the preface. Cabot ended the book noting:

> We are driven to the conclusion that though long distance planning under democracy is beset with many vicissitudes, nevertheless such plans must be made and, by dint of good temper and the laws of the cosmos, they may come to fruition.

Nowhere in the book does he mention George Bernard Shaw's play *The Doctor's Dilemma* of 1906, but the irony probably didn't escape Cabot.

Upon retirement from Mayo in 1939 and return to New England, Cabot engaged deeply in issues of medical reform. On the occasion of his 50th year since graduation from Harvard College, the Fiftieth Anniversary College Report summarized him as

> ... eminent surgeon and medical dean. Eloquent speaker and writer. Ardent crusader in war and peace, brushing aside all men and things if they block the way to truth.

Cabot's twin brother Philip died in 1941 and was reported in the *New York Times*, which described him as an economist, lecturer, and Harvard Business Administration School professor. The only sibling mentioned in the article was "Dr. Hugh Cabot of Needham" in a sentence including Philip's first wife, present widow, two daughters, and several grandchildren. How Richard Cabot could have been omitted from mention much less the other brothers must be ascribed to a rookie error for the reporter. Philip was noted as "an outspoken critic of the New Deal" and referred to the Social Security Act as "the most ridiculous document that ever was printed, although the idea is sound."[11]

Hugh Cabot died of a heart attack while sailing off the coast of Maine in Frenchman's Bay in 1945. He was buried in Brookline, Massachusetts, in the family plot. In his memory, friends raised money to establish a penicillin plant in Russia, although why this in particular seemed suitable remains to be known. The name, Hugh Cabot, persisted for several ensuing generations with his son, Hugh Cabot II (1905–1967), a professor of sociology at Harvard and grandson, Hugh Cabot III (1930–2005), a naval combat artist during the Korean War whose wartime scenes were exhibited in Tokyo after the war and praised by critics. He later became successful as an artist after the war, known for his distinctive stylized cowboys and Western landscapes. Hugh Cabot had three other children, Arthur Tracy Cabot (1916–1989) named for the celebrated cousin, John Boit Cabot (1909–1972), and Mary Anderson Cabot (1907–1924), who died at 16 in Italy and was buried in Brookline, Massachusetts.

Cabot's obituary was carried in the *New England Journal of Medicine*.[12] Sir Herbert Seddon, once Cabot's British rotator, wrote the memorial note for the *Lancet*.[13] While Cabot's last appearance with the Clinical Society, an organization he had helped start, had been in London in 1936, it was ironic that the 1946 meeting that included his memorial commentary, along with those of Hugh Young and Henry Bugbee, would be held in Ann Arbor. The Michigan Union was the headquarters, the very place Cabot had lived during his early weeks in Ann Arbor. The annual dinner and business meeting for the 19 attendees was held at the home of Dr. and Mrs. Reed Nesbit. The official meeting record noted simply that Cabot was "well known for his teaching abilities." As has been shown. he left behind so much more and his story is still quite incomplete, with much more to learn.[14]

Reed Nesbit was Cabot's heir in urology at Michigan for 38 years after Cabot left Ann Arbor. Nesbit's trainee, Jack Lapides, would follow for the ensuing 15 years and Ed McGuire for the next seven. Frederick Coller was Cabot's heir in general surgery at Michigan and his tenure as chair continued for 27 years (1930–1957). The Cabot-Coller-Nesbit era brought a medical school, that already was notable for its educational and research capacity, full throttle into the top league of clinical excellence. With the tripartite mission of education-research-clinical care largely fulfilled, the University of Michigan Medical School was indeed a full "triple threat" academic medical center under Cabot. Before him, clinical care in Ann Arbor was subordinate to education and research.

The twentieth century with its burgeoning technology, expanding specialties, economic contingencies, and public expectations have made the clinical part of the academic health center its moral, financial, and creative epicenter.

After Nesbit stepped down as Urology Section chief, his notes in preparation for return to Michigan as the Mayo lecturer in the Spring of 1968 were titled "Some Recollections of the Cabot-Coller Era." The eight pages of notes were written on University of Michigan Union stationary that Nesbit must have taken with him to Davis or perhaps prepared on a brief (and unaccounted for) visit to Ann Arbor before the talk. One can imagine him sitting in Davis, California, perhaps with a glass of wine, collecting his reminiscences on fitting stationary that he nostalgically had kept (below).

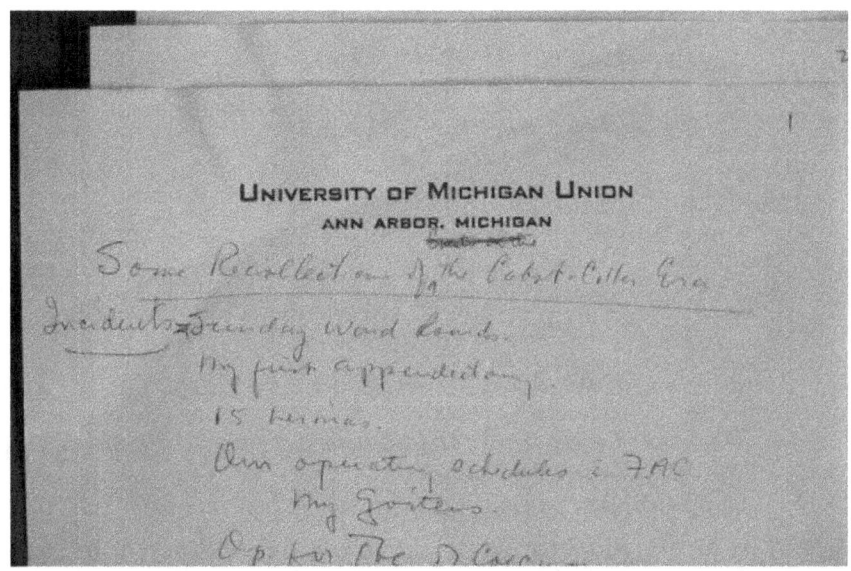

Nesbit's notes for Mayo lecture in Ann Arbor, 1968. Courtesy Nancy Nesbit and Reed Youmans.

The first seven pages, an almost random collection of "incidents," and observations, were in pencil except for the final typed page that began with the following paragraph.

> So an era in our department of surgery, The Cabot-Coller Era has passed and now is becoming part of the folk-lore of the institution. Those of us who were privileged to participate look back upon it with nostalgia. Nostalgia, as you recall, is a subjective and emotional remembrance of experience in our lives that we are happy and proud to have been associated with; most real but doubtless partly the creation of our imagination.[15]

A more accurate description of that referenced period of time would be the *Cabot-Coller-Nesbit Era*. The Nesbit notes offer some of his insights regarding Cabot in a randomly-ordered list:

> Family Tradition – Somber – Forceful person
> Life not a game – a challenge to meet head on
> Woodchipping, The Boat – Hermes Staebler, Walks in Winter – Tennis.
> Demanded Loyalty – gave trust + Confidence.
> "The Chief"
> Dynamic Teacher – admired + popular with students.
> Alcohol
> Acute Orchitis
> Butzel
> Litholapaxy – Bigelow – Holmes
> His Operating Style – Tension – again a challenge – Arthur Curtis
> Capacity for creating enemies
> No compromise – Black – White – no gray.

The Climax

> Many men of my generation owed him much for opportunities he gave them.
> Mayo Clinic Seminars – Dwight Wilbur
> Death – challenging a storm.
> [Reed M. Nesbit notes from Nancy Nesbit papers]

Some items and names are cryptic. For example, the "alcohol" mentioned by Nesbit under the *Dynamic teacher* and *students* section may point to a common problem in higher education that persists today. It may also relate to some family matters, possibly Cabot's attitude regarding the prohibitionist stance of his twin. Then, too, was the national constitutional ban on the production, importation, transportation, and sale of alcoholic beverages from 1920 to 1933. This period closely mirrored the Cabot era in Ann Arbor. The Volstead Act and Eighteenth Amendment of 1919, enacted in spite of President Wilson's veto, coincided with Cabot's start at the University of Michigan. Cabot was gone from Ann Arbor at the time President Franklin Roosevelt signed the Cullen-Harrison Act on March 23, 1933, legalizing beer up to 3.2 percent alcohol content. However, Cabot's visage had persisted in the yearly medical school class picture until the 1933 spring graduation when Nesbit's face was the only one representing urology. The Twenty-First Amendment repealed the frivolous Eighteenth Amendment that December. When Roosevelt signed Cullen-Harrison, he said, "I think this would be a good time for a beer."[16] While Nesbit's alcohol comment is unexplained, alcohol remains a problem in colleges, professional schools, and workplaces today, just as it was in Cabot's days as dean and Nesbit's time as Urology Section head in spite of the temporary constitutional ban. The *Acute orchitis* comment is even more mystifying, perhaps alluding to some clinical observation or treatment idea.

Deeper research into the life of Hugh Cabot awaits future historians, as some records remain missing or sealed. For example, certain records of Hugh Cabot (#158–164 at the Schlesinger Library, Radcliffe Institute, in the Harvard Library) remain "closed until January 1, 2062, at the request of the donor."

Hugh Cabot was a determined man, with progressive social and medical ideas that were out of step with many of his contemporaries but are far more widely accepted 100 years later. He rammed his ideas through organizational landscapes with little thought for consensus or compromise and he spent down political capital rather than accruing it, yet he brought Michigan into the mainstream of clinical medicine and the center stage of worldwide urology.

Notes

1 H. Cabot and R. M. Nesbit, "Coccus Infections of the Kidney: Their Frequency and Their Relation to the Upper Urinary Tract," *Annals of Surgery* 92 (1930): 766–773.
2 H. Cabot and M. D. Giles, *Surgical Nursing*, (Philadelphia, PA: W. B. Saunders, 1931).
3 I. Jones, Nephrostomy Paper, *New York Academy of Medicine* (1934), 197.
4 H. Cabot, *The Doctor's Bill* (New York: Columbia University Press, 1935), 66–67.
5 "Reviews," *Annals of Internal Medicine* 10, no. 10 (1937): 1600–1601.
6 "The American Foundation Proposals for Medical Care," *JAMA* editorial 109, no. 16 (1937): 1280–1281.
7 "Subsidized Medicine," *New York Times*, October 25, 1937.
8 "A Committee of Physicians for the Presentation of Certain Principles and Proposals in the Provision of Medical Care," *NEJM* 217, no. 20 (1937): 798–800.
9 L. W. Jones, P. C. Peters, & W. C. Husser, "The National AUA 1902-2002," *The American Urological Association Centennial History, 1902-2002 vol. 1* (Baltimore, MD: American Urological Association, 2002), 22.
10 Hugh Cabot, *Patient's Dilemma. The Quest for Medical Security in America* (New York: Reynal and Hitchcock, 1940).
11 *New York Times*, December 26, 1941
12 ELY. Obituary. Hugh Cabot (1872–1945). *New England Journal of Medicine* 233, no. 23 (1945): 706–707.
13 H. J. Seddon, "The Late Doctor Cabot," *Lancet* 2 (1945): 354.

14 W. W. Scott and H. M. Spence, *The Clinical Society of Genito-Urinary Surgeons. A Chronicle 1921–1990* (Baltimore, MD: Williams and Wilkins, 1991), 131; W. S. McDougal, H. Spence, D. Bloom, and G. Uznis, "Hugh Cabot 1872–1945: Genitourinary Surgeon, Futurist, and Medical Statesman," *Urology* 50 (1997): 648–654.
15 Nancy Nesbit papers.
16 J. E. Smith, *F.D.R.* (New York: Random House, 2007), 305, 316.

The Curious Connection of Howard Kelly to the University of Michigan

The University of Michigan and Johns Hopkins University, one public and the other private, had close links since the earliest days of the Baltimore institution, with particularly close connections between their medical schools. During the Cabot years at Michigan, the two medical schools were among the best to be found internationally. Then, the fields of gynecology and urology shared numerous mutual clinical interests and sometimes held joint sessions at their major societies. Major figures in each field usually knew their national counterparts and this was certainly true in the two institutions in Ann Arbor and Baltimore. Even though they came from different departments, it seems likely that Cabot would have known of Howard Atwood Kelly (1858–1943) and vice versa. Kelly's link to Michigan, however, came from one of his hobbies, the study of mycology, reptiles, and amphibians.

Kelly was born in Camden, New Jersey, to a family with no medical inclinations. His paternal great-grandfather, Michael Hillegas, was the first U.S. treasurer. Kelly's father, Henry, served in the Civil War and his mother, Louisa, took him to Chester, Pennsylvania, where he developed an interest in natural history with special attention to reptiles and mushrooms, in addition to bible studies. For the rest of his life, he would be deeply religious. At the University of Pennsylvania, he obtained a BA in 1877 and an MD in 1882. After commencement, he wrote in his diary,

> I dedicate myself-my time-my capabilities-my ambition-everything to Him. Blessed Lord, sanctify me to Thy uses. Give me no worldly success which may not lead me nearer to my Savior.[1]

Kelly began a 16-month rotating residency in the medical dispensary (clinic) of Episcopal Hospital northeast of Philadelphia (now Temple Health – Episcopal Hospital) where it was not unusual for him to see more than 80 patients in a day. He embraced the clinical work and learned avidly from the great clinicians of Philadelphia:

> Here at last my real medical education began in the dispensary and in the wards under the excellent and always kindly and sympathetic clinical chiefs—men of reputation, such as Morris Lewis, Louis Starr, and J. M. Anders in medicine, and C. B. Nancrede, John Hooker Packard, and William S. Forbes in surgery.[2]

This was also the time and place of Samuel David Gross and David Hayes Agnew immortalized in the iconic paintings of Thomas Eakins. de Nancrede, then using his simplified surname, would leave Philadelphia for a full-time job at the University of Michigan in 1889.

Kelly developed an interest in gynecology, which was then a part of general surgical practice, although some surgeons were becoming de facto specialists. After his training, Kelly's parents expected him to open an office near in their home in Philadelphia, while Kelly felt that a practice in Kensington would be more robust and needed by the community. He compromised with an office in each place, five miles apart. Over time his preference was for Kensington, although Episcopal Hospital didn't embrace the gynecological surgery. Most operative procedures, then, were performed at homes of patients after scrubbing floors, walls, and kitchen tables, but in time Kelly set up a house in Kensington for his operative procedures, hiring Helen Wood to help him in the operations and with postoperative care. Kelly began to build his personal library around this time and the collection became massive toward the end of his life. Later with philanthropic help, this two story facility transitioned to a formal clinic and operating room, eventually becoming the sixth women's hospital in the United States, the Kensington Hospital for Women, where he gained fame with his "Kelly Stitch" for stress incontinence. He traveled throughout Europe intermittently between 1886 and 1888 to watch other pelvic surgeons, including learning ureteral catheterization from Rudolf Virchow in Berlin and air cystoscopy from Parel Pawlik in Prague. He visited old bookshops and accumulated old editions of Hippocrates, Galen, Vesalius, and Paré, among others.

Returning to Philadelphia in 1888, Kelly became associate professor of obstetrics at the University of Pennsylvania, but in 1889, William Osler brought Kelly to the new Johns Hopkins School of Medicine as the first chair of gynecological surgery. With William Halsted and William Welch, they constituted "The Big Four."

While in Germany in 1889, Kelly married Olga Bredow, daughter of Danzig physician. After a honeymoon in Paris, they returned to Baltimore where they would raise nine children in a five-story, eight-bedroom house, full of books, dozens of cages of reptiles, and his mushroom collection. In 1892, Kelly founded the Howard A. Kelly Hospital where he collected substantial fees, which he didn't require at the Hopkins hospital.

Kelly's career as the initiating gynecologist at Johns Hopkins Hospital is well known and proudly celebrated. His role in ureteral investigations in the last years of genitourinary surgery and the early years of urology is documented previously in this text. Kelly's spiritual evangelicalism, described by H. L. Mencken, detracted from his clinical and scientific impact, but his skill as a physician and surgeon made him a wealthy man with freedom to indulge nonclinical scientific interests. Mencken, a respected journalist and "the sage of Baltimore," described Kelly as "the kind of friend who relieved him of the need for enemies" and furthermore, "the most implacable Christian I ever knew, at least among educated men." Kelly tried for years to convert the agnostic reporter but without success and their opinions diverged over many matters of contemporary interest from prohibition to the Scopes trial. In spite of their polar differences, Mencken retained deep respect for Kelly's clinical skills.[3]

Kelly collaborated with Max Brödel, whom he claimed to have brought to Baltimore from Leipzig. Brödel had also met Franklin Mall (UMMS 1883) from Hopkins in 1888, so Kelly's claim might be taken with a grain of salt. Brödel, known later as the father of medical illustration, collaborated extensively in urology with Young as well as with Halsted in surgery, Cushing in neurosurgery, and Kelly with his book *Operative Gynecology* in 1898. Years later, at Kelly's 75th birthday dinner, Brödel said,

> The planning of the picture therefore is the all important thing, not the execution. This is where we learned from Dr. Kelly. He had a way of making little modest outline sketches when he explained his operative procedure to his illustrators. . . . Dr. Kelly always permitted the artists to make original investigations to clear up the obscure point. . . . Without his sympathetic attitude we could not have learned our trade as we did.[4]

Kelly's interest in natural history, begun when he was a young boy in Chester, developed a keen focus on fungi and in wooded areas around Baltimore he began a serious study and collection. His biography, written by his long-time editorial assistant Audrey Davis, tells part of a story that created a curious link of Kelly to the University of Michigan:

> The best nearby collecting fields at this time were out beyond Towson and in the undeveloped properties along the rivers. One day some identification perplexities took him to Washington, and there he heard about the extraordinary artist-mycologist Louis C. C. Krieger,

whom Kelly persuaded to give up work with the government in order to come to Baltimore, help him build up a mycological library, and paint for him a series of plates from fresh specimens.[5]

Krieger spent 10 years with Kelly, whose library grew to 10,000 books, a card index of 400,000 references to the world literature in mycology, over 2,000 specimens, and 400 water-color plates painted from the natural specimens. In addition, botanical artist Eleanor C. Allen, of New York, made a number of deceptively realistic wax models displayed within glass cases. Kelly published a catalog of this collection in 1928. Davis explained how Kelly intersected with the University of Michigan:

> After careful consideration of a suitable depository, Kelly chose the University of Michigan because there, under Professor C. H. Kauffman, the most active interest was evidenced in mycology. Under no circumstances did Kelly wish the books, plates, and models to become absorbed in a general botanical library; they must go to a university with a progressive, working department of mycology. With appropriate ceremony the University of Michigan accepted this gift as the Louis C. C. Krieger Mycological Library, so named by Kelly as a tribute to Krieger's devoted labors. Shortly thereafter, in recognition of his wide scientific interests, Dr. Kelly was appointed an Honorary Curator of the Division of Reptiles and Amphibians of the University.[6]

Corresponding fragments of the story emerge in minutes of the regents of the University of Michigan, first in April 1920 when Regent Kraus announced a $300 gift from Kelly to study and photograph fungi under the direction of Professor C. H. Kauffman, curator of the Cryptogamic Herbarium. In March 1922, a gift of $550 was accepted to partially fund an expedition to Wyoming to be led by Kauffman, and in June 1922, Professor Ruthven noted that Kelly donated a portrait of the British Museum naturalist G. A. Boulenger to the university. The regents appointed Kelly Honorary curator of Reptiles and Amphibians in the Museum of Zoology in October 1923 on the recommendation of Professor Ruthven. The next reference to Kelly came in February 1927, acknowledging his contribution of $300 to help print a monograph for A. I. Ortenburger, described as a "former graduate student." The final cost of the monograph, $900, was covered by other sources. It was recorded in March 1928 that Kelly gave two rare editions to the university. The following month, Kelly is again acknowledged in reference to Kauffman. Then in May, Ruthven praised Kelly's donation of "elaborate, expensive, and rare works" to the library of the museum. In November 1928, Kelly contributed $500 toward the purchase of a large "lichen herbarium" from Dr. Fink in Ohio. Kelly gave 170 books and pamphlets to the museum library in February 1929. In April of that year, he devoted another $500 toward the Fink collection and in June made his last acknowledged gift of a monograph of *Genus salpa*. Kelly's illustrator, L. C. C. Kreiger, helped the gynecologist secure "what was probably the most extensive privately owned mycological collection in this country."[7]

The Kelly connection with Michigan or the Midwest seems to include no other academic, family, or geographic affinities. Kelly did vacation not very far away in the Parry Sound district of Ontario at Ahmic Lake, where he kept a microscope, small library, field glasses, and telescope. Whether Kelly ever visited Ann Arbor and intersected then with de Nancrede, Dean Cabot, or any of his gynecological peers at Michigan awaits discovery.

Notes

1 A. W. Davis, *Dr. Kelly of Hopkins: Surgeon, Scientist, Christian*, (Baltimore, MD: Johns Hopkins Press, 1959), 37.
2 A. W. Davis, *Dr. Kelly of Hopkins: Surgeon, Scientist, Christian*, (Baltimore, MD: Johns Hopkins Press, 1959), 37–38.
3 C. S. Roberts, "HL Mencken and the Four Doctors: Osler, Halsted, Welch, and Kelly," *Proceedings Baylor University Medical Center* 23 (2010): 377–388.
4 A. W. Davis, *Dr. Kelly of Hopkins: Surgeon, Scientist, Christian*, (Baltimore, MD: Johns Hopkins Press, 1959), 114.
5 A. W. Davis, *Dr. Kelly of Hopkins: Surgeon, Scientist, Christian* (Baltimore, MD: Johns Hopkins Press, 1959), 184–185.
6 A. W. Davis, *Dr. Kelly of Hopkins: Surgeon, Scientist, Christian* (Baltimore, MD: Johns Hopkins Press, 1959), 185–186.
7 B. Kanouse, "Doctor Howard Atwood Kelly," *Mycology* 35 (1943): 383–384.

Epilogue

Modern urology, in the larger sense that Cabot intended for his textbooks in 1918, 1924, and 1938, traced a long path from its pre-Hippocratic days of uroscopy, catheterization, horrific lithotomy, and other treatments for the common genitourinary dysfunctions that have always troubled mankind. Little changed from the most ancient days until the mid-nineteenth century when scientific ways of thinking and unprecedented technology began to assemble a verifiable conceptual basis for genitourinary function and disease, along with tools to investigate and repair dysfunctions. Professional expertise accrued, socialized, and coalesced into organizations, centers, teaching systems, and research units.

This book has followed that story of the formation of modern urology and its particular roots at the University of Michigan in greater detail than is customary for a departmental historical narrative. The richness of the stories of the specialty of urology and the University of Michigan, has been found so compelling that we were unwilling to reduce this work to a mere chronology of dates and names. The two stories, moreover, have been synergistic and neither can be understood in the absence of the other.

With the start of the Michigan Urology Centennial Year at the fall term of 2019, we intended this book to tell the conjoined tale of urology and Michigan up through the Cabot era. Hugh Cabot defined urology at Michigan. He transformed the University of Michigan Medical School, that was even then "not just any medical school" as Horace Davenport used the phrase, into a top league tripartite academic medicine center, although it is still a work in progress, a fragile house of cards like all other academic medical centers. Less fragile than most, we hope. The basis of its strength, moral epicenter, and resource engine is its clinical delivery system. Cabot recognized this better than most of his contemporaries and he also recognized its limits and inequities. His idea of a full-time salary model was ahead of its time but flawed and it proved transient. On the other hand, the raw commercialism that his contemporary, Ernest

Codman, lampooned in his famous cartoon was even more inadequate (see pp. 101n, 107, 127). The ideal balance remains to be found, but it appears closer to the model of the great medical clinics that have moved into the academic arenas, for example the Mayo Clinic, Cleveland Clinic, and closest to Ann Arbor, the Henry Ford Clinic. These bear particular relation to the Michigan Urology Story, although others are no less notable. If academic medical centers don't find a proper solution to the great pressing dilemma of health care in America, the government and the marketplace will produce answers, few of which are likely to optimally serve the public, the professions of health care, and the future generations of patients and learners.

The rest of the Michigan Urology story, from Nesbit through the inauguration of departmental status under Montie, last told by Konnak and Pardanani 20 years ago, will be revised, updated with terms of the next two chairs, and joined to this work as we begin the Second Centennial of Urology at Michigan.

Index

Note: Page numbers followed by "f" indicates figures; those followed by "n" indicates footnotes; and those followed by "t" indicates tables.

1918 Flu, 100 Years Later, 109n
AAGUS (*see* American Association of Genito-Urinary Surgeons)
Abbott, LeRoy, 148–9, 156, 165, 182
Abel, John, 79, 107–8
Abulcasis of Córdoba, 5
Academy, The, x, 91
ACMI (*see* American Cystoscope Makers Inc.)
ACS (*see* American College of Surgeons)
Act to establish the Catholepistemiad (Woodward), 18–20
Adams (Wirt) Regiment Mississippi Volunteer Cavalry C.S.A., 35
Adams, Zabdiel Boylston, 9n
Adie, George, 175, 180
AEF (*see* American Expeditionary Forces)
African American Students, 28, 36, 43, 179
Agnew, David Hayes, 222
Alberran, J., 73
Alexander, John, 148, 149, 156, 171n, 182–3, 194, 197, 204
Alexander, Samuel, 64
Alice in Wonderland, 214
Allen, Danielle, 17
Allen, Eleanor C., 224
Allen, John Adams, Jr., 24
  dismissal of, 29
Alumni Hall, 88
AMA (*see* American Medical Association)

American Ambulance Hospital, 104, 105
  University Service of, 128
American Association of Genito-Urinary Surgeons (AAGUS), 36, 70–1, 71t–2t, 103, 122, 124–7, 132, 208, 210, 213
  genitourinary surgery origin claim, 70–1
  papers presented by Cabot, Arthur and Hugh, 71t–2t
American Board of Medical Specialties, xi
American College of Surgeons (ACS), 101, 101n, 115, 147, 151, 175, 203, 208
American Cystoscope Makers Inc. (ACMI), 70
American Expeditionary Forces (AEF), 105n, 106, 132
American Foundation Studies in Government, 210–211
American Gynecological Society, 115, 127
American Institute of Homeopathy, 42n, 54
American Journal of Dermatology and Genitourinary Diseases, 35
American Journal of Medical Sciences, 64, 125, 182
American Journal of Obstetrics and Gynecology, 168
American Medical Association (AMA), 11, 38, 55, 90, 101, 210

Index 229

Council on Medical Education, 89–90
American Red Cross, 103, 128, 128n, 214
American School of Osteopathy, 55
American Statistical Society, 30n
American Surgical Association (ASA), 36, 70, 81, 83
American Urological Association (AUA), 60–1, 66n, 73, 89, 101, 124, 139, 208, 214
American Urological textbooks, 110f
American Women's Hospital in Devon, 148
Americans Abroad, 11, 32n
Amory, Elizabeth Cole, 213, 214f
Amory, Walter, 213
Andania, 129
Anatomical laboratory building, 81
Anders, J. M., 222
Anesthesia, 3, 14, 15, 32n, 35, 60, 64, 67, 68, 82, 85, 101, 108, 126, 167, 180, 191, 195
Angell, James, 38, 42, 43, 46, 48, 50, 52, 77–8, 82, 88, 100, 102n, 140, 143, 145, 147
  alumni cohort, 53
  Blouin on, 43
  Fishery Commission, 52
  MD program under, 45
  minister to China, 45
Annals of Internal Medicine, 210
Annals of Surgery, 61, 195
Ann Arbor
  city of and University of Michigan, 22–4, 33, 36, 59, 103
  citizens of, 33, 36, 103
  draft, 36
  draftees, 106, 109
  population, 22, 24
Ann Arbor Courier, 46
Ann Arbor Daily News, 193
Ann Arbor Gazette, 84
Ann Arbor Land Company, 22
Ann Arbor Observatory, 48, 176f
Archives of Internal Medicine, 124
Argus, 33
Armistice 104n, 106, 110
Army Medical Department, 34
Army of the Potomac, 34
Arnold Gold Foundation, 68n
Arrowsmith (Lewis), 116–117, 173

ASA (*see* American Surgical Association)
Association of American Medical Colleges (AAMC), 180
  Thirty-Third Annual Meeting, 162–4, 162f–4f
Astronomia, 10n
Athletics, 53, 172, 189
Atlantic Magazine, 32n
AUA (*see* American Urological Association)
Averell, Mary Williamson, 182n
Avicenna, 5
Ayurvedic medicine, 3, 31

Bachelor of science degrees, 25
Bacon, John U., 106–7
Bacon, Robert, 105, 128
Bacteriology curriculum, 180
Badgley, Carl, 165, 182
Baghdad, 4
Baltimore, 60–3
Banting, Frederick, 40n, 151
Bard, Samuel, 68n
Barney, J. Dellinger, 126–7
Barrows, David, 158f
Barry, John M., 109
Barry Guards, 33
Bartlett, Robert, 195n
Bates, Elizabeth, 54
  Endowment, 54, 115
Bates, Frederick, 18
Bates Street, 20, 21
Battle of Bull Run, 9n, 34
Battle of Las Guasimas, 83
Baxter, Katie, xv
Beal, Harold W., 132
Beal, Rice, 46, 46n, 171, 185
Beaulieu, Jacques, 8
Beauregard, P. G. T., 34
Beer, Edwin, 151
BEF (*see* British Expeditionary Forces)
Bell, Alexander Graham, 15, 182n
Bellevue Hospital, 12, 44, 66–7
Best, Charles, 40n
Bigelow, Henry Jacob, 14, 64, 70, 122, 128, 129, 147, 218
"The Big Four," 61–2, 222
Bill of Rights, 142
Billi, Jack, xiii
Bimaristan Argun in Aleppo, Syria, 5

Bimaristans, 4
Birds of America (Audubon), 23
"Black Thursday," 187
Blackwell, Elizabeth, 29
Bladder stone surgery
  (see lithotomy), 10
Bliss, Willard, 15n
Bloom, Martha, xv
Blouin, Fran, xi, xv, 43
Bogart, Humphrey, xv
Boggs, Thomas, 154–5
Boit, Mary Anderson (see Cabot), 123, 209
Bollinger, Lee, 68n
Bond, Thomas, 9–10
Bossidy, John Collins, 125
Boster, Joel and Dea, xi
Boston, 17, 30, 32n, 60, 61, 64, 70, 73, 80, 89n, 101, 101n, 103, 104, 105, 106, 107, 113, 114, 117, 121, 121n, 122, 124, 125, 127, 128, 129, 131, 132, 133, 136, 137, 139, 142, 143, 147, 212, 214
Boston Brahmin, 32n, 121, 121n, 209n
Boston Daily Globe, 105, 126–7, 129, 131, 132, 133, 136, 136f, 145, 166, 192, 193
Boston Herald, 174
Boston Medical and Surgical Journal, 110, 124, 125, 126, 128
Boston News-Letter, 9
Boston Society for Medical Improvement, 30, 59, 122
Boston Surgical Society, 128, 147
Bostwick, Homer, 11–2, 13f
Botanical therapies, 31
Bottini, Enrico, 89
Boulenger, G. A., 224
Bovie, William T., Jr., 29–30
Bovie, William T., Sr., 29
Bowditches, 129
Bowlby, Anthony, 139, 184
Bowles, Charles, 190
Boyer, Alexis, 63
Boylston, Zabdiel, 9–10, 59, 74
Braasch, William, 151
Bradley, Alfred E., 106
Brady, Diamond Jim, 63
Brady Institute, 63
Brandeis, Louis, 209n
Breakey, William F., 94

Bredow, Olga, 222–3
Brian, Thomas, 8
Brieger, Gert, 205n
British Clinical Society of Urology, 209
British Expeditionary Forces (BEF), 105, 106, 128, 129, 131, 132, 56, 170, 184
British General Hospital in France, 128n–9n, 148
British Medical Journal, 14, 69, 171n
Brödel, Max, 223
Bruce, James, 172, 179, 186, 188, 192–197, 201
Brünnow, Franz, 35, 48
Bryson, John, 64
Budd, William, 30n
Buerger, 69
Bugbee, Henry, 216
Bumstead, Freeman, 12, 67
Bunker Hill Monument Association, 132–3
Burton, Marion Leroy, 141–2
  Cabot and, 143–9
  Cabot's letters to, 152
  Coolidge nominating speech, 167
  death, 167, 171, 174
  fellowship in creative art, 155
  homeopathic issue, 158, 161–162
  Hutchins' letter to, 146
  letters to Hutchins, 145–6
  letter to Boggs, 154
  letter to Goodnow, 153
  letter to Hadley, 153–4
  letter to Regent Clements, 143
  Mayo's letter to, 149–50, 153
  as presidential phenotype, 147
  recommendation for Cabot as dean to, 155
  Sawyer's letter to, 102n, 154
Burton Memorial Tower, 183
Burton, Theodosia, 141
Buss, Sarah, xii–xiv

Cabot, Arthur Tracy, 64, 101, 113, 122
  AAGUS and, 70, 71, 71t–2t, 103, 122, 124
  book dedication, 129, 168, 210
  death, 126
  family, 122–3, 125, 184, 216
Cabot, Charles Mills, 122–3
Cabot, Edward Twiselton, 122–3
Cabot, Elizabeth, 122
Cabot, Elizabeth Cole Amory, 213

Cabot, Hugh, 32n, 43, 64, 266–7
 AAGUS and, 71, 71t–2t, 124–7, 208, 210
 as president of AAGUS, 103
 academic productivity, 124
 appointment as chief of surgery, 97–8, 113, 135–41
 Ann Abor, comes to, 135–42
 Ann Arbor campus, 74
 on athletics, 172
 AUA and, 124
 as president of AUA, 100–1
 as president of New England Section of AUA, 208
 being troublesome for the university, 139–41
 birth, 122–3
 Boston and, 103
 Boston Brahmin, 121, 121n
 Burton and, 143–50
 children, 123
 Clinical Society (of Genito-Urinary Surgeons), 151, 185, 195, 207–10, 213, 216
 Coller and (see Coller, Fredrick)
 curricular reform, 163–4
 as dean, 80, 151–9, 173
 death, 216
 Doctrine of the prepared soil, 127, 157
 The Doctor's Bill, 208–9
 European experience, 139
 faculty discontent with, 182, 187–8
 family and early career, 121–33
 financial resources, 133
 full-time faculty/salary model, 97, 112, 113, 115, 133, 135, 139, 141, 144, 148–9, 151, 153, 154, 155–6, 160–1, 165, 176, 187, 191, 196–7, 198, 204, 226
 geographic fulltime clinical faculty, 137
 Harvard Surgical Unit, 129–31
 Journal of Urology, 107
 leadership support for, 188
 letter from Regent Clements to, 157, 158f
 letter to colleagues on Principles and Proposals, 211
 letter to Hutchins, 137–9, 138f
 marriage, 123, 213
 Mayo Clinic and, 197–8, 208, 212–13, 214f, 215

Mayo's letter to Burton, 149–50
 Mayo's letter to Vaughan, 141
 MGH and, 123, 125–6
 Modern Urology, 64, 89n, 109–10, 131, 156, 167–8, 173, 210
 as naturalist, 123
 Nesbit's insights regarding, 218
  from 1922 to 1926, 160–78
  from 1927 to 1930, 179–200
  from 1931 to 1939, 207–14
  from 1940 to 1945, 214–19
 Phenolsulphonephthalein test, 72t, 125
 Post-Flexnerian decade and, 100–17 practice, 123
 President's House and, 139–41, 143–7
 psychological safeguards for patients, 157
 publication, 124
 quotas for ethnic groups and, 179–80
 reading habits, 173
 recommendation for dean, 155
 reputation and mentorship, 124
 Smith's letter to, 140–1
 social events, 181
 termination, 102n, 201, 207, 214–5
 trainee first as house surgeon, 126
 tripodal capacity, 126
 UMMS Class Picture, 207f
 University Hospital, 114
 on venereal disease, 126–7
 White Cross in Boston, 214
 World War I and, 103–11, 128–33
Cabot, Hugh, II (Jr.), 123, 165, 184–5, 216
Cabot, Hugh III, 216
Cabot, J. Elliott, 32n, 122
Cabot, John, 121
Cabot, Joseph, 121
Cabot, Mary Anderson (daughter), 123, 166, 166f, 169, 216
Cabot, Mary Anderson Boit (wife), 123, 133, 136–137, 144, 161, 166, 172, 175, 208, 209
Cabot, Philip, 122, 123, 215–216
Cabot, Richard Clarke, 122–4, 172, 210, 213–16
Cabot, Samuel, III, 122
Cabot, Samuel, Jr., 121
Caboto, Giovanni, 121
The Canon of Medicine (Avicenna), 5
Capener, Norman, 170, 184

232 Index

Carnegie Foundation for the
   Advancement of Teaching, 90, 169
Carrow, Flemming, 79
Casablanca, xv
A Case of Priapism (Gross), 28
Cass, Lewis, 20–21
Cassatt, Mary, 174
Catgut, 110, 124
Catheterization, 3, 5, 15n, 51, 59,
   61–3, 65, 222, 226
Caulk, John, 151, 208
Centenary of Urology at the
   University of Michigan, 117
Chang family, 203
Chemical analysis, 12, 31, 45, 92
Chemical Laboratory Building, 25,
   30–1, 36, 92
Chemistry (Barker), 48
Chetwood, Charles, 89
Chiang Kai-shek, 203
Chicago, viii, 52, 79, 94, 100–1,
   126, 146
   Cholera Epidemic, 25
   Gunn, Moses, viii, 36, 70, 77, 122
   Huggins, Charles Brenton, 183
   Origin to American urology, 60, 66
   Palmer, Alonzo, 25
   Peterson, Reuben, 114
   Rush Medical College, viii, 36, 70,
      77, 114, 122
   University of Chicago, 100, 166–7,
      175, 183
Chicago Daily Tribune, 184
Chinese medicine, 3
Cholera, 20–1, 25
Churchill, Edward, xii, xiv
Churchill Project, xivn
Churchill, Winston, xiv, 181n
*Civilization in the United States: An
   Inquiry by Thirty Americans*
   (Stearns), 116–17
Civil War, viii, 9n, 27–38, 40–1, 48,
   55–6, 65, 122, 203, 221
   slavery and, 35
Clements (Regent), 143–6, 145n, 157,
   165, 171, 185–6
Clements Library, 144–5, 145n, 183
Cleveland Clinic, 151, 227
Cleveland Medical College, 28
Cleveland Plain Dealer, 92n
Clinical care, 61, 88, 92, 160, 190,
   198, 216

Clinical Congresses of Surgeons of
   North America, 101
Clinical demonstrations, 29–31
Clinical Practices Conferences, 124
Clinical Society of Genitourinary
   Surgeons, 151, 185, 195, 207,
   208, 209, 213, 216
Cobb, Ty, 174
"Cocaine and its derivatives" (Novy),
   79, 79–80n
Code of Hammurabi, 3
Codman, Ernest, 101n, 107, 127,
   226–227
Coffey, Don, vii
Colclazer, Henry, 22
Coleman, Bessie, 174
"A Collection of Ten Sermons of
   Religion" (Parker), 92n
College of Engineering, 109 College of
   Physicians and Surgeons (P&S),
   22, 22n, 25, 38, 68, 68n, 90
Coller, Fredrick, 95, 128–129, 148,
   156, 165, 167, 170, 172, 175,
   182, 183, 184, 188, 194, 197,
   202–4, 205, 212, 216–18
Collip, James, 40n
Colorado Medicine, 169
Colston, J. A. Campbell, 213
Columbia College, 68n, 90
Columbia University Roy and Diana
   Vagelos College of Physicians and
   Surgeons, 68n
Columbus, Christopher, 121
Columbus and Amsterdam
   Avenues, 68n
A Complete Practical Work on
   the Nature and Treatment of
   Venereal Diseases, and Other
   Affections of the Genitourinary
   Organs of the Male and Female
   (Bostwick), 12, 13f
Committee of Physicians for the
   Presentation of Certain Principles
   and Proposals in the Provision of
   Medical Care, 212, 213f
Confederate Army, 34
A Congressional Act, 18
Contagious Hospital, 114, 157
Continuing medical education, vii, 81,
   101, 172
Cooley, Thomas M., 48
Coolidge, Calvin, 165, 167, 174, 180

Cooper Medical College, 116
Corbett, Rupert, 170, 184
Cosy Corner Tea Room, 161, 175–6
Council on Medical Education
  (AMA), 89–90
Courthouse Square, Ann Arbor, 33f
Cowie, David Murray, 113–4, 155,
  157, 187–188
Cowie Hospital, 114
Crabtree, E. Granville, 126, 131
Crile, George, 104, 151–2
Crookes tube, 82
Crosby, Alpheus Benning, 38, 77
Cuba, 83, 103n
Cullen-Harrison Act, 218–19
Cummings, Miss, 193
Cunningham, John H. Jr., 64, 89n,
  108, 151
Curriculum
  bacteriology, 180
  clinical education, 40–1
  Ford and, 30
  scientific, 25, 50–1
  Tappan and, 25
  Woodward and, 19
Curtis, Arthur, 180, 186, 193, 196n, 218
Cushing, Harvey, 29, 105, 106, 148,
  155, 205, 223
Cushny, Arthur, 79, 108
Cutler, Elliott Carr, 105, 129
  BEF and, 128
  Henry Jacob Bigelow Award, 128
Cystoscopes, 61–2, 62f, 69–70, 96–7,
  101, 126
Cystourethroscopy, 14, 67

Darling, Cyrenus, 94–9, 103, 112,
  136–9
  Cabot's appointment as chief of
    surgery, 97–9, 136
  Catholic hospital, 84–5
  Coller on, 95
  cystoscopy, 94
  death, 98–9, 204
  de Nancrede and, 81–2
  as dental school dean, 95
  general surgical practice, 83, 84
  Loree and, 95–7
  Lyons and, 94–5
  oral surgery, 95–6
Daguerre, Louis-Jacques Mandé, 11n
Daguerreotype, 11n

Darwin, Charles, 22n, 23, 181n
Darwin, Leonard, 181n-2n
Darwinian, 60
Davenport, Charles, 181, 182n
Davenport, Horace, xi, 8n, 29, 78,
  182n
  on Cabot, 139, 179, 187, 202,
    204–205
  on diversity, 36
  on the hospital, 82
  Not Just Any Medical School,
    190–1, 226
  on Peterson, 176
  on toxicology, 31–2
  University of Michigan Surgeons, 35
  on Vaughan, 50, 78, 195n, 205
Davidson, John Summerfield, 36
Davis, Audrey, 223–4
Davis, Fenimore, 204
Davis, Laura, 167, 191, 204
  (see also Dunstone)
Declaration of Independence, 17
De Humani Corporis Fabrica
  (Vesalius), 7
De Kruif, Paul, 116–17, 173
de Nancrede, Charles, 15, 28,
  53, 77–85, 84n, 103, 204,
  222, 225
  Darling and, 81–2, 94, 97, 139
  death, 85, 155
  general surgical practice, 82–5
  on Gunn, 70
  illness, 85
  Listerian principles, 81
  Spanish-American War and, 83–4,
    105–6
de Nancrede, Paul J. G., 84
Deane, Archie, 213
Dental Department, 44, 82
Denton, Samuel, 24, 25
De Regge, G., 121
Desnos, E., 73
Detroit, 20
  cholera epidemic, 20–1
  hospitals, 24
  population, 22, 24
  taxation law, 20
The Detroit Free Press, 35, 157, 160,
  161, 165, 181, 184, 185
Detroit Gazette, 18–19
Detroit Medical Journal, 38, 96
Detroit Observatory, 25

Detroit Tigers, 174
Devil in the White City (Larson), 52
DeVos, Richard, 174
Dictionary of Practical Surgery (Dorsey), 63
Dingell, John, Jr., 174–5
Dioscorides, Pedanius, 31
Diphtheria antitoxin serum, 173
Diphtheria epidemic, 173
Diseases and Surgery of the Genito-Urinary System (Watson), 64
Diseases of the Urinary Organs Including Stricture of the Urethra, Affections of the Prostate and Stone in the Bladder (Gouley), 67
Diversity, 36, 179–80, 195
Dixon, Edward, 11
Dock, George, 79, 80, 80n, 96, 113–5, 155
Doctor Dock (Davenport), 80n
The Doctor's Bill (Cabot), 208–9
The Doctor's Dilemma (Shaw), 131, 215
A Doctor's Memories (Vaughan), 49n, 190
Doctrine of the prepared soil, 127, 157
Dodd, Walter J., 72f, 168
Donabedian, Avedis, 101n, 127
Dorsey, John Syng, 63
Douglas, Silas, viii, 23, 24, 31, 37, 45, 46, 46n, 48, 49, 50
Dow, Herbert, 87–8, 198, 201
Dow-Jones, 190
Doyle, Arthur Conan, 32
Duderstadt, Anne, xv, 139–40
Dupin, C. Auguste, 32
Dupont, 198
Dunstone, Laura Davis, 167, 191, 204 (See also Davis, Laura)

Eagle River, 23
Eakins, Thomas, 222
Eberbach, Carl, 182
Edison, T., 14, 61, 67, 88
Edmunds, C. W., 161, 188
Edwin Smith Papyrus, 3
Effinger (Dean LS&A, Michigan), 146–7
Eighteenth Amendment, 142, 218–9
Einstein, Albert, 151
Elements of Surgery (Dorsey), 63

Elliot, Charles, 122–3
Emerson, Ralph Waldo, 32n, 122, 123
"Employment of a New Agent in the Treatment of Stricture of the Urethra" (Bigelow), 64
Endoscope (Fisher), 67
Ennoeica, 19
Enrollment, 36, 42, 53, 54, 100, 187
Episcopal Hospital, 221–2
Essentials of Anatomy and Manual for Practical Dissection (de Nancrede), 81
Ethnic groups, quotas for, 179–80
Ethylene anesthesia, 167, 180, 187
Eugenics, 60, 179, 181, 181n-182n, 195n
Executive Committee, Medical School, 96, 187, 191–7, 196f, 201, 204, 205–6
Exercitatio Anatomica de Motu Cordis et Sanguinis in Animalibus (Harvey), 8

"Faculty-Student Debate Held on Athletic System," 172
Fairfield Medical College, New York, 22
Farr, William, 30n
Fasquelle, Louis, 48
Faulkner, William, 131
Fellowship in creative art, 155
Fibiger, Johannes, 180
The Fighting Fifth 34–5
Fin de siècle, 54, 87–8, 90, 113
First Amendment, 109
Fisher, Irving, 181
Fishery Commission 52
Fitzbutler, W. Henry, 43
Fitzbutler Jones Society, 43
Fitzpatrick, S., 60n
Flexner, Abraham, 90–1, 100, 101, 102, 103, 111, 114
Flexner's Report, 90–1, 100–2
Folkman, M. Judah, xii, xiv
Forbes, William S., 222
Ford, Corydon La, 25, 29–30, 37, 52, 78–9, 90, 152
Ford, Edsel, 142
Ford Motor Company, 174
Forestus, Petrus, 7
Fort Sumter, 33
Foster, Nellis B., 107, 107–8n, 112
Fowler, H. A., 125
Fox, G. H., 68

Franklin, Benjamin, 5, 9n, 10, 63
Franklin, John, 63
Fraser, Catherine M., 140
Frazier, Charles Harrison, 182–4
Freer, Paul, 79
Freyer, Peter, 69
Frieze, Henry, 41, 45, 48, 53, 140
Frost, Robert, 156
Frothingham, George, 52, 77, 78, 80
Fuller, Eugene, 65, 68–9, 73, 89
Full-time employment/salary model, 52, 153–4, 203
   Cabot and, 97, 112–3, 115, 133, 135, 139, 141, 144, 148–9, 151, 153, 154, 155–6, 160–1, 165, 176, 187, 191, 196–7, 198, 205, 226
   de Nancrede, 80–1, 84, 113
   Mall and, 90
   Marketplace incomes and, 97
   Peterson on, 115
   Phemister on, 112
Furstenberg, Albert Carl, 190, 201–2, 202n, 205
Furstenberg Study Center, 190

Galen, 4, 8, 74, 222
Galenic, 7
Galton, Francis, 181n
Gardner, Faxton E., 125
Garfield, James, 15n
Gastric cancer, 180, 214
Gender Reporting, 92
General anesthesia, 60, 64, 67
Geneva Medical College, 25, 27, 29, 37
Genito-Urinary Diseases (Watson and Cunningham), 89n
Genito-Urinary Diseases and Systems (Keyes and Van Buren), 44
Genitourinary surgery, origin claims, 11, 59–74
Geological Survey, 23
Geraghty, John, 125
Germ theory, 32n, 55, 59–60, 170
Gessel, 180
Goddard, Robert, 174
Golden Age of Islamic Medicine, 4
Goldsmith, Alban, 12
Gomberg, Moses, 109
Gonorrhea, 77, 107, 127
Goodnow, 153
The Gospel Messenger, 92n

Gottlieb, Max, 117
Gouley, John, 12, 67, 71
Graduate Library, xi, 183
Graduate medical education, vii, 87
Gram, Hans Birch, 42n
Grammatica, 10n
Gray, Asa, 22–3
Great Depression, 169n, 182, 187, 190, 199
Great Influenza (Barry), 109
Great Trilogy, 31
Green, Fred, 190
Green, Robert, 89
Greene, William Warren, 37–8, 77
Greenfield, Lazar, ix
Griffin, John, 18
Grosbeck, Alex, 174
Gross, Samuel David, 12, 30, 44, 63, 64, 71, 80, 81, 82, 222
   A Case of Priapism, 28
   genitourinary disorders and injuries, 28
   A Practical Treatise, 12, 28, 63
   published papers, 28
   A System of Surgery, 27–8
Guiteras, Ramon, 64, 66, 69, 71, 73, 89, 101, 124, 139
Gunn, Moses, 9n, 24, 27–8, 40, 41, 70–1
   AAGUS membership, 122 case reports of, 36
   clinical demonstrations, 35
   as dean, 30
   fellow faculty members, 29–30
   Michigan Volunteer Infantry, 33–4
   professor of surgery at Rush Medical College, 36
   as regimental surgeon, 34
   reputation, 29, 36, 39, 84
   surgery lectures, 30, 34
   surgical practice, 28, 29
   Vaughan on, 36–7
Guy, William, 30n
Guyan, Felix, 73

H1N1 virus, 109n
Hadley, 153
Hagner, Francis, 151
Hahnemann, Samuel, 42n
Haight, Cameron, 182
Hale, William, 107n
The Halifax Disaster (Bacon), 106–7

236 Index

Halsted, William, 103, 222, 223
Hamer, Homer, 66
Hamilton, Alice, 53, 53n
Hanchett, Ben, 186
Hand-Book of Toxicology (Rose), 31
Hapgood, Lyman Sawin, 130f
Harding, Warren G., 150, 165
Hargo, Gabriel Franklin, 36
Harley, George, 45, 45n
Harper Hospital, 24, 38
Harvard, xv, 23, 29, 32n, 53, 53n, 64, 68, 83, 100, 101n, 104, 107, 108, 109, 112, 122, 123, 128, 132, 133, 141, 148, 155, 162, 165, 166, 167, 170, 171, 174, 175, 183, 202, 208, 209n, 215, 216, 219
Harvard Cancer Commission, 29
Harvard Corporation, 131
Harvard Surgical Unit, 105, 129–31
Harvey, William, 8, 10
Haven, Erastus, 36, 41, 140
Hayes, Rutherford, 45
Health services research, 127, 213f
Haynes, Harley, 172, 176, 195–7, 201
Hemingway, Clarence Edmonds, 94
Hemingway, Ernest, 94
Henry Clay (steamer), 20
Henry Ford Clinic, 227
Henry Ford Hospital, 182
Henry Jacob Bigelow Award, 128
Henry IV (King), 7
Henry VII (King), 121
Heskett, Sandra, xv
Hewlett, Albion Walter, 80, 96, 103, 107, 112, 113, 115, 116, 155
Hickey, Preston, 172
Higher education, 9–10n, 20, 43, 94, 143, 147, 218,
Hill, Henry, 9
Hill Auditorium, 103, 104n, 106, 183, 189
Hillegas, Michael, 221
Hinckley, Miss, 194
Hinman, Frank, Sr., 151, 203
   son (Frank, Jr.), 203
Hinsdale, W. B., 54, 147, 158, 160
Hippocrates, 4, 5, 59, 222
Hippocratic Oath, 4
Hippocratic School, 3–4
"Historical Sketch of Genito-Urinary Surgery in America" (Watson), 64, 168

History of the American Association of Genito-Urinary Surgeons 1886–1982 (Spence), 71
The History of Urology (Keyes), 60–1, 66n, 73
History of Urology at the University of Michigan (Konnak and Pardanani), xi
Hitler, Adolph, 151
Hodges, Clarence, 183
Holmes, Henry Howard, 52
Holmes, Oliver Wendell, 14, 30, 30n, 32, 32n, 42n, 59, 121n, 122, 170, 218
Holmes, Sherlock, 32, 45
Homeopathic College, 42, 45, 90–1, 102, 137, 147, 149, 151, 158, 160, 161, 174
Homeopathic Medical College of Pennsylvania, 42
Homeopathy, vii, 25, 36, 41, 42, 42n, 54, 55, 60, 82, 160, 162
Homoeopathy and Its Kindred Delusions (Holmes), 42n
Hoover, Herbert, 167, 190, 199
Hortus Sanitatis (Meydenbach), 5, 6f
Houdini, Harry, 175
Houghton, Douglass, 23
Howard A. Kelly Hospital, 223
Howell, Joel, xi
Howell, William H., 79
Huang Ti Nei Ching Su Wen, 3
Huber, G. Carl, 135, 152–3, 155, 171, 180, 186, 188, 192–4
Huggins, Charles, viii, 117, 167, 172, 173, 175, 183, 203
Hull, William, 18
Hume, Basil, 170, 184
Hunter, John, 10, 63
Hurd, Henry M., 79
Hutcheon, Sarah, xv
Hutchins, Harry B., ixf, 100, 102n, 105, 106, 111, 112, 137–42, 143–7, 171, 174, 191
   letter from Regent Clements to, 143–4
   letters from Burton to, 145–6
   letter to Burton, 146
   letter to Clements, 144
Hutchins, Willard H., 96

Iatrica, 18, 19, 20
Indianapolis City Hospital, 65
Indiana Territory, 18

Influenza epidemic, 109, 133, 145
Interim Executive Committee, 201
Internal medicine (*see* Warfield, Louis M)
International Eugenics Congresses, 181, 181n-2n
Iowa (medical school), 162, 166, 204
Irish Free State, 151
Isaacs, Raphael, 177, 179
Ivy Towers vs. Ivory Towers, x, xn

Jackson, 129
Jackson, Andrew, 21
Jackson, Roscoe B., 185
Jacques, Frère, 8, 74
Jarvis, Edward, 30n
Jefferson, Thomas, 17–18
Jenner, Edward, 59
Johns Hopkins School of Medicine, vii, 61–2, 79, 83, 90, 128, 155, 222–3
Johns Hopkins University, 221
Jones, John, 68n
Jones, Samuel, 42
Jones, Sophia Bethena, 43
Jordan, David Starr, 181
Journal of Cutaneous and Genito-Urinary Diseases, 70–1,
Journal of Laboratory and Clinical Medicine, 102
Journal of the American Medical Association, 109, 210–12
Journal of Urology, 107
The Journal of Urology, Experimental, Medical, and Surgical, 107

Kahn, Albert, 177, 183
Kahn, Eddie, 175, 197
Kahn, Edgar, 116, 183, 188, 202
Kahn, Reuben, 182
Kampmeyer, Dr., 195
Kansas, as slave state, 29
Kansas-Nebraska Act, 29
Kauffman, C. H., 224
Kazanjian, Powell, 131n
Kazanjian, Varaztad, 131
Keane, Jefferson R., 128, 128n
Kellogg, John Harvey, 21, 21n, 44, 48, 181
Kellogg, John Preston, 21
Kellogg, Will Keith, 21
Kelly, Henry, 221
Kelly, Howard Atwood, 61–3, 63n,184, 221–5

Brödel and, 223
Davis on, 223–4
donation made by, 224–5
education, 221
family background, 221
gynecology, 222
Howard A. Kelly Hospital, 223
Mencken on, 223
as naturalist and collector, 62, 62n
Operative Gynecology, 223
personal library, 222, 224
speculum, 62
spiritual evangelicalism, 223
"Kelly Stitch," 222
Kelly, Louisa, 221
Kensington Hospital for Women, 222
Keyes, Edward Lawrence, 12, 21n, 34, 44, 64, 65, 66, 67, 68, 70–1, 108n, 122
Keyes, Edward Loughborough, 64, 66, 66n, 71, 73, 106, 108, 108n, 132, 151, 183
Keyes, Erasmus Darwin, 34
Khrushev, Nikita, 60n
Kiefer, Herman, 54, 88, 102, 102n
Kin, Jeanne, xiii
King Ferdinand, of Spain, 121
King George, 131, 133
King Henry IV, 7
King Henry VII, 121
King, Martin Luther, 92n
King's College, 68n
Kleb, Margaret, 14
Kohn, Rabbi Jacob, 92n
Konnak, John W., viii, xi, xiv, 227
Korean War, 216
Kraft, R. W., 96
Kraus (regent), 224
Kreiger, L. C. C., 223–5
Kretschmer, Herman, 66, 132, 151

Labardini, Mario, 121
Laennec, René, 30
La Ford, Corydon (see Ford, Corydon La)
Lake Saranac Sanitarium in New York, 182
Lake Superior, 23
Lancet, 14, 184, 216
Langerhans, Paul, 40, 40n
Lapides, Jack, 22n, 107, 216
Larder, Ring, 116
Larson, Erik, 52
Lasker Awards, 201

238 Index

l'Association Internationale
  d'Urologic, 73
Law School, 37
League of Nations, 104n, 132, 150,
  175, 209n
Lectures on Lithotomy (Stevens), 11, 74
Lectures on the Principles of Surgery
  (de Nancrede), 81
Lee, Robert E., 34
Leprosaria, 4
Lewis, H. B., 161
Lewis, Morris, 222
Lewis, Sinclair, 116–7, 173
Lichter, Allen, viii–ix
Lincoln, Abraham, 33–6
Linnaeus, Carl, 31
List, Carl, 205
Lister, Joseph, 14, 15, 38, 60, 77, 170
Listerism, 81
Lithotomy, 3–5, 8–10, 10n, 12, 59,
  63, 66–7, 226
Little, Clarence, 102n, 171, 173–4, 176,
  179, 180, 181, 184–5, 192, 193
Lloyd, Alfred Henry, 155, 171, 174
Lodge, Henry Cabot, 103, 103n-4n,
  209n
Lombard, Warren Plimpton, 161
Longfellow, Henry Wadsworth, 32n
Loree, Ira Dean, 84, 85, 94, 95–9,
  112, 138–9
  as clinical associate professor of
    genitourinary surgery, 96
  Darling and (*see* Darling, Cyrenus)
    death, 204
  as demonstrator in oral surgery,
    95, 96
Lottmann, Henri, 110n
Louis, Pierre Charles Alexandre, 30, 30n
Louisiana Purchase, 17–18
Lowell, A. Lawrence, 128, 208, 209n,
Lowell, Hanna, 122
Lowell, James Russell, 32n
Lower, William, 151–2
Lum, Harpin, 139
Lyceum of Natural History, 22
Lyons, Chalmers, 94–5, 95n, 98, 139
Lysenko, Trofim, 60n
Lysenkoism, 60, 60n
Lyster, Henry, 38, 77

Maclean, Donald, 38–9, 44, 51, 52,
  77–8
Macleod, J. J. R., 40n

Main Street (Lewis), 173
*The Making of the University of
  Michigan 1817–1992* (Peckham,
  see Steneck), ix, 46n, 91
Mall, Franklin, 79, 90, 223
Malpighi, Marcello, 8
Markel, Howard, xi, 21n, 44, 195n
Marshall, John, 10n, 63
Martin, Clarence, 35
Martin, Franklin H., 101
Martin, S. C., Jr., 35
Martin, Solomon Claiborne, 35, 65
Mason, Stevens T., 21, 22
Massachusetts General Hospital
  (MGH), xii, 12, 122, 123, 127
Massachusetts Quarterly Review, 122
Mastin, Claudius, 70
Materia medica, 31, 87, 108
Mathematica, 10
Mather, E. J., 174
Maumee River, 21
Mayo, Charlie, 89
Mayo, William, 51, 90, 145, 147, 153,
  165, 168–9, 172, 197–8, 215
  letter to Burton, 149–50
  letter to Vaughan, 141
Mayo Clinic, 197–8, 208, 212–13,
  214f, 215, 218, 227
McClellan, George, 34, 36
McCotter (requestor), 165n
McCotter, Rollo Eugene, 165n
McCullough, David, 32n
McDonald, Terry, x
McGraw, Theodore, 38, 77
McGuire, Ed, 107, 216
McLellan, Frederick, 107
McMurrich, James, 79
*Medical Education in the United
  States and Canada* (Flexner),
  90–1
Medical Reserve Corps, 112, 148
Medical School, Michigan, 24, 51f,
  52, 78, 87, 88, 90–2, 94, 101–2,
  106, 112, 117, 135,137, 144,
  148, 151–2, 156–8, 162, 171,
  173
  Class picture, 207f
Medical specialty boards, 87
Medical students, xi, 24, 28–9, 31–2,
  34, 49, 51f, 53, 56, 82, 103, 137,
  156, 160, 181, 194, 195n, 197
Medicinal plants, 31
Medicine at Michigan (Boster), xi

Medicine, Department of, Michigan, 157, 195
Medicine and Surgery, Department of, Michigan, 24, 24n, 27–39, 53, 87, 90
Melanson, Louise, 184
Mencken, H. L., 62, 116, 223
Mental illness, 4
Mering, Joseph von, 40n
Mertz, Henry, 66
Mettauer, John Peter, 11
Meydenbach, Jacob, 5
Miami Medical College, 65
Michigan Alumnus, 174–5
Michigan Daily, 98f, 99, 104f, 136, 137f, 145, 157, 161, 166, 166f, 172, 175
Michigan Hospital Association, 156
Michigan Stadium, 184
Michigan Territory, 18
   Geological Survey, 23
   land dispute with Ohio, 21
   population of, 21–2
   state constitution, 21
Michigan Union, 88, 137, 140, 162, 185, 216, 217, 217f
Michigan Volunteer Infantry, 33–4, 38
Microscopy, 12, 50, 60
The "Middle West," 64–6
Milestone Mo-Tel, 173
Millard, Candice, 15n
Mill tax, 43, 52, 187
Millin, Terence, 89
Milne, A. A., 175
Minkowski, Oscar, 40n
Minnesota (Med Sch/University), 127, 141, 149, 162, 166, 173, 189
Mississippi Valley Medical Association, 127
Modern Urology (Cabot), 64, 89n, 109–10, 131, 156, 167–8, 173, 208, 210
Monteith, John, 20
Montie, Jim, viii, xi, xiv, 227
Montreal (Medical School), 166
Monument Association (*see* Bunker Hill Monument Association)
Moral universe, 91, 92n
Morbidity and mortality/conferences, 3, 101n, 109n
Morgan, John, 9n, 42
Morland, William, 12
Morton, Dr., 13, 14

Mott, Alexander, 66–7
Mott Children's and Women's Hospital, 88
Mudgett, Herman Webster, 52
Multiversity, x, 91
Mumford, Lewis, 116
The Murders in the Rue Morgue (Poe), 32
Murfin (Regent), 140, 146,
Mustard, Russell, 175, 202

Nancrede, Charles de (see de Nancrede)
Natural History Club, 51
Nelson, Henry Philbrick, 170, 171n
Neoprene, 198
Nephrectomy, 14–15, 66, 71, 83
Nesbit, Mabel, 183
Nesbit, Nancy, 176, 202, 217f, 218
Nesbit, Reed, viii, 22n, 70n, 117, 172, 173, 175–6, 183, 187, 197, 202–5, 207–8, 207f, 213, 216–18, 217f, 219, 227
Newburgh, Louis Harry (L. H.), 112, 155, 205
New Deal, 123, 216
New England Journal of Medicine, 124, 212, 216
New York Academy of Medicine, 208
New York Academy of Sciences, 22
New York City, 66–70
New York Genitourinary Society, 89
New York Medical Journal, 125
New York's Mt. Sinai Hospital, 151, 166
New York Postgraduate Hospital, 89
New York State Medical Society, 210
New York Times, 99, 194, 212, 215
Nichols, Walter, 88
1918 Flu, 100 Years Later, 109n
Nineteenth Amendment, 142
Nitze, Maximilian, 61, 67, 69, 88
Nobel prize, viii, 40n, 60n, 151, 167, 175, 180, 183, 201
Noble, Miss, 193
Northern Tri-State Medical Association, 96
Northwest Ordinance of 1787, 17
Northwest Ordinance of 1789, 17
Northwest Territory, 17
Not Just Any Medical School (Davenport), 190–1, 205n, 226
Novy, Frederick George, 79–80, 80n, 98, 116, 117, 131n, 135, 152,

153, 155, 161, 173, 180, 188, 192, 194, 195, 196, 196f, 196n, 197, 201
Nuri Hospital, Damascus, 4

Obama (president), 92n
Obetz, Henry Lorenz, 54
Ohio, land dispute with Michigan, 21
Ohio University, Athens, Ohio, 20
O'Neill, Richard, 126
Operative Gynecology (Kelly), 223
An Ordinance for the Government of the Territory of the United States, North-West of the River Ohio, 17
"Organic Act," 18, 19f
Organizations, 70–4
Origin claims of genitourinary surgery, 59–74
Osborne, Chase, 156
Osgood, Robert B., 129n, 211–2, 211n
Osler, William, 105, 113, 128, 157, 197, 222
Osteopathic manipulation therapy (OMT), 55
Osteopathy, 55
Otis, Fessenden Nott, 67–8, 69f, 70
Otis Urethrameter, 68, 69f
Our Declaration (Allen), 17

Packard, John Hooker, 222
Paine, George, 198–9
Palapattu, Ganesh, xv
Palmer, Alonzo, 25, 29, 30, 34, 78, 88, 114, 157
Palmer, Daniel David, 55
Palmer College of Chiropractic (D. Palmer), 55
Pardanani, Dev. S., viii, xi, xiv, 227
Pardon (superintendent), 141, 145–6
Paré, 222
Park, Roswell, 70, 71
Parke-Davis, 54
Parker, Theodore, 92n
Parkman, George, 32n
Parnall, Christopher Gregg, 140, 144, 153, 153n, 156, 165
Parry, Bill, 22n
Parry, Charles Christopher, 22n
Pasteur Institute, 88
Pasteau, O., 73
The Patient's Dilemma (Cabot), 214–17

Pawlik, Parel, 222
Peckham, Howard (see Steneck), ix, 46n, 91, 187
Pediatrics, Department of, Michigan, 157
Peet, Max, 116, 183, 194
Penicillin, 198, 216
Pennsylvania Hospital, 9–10, 9n-10n, 63
Perkins, Thomas Handasyd, 121–2
Pershing, John J., 105n, 106
Peter Bent Brigham Hospital, 106, 155, 179
Peterson, Reuben, 102, 113, 114, 152, 155, 157, 176, 180, 187, 188
  full-time employment/salary model and, 115
  hospital, 115, 115n
  retirement, 176
Phemister, Dallas, 112
Phenolsulphonephthalein test, 72t, 125
Philadelphia [origin claims], 63
Philanthropy, viii, 5, 19, 25, 46, 53, 54, 88, 156, 157, 165, 168–9, 177, 224–5
Philosopica, 10n
Physick, Philip Syng, 10, 10n, 63
Pinkus, Herman, 205
The Pisse-Prophet (Brian), 8
Pitcher, Zina, 23
Podolsky, Scott, xv
Poe, Edgar Allen, 32, 45
Polyclinic Medical School, 65–6
Pond, Elihu, 33
Porter, George, 21
Posner, Karl, 73
Post-Flexnerian decade, 100–17
Postgraduate Medicine, Department of, 195–6, 196n, 197
Postgraduate medical education, viii
  department of, 172
Potter, Eugene, 197
A Practical Treatise on the Diseases and Injuries of the Urinary Bladder, the Prostate Gland, and the Urethra (Gross), 12, 28, 63,
A Practical Treatise on the Surgical Diseases of the Genito-Urinary Organs, Including Syphilis (Van Buren and Keyes), 12, 67
Presbyterian Hospital, 68n
Prescott, Albert B., 48
Priapism, 28
Private hospitals in Ann Arbor, 157

Professors, hiring based on scholarship rather than religious affiliation, 30
Prostatic surgery, 66
Public primary schools, 20
Pulitzer Prize, 117, 173
Pulse rate measurement, 30

Qualitative Analysis (Douglas and Prescott), 48
Quinby, William, 151
Quotas for ethnic groups, 179–80

Race Betterment Conference, 181
Race Betterment Foundation, 181
Radiology, 87–8, 124, 172
Rains, Claude, xv
Ransom, Henry, 180, 184, 194, 197
Ravitch, M. W., 84
Readings from Great Authors, 92n
Red Scare, 150
Reed, Thomas, 189
Reed, Walter, 83
Reeve, 171
Regents-University of Michigan
 board of, 22–5, 24n, 29, 35–6, 41–2, 45–6, 46n, 52, 54, 77–82, 88, 94–8, 100, 102, 102n, 135, 137, 139–42, 146, 148, 152–3, 155–6, 166, 174, 176, 184, 185–6, 188, 191–3, 193n, 196, 196f, 201, 204, 207
 proceedings, 96, 98, 185, 196n, 224
 bylaws, 190
 Beal, 171
 Clements, 143–6, 145n, 157, 165, 171, 185–6
 Hanchett, Ben, 186
 Kraus, 224
 Murfin, 146
 Osborne, Chase, 156
 Sawyer, Walter, 96–8, 102, 102n, 115, 144, 152–5, 155, 164–6, 171, 185–7, 190–1
 Stone, Ralph, 186
"Regular medicine", 55, 82
Rensselaer School, 23
Report of Committee on Education and Pedagogics, 163
Republican Party, 29, 33, 35, 190
Respiratory rate measurement, 30
Rhetorica, 10n
Richard, Father Gabriel, 20
Richardson, Allen, 83

RMS Lusitania, U-boat sinking of, 105
Robinson, Carl, 130f
Rockefeller, John D., 88
Rockefeller – fellowships for advanced medical research, 88, 114, 170
Rockefeller Institute, 116
Roentgenological laboratory, 82
Roosevelt, Eleanor, 210
Roosevelt, Franklin, 218–19
Roosevelt, Theodore, 105n
Root, Elihu, 132–3
Root, William, 132–3
Rose, Preston B., 31–2, 45–6, 46n, 49, 50
Rose-Douglas, viii, 46, 49
Rough Riders 83, Regiment, 105n
Route 66, 175
Rowntree, Leonard, 125
Royal Medical Corps, 131
Runge, Marshall, xv, 194
Rush Medical College, viii, 36, 70, 77, 114, 122
Russian Academy of Sciences, 60n
Ruth, Babe, 142
Ruthven, Alexander, 98, 102n, 185, 186, 187, 188, 190–4, 195, 196, 201, 224
Rutkow, Ira, 11–12, 67, 68n

Sadler, 171
Sager, Abram, 23, 24, 30, 35, 37
Sakharov, Andrei, 60n
San Francisco (Medical School), 166
Sanitary Corps, 116
Sawyer, Walter H., 96–8, 102, 102n, 115, 144, 152–5, 164–6, 171, 185–7, 190–1
Scardino, Peter L., 14, 15
Schirm, Mary Helen (Williams), 14–15
Schlesinger Library, Radcliffe Institute, xv, 219
Schoolcraft, Henry R., 23
School of Homeopathy, 41, 42–3
The Scientific Club, 51
Scientific crime solver meme, 32
Scott (General), 33
Scudder, Charles Locke, 129
Secretion of the Urine (Cushny), 108
Seddon, Herbert J., 170, 182, 184, 216
The Seevak Website Competition, 60n
Selective Service Act of 1917, 106
Semmelweis, 170
September Revenue Classification, 187

242 Index

"Sex Knowledge Essential," 126–7
Sex reassignment surgery, 198
Shakespeare, Edward, 83
Shakespeare, William, 7, 8n
Shattuck, George, Jr., 30n, 131
Shattuck, Susan, 122
Shaw, George Bernard, 131, 215
Sheahan, George, 130f
Sheehan, Mrs., 144
Shoenfield, Allen, 185–6
Showboat, 181
Sidney, Albert (General), 35
Silver catheter technology, 5, 10, 63
Simon, Gustav, 14–15
Simpson Memorial Institute, 169, 176–7, 176f, 179, 183
Simpson, Mrs., 165
Simpson, Thomas Henry, 165, 177
Sims, James Marion, 11
Sinclair-Sheehan house, 144
Slavery, 11, 29, 35
Slemons, Clyde C., 212
Smith, George Gilbert, 126
Smith, John, 174
Smith, Shirley W., 140–1, 147
Smith, William H., 49, 50
Social worker, 215
Society for Medical Observation, 30
Society of Pediatric Urological Surgeons, 110n
Spanish-American War, 56, 83–4, 105, 105n, 106
Spanish flu, 109
Special Executive Order, 145
Speculum, 61–62
Spence, Harry, 71, 123
Squier, J. Bentley, 108, 151
SS *Imo*, 106
SS *Mont-Blanc*, 106
Stalin, Joseph, 60n
Stanford, 80n, 112, 116, 172, 181
Starr, Louis, 222
State Board of Health, 38, 52
State Homeopathic Medical Society, 147
Statistical Society of London, 30n
Steere, Joseph, 46n
Steneck, Margaret and Nicholas, ix-x, xiv, 19, 91, 150
Sterns, Harold, 116
Steuben Guards, 33
Stethoscope, 30
Stevens, Alexander Hodgdon, 11, 74
Still, Andrew Taylor, 55

St. Joseph Mercy Hospital, 84, 97–9, 139, 151, 196, 201, 203–4
St. Louis Medical Era, 35
St. Mary's Hospital, 24, 38
Stock market crash, 169n, 187, 190
Stone, Ralph, 186
Straffon, Ralph, 208
Streit, Sarah, xv
Stricture of the Male Urethra, Its Radical Cure (Otis), 67–8
Student Affairs, Committee on, 195
Students' Army and Navy Training Corps, 106
A Study in Hospital Efficiency (Codman), 101n
Sturgis, Cyrus, 169, 179, 195
Sturgis, Frederic R., 66
Subsidized Medicine, 212
Sullivan, John L., 73
Suprapubic prostatectomy, 68, 69, 89, 126, 205
Supreme Court, Michigan, 25, 42, 46, 54
Surgery, Gynecology and Obstetrics (SG&O), 101, 110, 111f, 132
The Surgery of Pulmonary Tuberculosis (Alexander), 182
Surgery training program, 167
Surgical centers, 17
Surgical Nursing (Cabot), 208
Surgical procedures, 30
Sushruta Samhita, 3
Syme, James, 38, 77
A System of Surgery (Gross), 27–8
A System of Universal Science (Woodward), 18

Taft, William, 105n, 132–3
Tappan, Henry, 25, 30, 33, 35, 140
Taxation law, 20
Teachers Insurance and Annuity Association of America (TIAA), 169, 169n
Territorial Law, 18
Terry, Jane Augusta, 27
Theologica, 10n
Third Harvard Surgical Unit, 105, 129, 130, 130f
Thoreau, Henry David, 122 TIAA (*see* Teachers Insurance and Annuity Association of America)
Toledo War, 21
Torrey, John, 22, 22n

Index   243

Toxicology, 31–2
Transactions of the American Association of Genito-Urinary Surgeons, Volume 2, 125
Transylvania University, Lexington, Kentucky, 20
A Treatise on Diseases of the Sexual System: Adapted to Popular and Professional Readings and the Exposition of Quackery (Dixon), 11
A Treatise on the Nature and Treatment of Seminal Diseases, Impotency, and Other Kindred Affections: With Practical Directions for the Management and Removal of the Cause Producing Them; Together with Hints to Young Men (Bostwick), 12
The Treatment of Fractures (Scudder), 129
Treaty of Versailles, 104n, 110, 150
Trendelenburg, Friedrich, 89
Tripodal capacity, 126
Tschanz, D. W., 5
Tuberculosis (BCG vaccination), 151, 182
Tucker, Robert, 68n
Tupper, C. J., 190
TURP (transurethral resection of prostate), 203
Twenty-First Amendment, 218

U-boat sinking of RMS Lusitania, 105
United Kingdom Mental Treatment Act, 198–9
The University Encyclopedic Survey, 85, 155
University Hospital
  Administrator, director, 102, 115, 145, 156, 172, 176, 195–196, 197
  North University Avenue (1869), 24, 40, 44, 52, 53, 92
  new hospital opened under Dean Cabot (1925), 114, 137, 172, 182, 183, 196, 201, 203–4
  on Catherine Street (1892), 40, 40n, 53–4, 84, 92, 95, 102, 138, 140, 151, 155, 157, 165, 182
University of Chicago, 100, 166–7, 175, 183
University of Edinburgh, 10, 38, 51, 63
University of Louisiana, 35, 65
University of Michigan, 18–20
  bachelor of science degrees, 25
  board of trustees, 20
  college classes, 24
  curriculum, 19
  hospital, 24
  library acquisition, 23
  philanthropy (see philanthropy)
  professors/professorships, 19, 20, 22–3
  relocation, 22
  remodeling, 25
  reorganization, 20
  research and teaching, 25
  state legislature and, 22, 23–4
University of Michigan Surgeons (Davenport), 35
University of Michigania, 18–9
University of Pennsylvania, 10, 10n, 11, 63, 83, 105, 113, 149, 162, 182, 184, 221, 222
University Service of American Ambulance Hospital, 128
Upjohn, William, 25
Upper Peninsula, 21
Urinary tract catheterization, 5
The Urine and Its Derangements (Harley), 45
The Urologic and Cutaneous Review, 35
Urology (origin), vii–xv, 4, 11, 44–5, 60–1, 63–8, 70–1, 73–4, 87–99, 89n, 97, 100–1, 103, 108, 108n, 110, 113, 117, 124, 126, 132 148, 151–2, 156, 173, 202
  Centennial, 226–7
Uromancy, 7, 108
Uroscopy, 3–5, 7–8, 30, 59, 63, 108, 226
Uroscopy Chart, 6f
U.S. Army (medical corps), 83, 106, 128, 131, 149
U.S. Marine Hospital, 24
U.S. Mexican Expedition, 116
U.S. Numbered Highway System, 175
U.S. Regular Cavalry, 10th (Buffalo Soldiers), 83
U.S. Volunteer Cavalry, 1st (Rough Riders), 83

Valentine, Ferdinand, 69–70, 70n
Van Buren, William, 12, 44, 65, 66–7, 68

van Calcar, Johan, 7
Vanderbilt, William, 68n
Vanderpoel, John, 73
Van Zwaluwenburg, J. G., 155
Vaughan, Victor, 22, 36–7, 44, 48–56, 62, 77–80
  appointment of Cabot as chief of surgery, 97, 135–6
  autobiography, 48
  chemistry and, 48–9
  Cushny and, 108–9
  Davenport on, 205
  as dean, 55, 79
  death, 190
  A Doctor's Memories (Vaughan), 49n, 190
  early life, 48
  education, 48–9
  on Gunn, 36–7
  on homeopathy, 42
  letter to Sawyer, 144–5
  Mayo's letter to, 141
  medical student teaching, 46, 49–50
  retirement, 152
  The Scientific Club, 51
  Spanish-American War and, 83
  teaching, 46
Victor Vaughan Society, 195n
Vaughan, Warren, 155
Venereal disease, 107, 126–7
The Venereal Diseases, Including Strictures of the Male Urethra (Van Buren and Keyes), 68
Venereology, 88
Vesalius, 7, 10, 222
Virchow, Rudolf, 40n, 90, 222
Volstead Act (see Eighteenth Amendment), 218
Visick, Arthur, 170, 184
von Mering, Joseph, 40n

Wappler, Reinhold, 68, 69–70, 97
Wappler Electric Controller Company, 70
Warfield, Louis M., 112
Waring, Holburt, 170
Warthin, Aldred, 152, 155, 180
Warren, 129
Washburne, Charles, 95, 138
Waterman, Joshua, 53
Watson, Francis S., 64, 73–4, 89n, 168

Watson, James Craig, 48
Watson, Samuel Codes, 28, 36
Wax models, 224
Webster, George, 32n
Weimar Republic, 175
Weiss, Joseph, 8n
Welch, William, 62, 90, 155, 222
West Point, 22n, 25
Western Front, 103, 106, 109, 113, 128, 139, 148, 182
White, Ellen, 44
White, James, 44
White Coat Ceremony, 68n
Whiteside, George, 125
Wilbur, Ray Lyman, 116
Wile, Udo, 109, 155, 165, 186, 188, 191–2, 193–4, 195, 196, 196f, 197, 201
Wilkins, Mabel Ophelia, 176
Williams, Brian, xi
Wilson, E. O., 4
Wilson, Frank, 188, 205
Wilson, Woodrow, 100, 103, 103n-4n, 105, 105n, 128, 142, 150, 209n, 218
Winnie-the-Pooh (Milne), 175
Wishard, William, 64–6, 132
Wolaver, 99
Women medical students, 29
Women's suffrage, 142
Wood, Helen, 222
Wood, Leonard, 83, 83n, 105, 105n
Woodward, Augustus, 18–20, 51
World War I, 56, 83n, 84, 103–11, 128–31, 205, 211n
  civilian medical practice and, 148–9
World War II, 198n, 205

X-ray, 87, 88

Yamagiwa, Katsusaburo, 180
Youmans, Reed, 217f
Young, Edward, 126
Young, Hugh, 61, 62, 63, 69, 73, 89, 106, 107, 109, 132, 151, 168, 173, 216, 223

Zentmayer microscopes, 50
Zuzow, Nancy, 8n
Zwerdling-Darling Block, 95
Zwerdling, Osias, 95

www.ingramcontent.com/pod-product-compliance
Lightning Source LLC
Chambersburg PA
CBHW050105170426
43198CB00014B/2470